Medical Rehabilitation

Medical Rehabilitation

Editors

Lauro S. Halstead, M.D.
Associate Professor
Departments of Rehabilitation,
Physical Medicine, and Community Medicine
Baylor College of Medicine, and
Attending Physician
The Institute for Rehabilitation and Research
Houston, Texas

Martin Grabois, M.D.
Associate Professor
Departments of Physical Medicine
and Rehabilitation, and
Chairman, Department of Physical Medicine
Baylor College of Medicine
Houston, Texas

Consulting Editor

Carol A. Howland
Department of Physical Medicine
Baylor College of Medicine
Houston, Texas

Raven Press ■ New York

Raven Press, 1140 Avenue of the Americas, New York, New York 10036

Made in the United States of America

Library of Congress Cataloging in Publication Data
Main entry under title:

Medical rehabilitation.

   Includes bibliographies and index.
   1. Rehabilitation. I. Halstead, Lauro S., 1936-
II. Grabois, Martin. [DNLM: 1. Rehabilitation.
WB 320 M4892]
RM930.M43   1985   617   85-2383
ISBN 0-88167-085-5

ACKNOWLEDGMENTS: We wish to express our special gratitude to Dorothy L. Gordon, R.N., D.N.Sc., from the University of Maryland, and Laura C. Campion, M.S., R.N., from the Institute for Rehabilitation and Research, for their recommendations on the nursing care of disabled patients. We also thank Adrian Balch for her excellent secretarial support and Laurie Boyd for typing the manuscripts into the word processor. Charlotte Holden and Gordon Stanley, of the Institute for Rehabilitation and Research, provided many of the line illustrations and photographs, respectively, in the text. We are grateful for their efforts to enhance the appearance of this work.

                                                                    Lauro S. Halstead
                                                                    Martin Grabois

Preface

Rehabilitation medicine is a relatively new specialty, especially in the United States. The number of practitioners is small and the presence of a rehabilitation medicine curriculum in medical schools remains limited. As a consequence, the philosophy, techniques, and contributions of rehabilitation medicine are widely misunderstood or simply unknown to many private practitioners and other health care professionals. This is particularly ironic as the major concerns of rehabilitation medicine involve long-term physical disabilities, which represent a large and steadily increasing percentage of health care problems in all age groups. In response to this growing need, this volume provides a comprehensive yet basic overview of rehabilitation medicine to help primary care and specialty physicians in managing patients with long-term disabilities.

The authors represent a variety of rehabilitation specialists who provide rehabilitation service as individuals. However, they also provide comprehensive health care as an interdisciplinary team, affiliated primarily with Baylor College of Medicine. The private practitioner is the other member of that team, and this book aims to better equip him or her for working with one or more rehabilitation specialists in managing the complex patient problems that typically accompany chronic illness.

The book's organization enables the reader to approach patient management from three different perspectives: Part I: Principles of Rehabilitation Medicine, Part II: Rehabilitation Management of Specific Disorders, and Part III: Rehabilitation Management of Special Populations and Complications.

Part I provides an overview of general rehabilitation principles, the therapeutic modalities employed, and the specialists who provide them. The similarities and differences between evaluating and treating *medical problems* and *disability problems* are also emphasized. This section assists the reader in deciding which aspects of patient care to provide themselves, and which aspects are best performed by one or more of the rehabilitation specialists.

Part II discusses those injuries and diseases that are most likely to be encountered in private practice, result in chronic or progressive physical disabilities, benefit from an interdisciplinary approach to management, and require long-term management. In this section, the principles of evaluating and treating disability problems are put into practice. An illustrative case report in each chapter of Part II applies the problem-oriented approach presented in Part I to the management of a lost valued function, such as ambulation or vocation.

Disabled people suffering from one of the disorders described in Part II commonly experience complications such as pressure sores and the effects of immobilization. The management of these and other complications that may interfere with recovery and resumption of independent activities is discussed in Part III. Disabled elderly people and children have special needs that are considered in this section.

Supplementing the text are nearly 400 illustrations, tables, and graphs that facilitate a rapid and clear communication of key concepts and management techniques. A generous number of topic headings and cross-references serve as guideposts to locating specific areas of inquiry, as does the cross-referencing. The Appendix refers the private practitioner to patient education materials; patient-sponsored periodicals; manufacturers of prostheses, orthoses, and other adaptive aids.

While written mainly for primary care physicians in private practice (general practitioners, family practitioners, and internists), *Medical Rehabilitation* is also useful for neurologists and orthopedists. In addition, it provides practical advice for house officers, medical students, nurses, vocational counselors, and other health care professionals who deal with chronically disabled persons. The practical techniques described can be applied to managing patients at home, in the office, and in the general hospital. This volume is not intended to be encyclopedic or basic science-oriented, nor will it replace standard textbooks in the field of physical medicine and rehabilitation; it is a practical, concise, easy-to-use reference that emphasizes the major and most common problems the private practitioner is likely to encounter.

Lauro S. Halstead
Martin Grabois

Contents

Contributors

William P. Blocker, Jr., M.D., F.A.C.P.
Rehabilitation Medicine and Cardiac Rehabilitation Program
Veterans Administration Medical Center, and
Departments of Physical Medicine and Rehabilitation
Baylor College of Medicine
Houston, Texas 77030

Rogelio M. Borrell, M.D.
St. Anthony Center
Houston, Texas 77030

Barry L. Bowser, M.D.
Departments of Physical Medicine, Rehabilitation, and Pediatrics
Baylor College of Medicine, and
The Institute for Rehabilitation and Research
Houston, Texas 77030

Randall L. Braddom, M.D.
Department of Physical Medicine and Rehabilitation
University of Cincinnatti Medical Center
Cincinnati, Ohio 45230

R. Edward Carter, M.D.
Departments of Rehabilitation and Physical Medicine
Baylor College of Medicine, and
The Institute for Rehabilitation and Research
Houston, Texas 77030

Thorkild J. Engen, C.O.
Departments of Physical Medicine and Rehabilitation
Baylor College of Medicine, and
Orthotics Department
The Institute for Rehabilitation and Research
Houston, Texas 77030

Martin Grabois, M.D.
Departments of Physical Medicine and Rehabilitation
Baylor College of Medicine
Houston, Texas 77030

Kris M. Halstead, M.S., C.C.C.
Speech-Language Pathologist
Private Practice
Houston, Texas 77005

Lauro S. Halstead, M.D.
Departments of Rehabilitation, Physical Medicine, and Community Medicine
Baylor College of Medicine, and
The Institute for Rehabilitation and Research
Houston, Texas 77030

Katie D. Irani, M.D.
Physical Medicine Service
Ben Taub General Hospital, and
Department of Physical Medicine
Baylor College of Medicine
Houston, Texas 77030

Laxman Kewalramani, M.D.
Louisiana State University
New Orleans, Louisiana 70112

Vincent J. Kitowski, M.D.
Departments of Physical Medicine and Rehabilitation
Baylor College of Medicine
Houston, Texas 77030

Michael A. Krebs, M.D.
Veterans Administration Medical Center, and
Departments of Physical Medicine and Rehabilitation
Baylor College of Medicine
Houston, Texas 77030

Janice Ledebur, L.P.T.
Department of Physical Medicine and Rehabilitation
Philadelphia Geriatric Center
Philadelphia, Pennsylvania 19104

Shelly E. Liss, M.D.
*Department of Physical Medicine
Memorial Hospital, and
Department of Physical Medicine
Baylor College of Medicine, and
Department of Family Practice
University of Texas Medical School
Houston, Texas 77030*

Ralph M. Mancini, M.D.
*Rosewood Rehabilitation Center, and
Department of Physical Medicine
Baylor College of Medicine
Houston, Texas 77030*

Robert H. Meier, M.D.
*Departments of Rehabilitation, Physical Medicine,
and Orthopedic Surgery
Baylor College of Medicine, and
Houston Center for Amputee Services
The Institute for Rehabilitation and Research
Houston, Texas 77030*

Mary Joyce Newsom, M.A., O.T.R.[1]
*Department of Occupational Therapy
The Institute for Rehabilitation and Research, and
Department of Rehabilitation
Baylor College of Medicine
Houston, Texas 77030*

Dan K. Seilheimer, M.D.
*Private Practice, and
Department of Pediatrics
Baylor College of Medicine
Houston, Texas 77030*

Paul C. Sharkey, M.D. F.A.C.S.
*Departments of Neurological Surgery and
Rehabilitation
Baylor College of Medicine
Houston, Texas 77030*

Itzel S. Solis, M.D.
*Departments of Physical Medicine and
Rehabilitation
Baylor College of Medicine, and
Texas Children's Hospital
Houston, Texas 77030*

Thomas E. Strax, M.D.
*Department of Rehabilitation Medicine
Temple University School of Medicine, and
Moss Rehabilitation Hospital
Philadelphia, Pennsylvania 19141*

Roberta B. Trieschmann, Ph.D.
*Consulting Psychologist
Private Practice
Scottsdale, Arizona 85261*

Carlos Vallbona, M.D.
*Department of Community Medicine
Baylor College of Medicine, and
Community Medical Service
Harris County Hospital District, and
The Institute for Rehabilitation and Research, and
Family Practice Service
St. Luke's Episcopal Hospital,
Texas Children's Hospital, and
Rehabilitation Medical Service
Veterans Administration Medical Center
Houston, Texas 77030*

Raul Villaneuva, M.D.
*University of Texas Medical School, and
Private Practice
McAllen, Texas 78501*

[1]Deceased.

Medical Rehabilitation,
edited by L. S. Halstead et al.
Raven Press, New York © 1985.

CHAPTER 1

Philosophy of Rehabilitation Medicine

Lauro S. Halstead

Departments of Rehabilitation, Physical Medicine, and Community Medicine, Baylor College of Medicine, and The Institute for Rehabilitation and Research, Houston, Texas 77030

DEFINITIONS

Traditionally, the central concern of rehabilitation has been the restoration of function so that persons can perform to their fullest physical, emotional, social, and vocational potential. From another perspective, rehabilitation involves behavioral changes and emphasizes coping with a physical impairment caused by disease or injury and learning to adapt in one's own environment.

The terms "rehabilitation" and "physical medicine" are often used synonymously. In fact, they share much in common but are not identical. Physical medicine traditionally has been concerned with the diagnosis and treatment of physical disorders, with special emphasis on the use of neurodiagnostic techniques such as electromyography and the therapeutic application of physical agents such as heat, cold, water, and electricity. Rehabilitation, a broader term, has been associated more with the diagnosis and treatment of functional disorders, with emphasis on the practical, functional assessment of motor, sensory, and cognitive skills and treatment aimed at enhancing function and altering behavior.

Over the years, physical medicine has greatly expanded to include many of the techniques and strategies associated with the rehabilitation process. Although persons who enter the field of physical medicine and rehabilitation are called physiatrists (literally, a physical physician), the training programs combine knowledge and skills in the application of physical agents with those used in the evaluation and treatment of physical, psychological, social, and vocational problems.

Other terms associated with rehabilitation include impairment, disability, and handicap. Impairment is the residual limitation resulting from disease, injury, or a congenital defect. Disability is the inability to perform some key life function. Handicap is the interaction of a disability with the environment. With mild impairment, no disability or handicap may exist. The estimated number of noninstitutionalized persons with severe disabilities in the United States in 1975 was over 8 million.

For the most part, rehabilitation deals with persons who have long-term physical disabilities or chronic illnesses. Infatuated with youth and good health, our society often shuns or neglects chronic illness. This attitude is reflected in medical schools, where there is relatively little training in managing persons with chronic illness and recognizing the special challenges inherent in their care.

Influences on Patient Management

Modern medicine has been very effective at eliminating or devising cures for many of the acute diseases. The trend, however, is toward an increasingly older population with more complex, chronic disease processes that require ongoing, restorative care. The challenge, therefore, is enormous and the cost to the nation is staggering in terms of lost productivity, yet the number of rehabilitation professionals available to meet this growing need is relatively small.

Defining the scope of rehabilitation problems in our society requires going beyond simply

TABLE 1–1. *Factors influencing the management of patients with chronic illness*

Lesion	Stable	Progressive
Age at onset	Congenital, prepuberty	Adolescence, postadolescence
Extent	Limited	Systemic, multisystem
Visibility	Not apparent	Readily apparent

counting the number of persons with stroke, heart disease, or degenerative disorders. In developing programs tailored to the individual needs of patients with chronic illness, the primary care physician must consider a number of other factors that will influence the management of these persons (Table 1–1).

For example, the issues involved in managing a 45-year-old male executive who has a traumatic below-knee amputation are quite different from those involved in managing a 5-year-old child who has a below-elbow amputation for metastatic bone cancer in his dominant hand. The man's lesion is stable and he has passed through crucial periods of psychosocial development and maturation. With a good prosthetic fit and proper training, this patient's limb loss would not be readily apparent, and within certain limitations, he should be able to return to his previous occupation with little or no change in productivity. The child's lesion, however, is likely to be progressive, the rate depending on the cell type and availability and response to therapy. This patient is in a crucial stage in his physical, psychological, and social development. Even if there is a significant remission, the child and his parents, classmates, and teachers will be dealing with a readily apparent disability that will affect his body image, ability to participate in usual activities, interaction with others, and eventually, choice of careers. These issues are discussed in greater detail in Chapter 7.

TRADITIONAL MEDICAL MODEL VERSUS REHABILITATION MODEL

Problem Orientation

Table 1–2 compares some of the characteristics that distinguish the medical model from the rehabilitation model of health care in this country in the 1980s. The general orientation of the medical model is toward disease, while that of rehabilitation medicine is toward disability, or more broadly, illness. Disease is defined as the interaction of a pathological process with individual molecules, cells, and organs. It is essentially a biological event. Disability or illness, however, is essentially a human event. It represents the resulting interaction of a person with a disease.

Physician's Role

In the medical model, the physician's role tends to be active. It is a physician who does the examination, orders the tests, makes a diagnosis, and prescribes appropriate medications. The physician's role in the rehabilitation model also encompasses these functions but extends to include helping the patient adjust to the disability and problem solving to minimize the functional loss from a long-term, chronic condition. To accomplish this, the physician needs the help of allied health professionals who are trained to teach patients new skills in homemaking, child care, vocational training, driving, and coping with emotional stress. Often, a crucial role for the physician is to help facilitate or coordinate the accessibility to these services and their implementation. Along with other health care providers, the physician plays an active role in teaching the patient about his or her illness.

Patient's Role

In the medical model, the patient's role is often passive and uninformed, with diagnostic and therapeutic measures done or given to him. By contrast, in the rehabilitation model, the patient is encouraged to be an active, informed participant. Since an important part of rehabilitation is achieving behavioral changes and helping the patient to adjust physically and emotionally, the patient needs to know what to expect and have enough information to assist in problem identification and resolution.

TABLE 1–2. *Comparison of the medical and rehabilitation models of health care*

	Medical model	Rehabilitation model
Problem orientation	Disease	Disability and illness
Physician's role	Doer, knower	Teacher, facilitator
Patient's role	Passive	Active
Care orientation	Staff oriented	Patient oriented
Organization	Fragmented, no formal team	Team approach
Therapeutic approach	Treatment of disease	Management of disabilities
Objectives	Cure, enhance physical function	Healing, coping, adjusting, enhance functional performance

Care Orientation and Organization

In the medical model, patient care is organized for the convenience of the staff or care providers. Frequently there is no formal, organized team (except in surgery) and care is often fragmented, being dispensed in isolated units. In the rehabilitation model, care is organized more for the convenience of the patient or consumer. Teams are a formal and intentional part of the health care provision. Perhaps because the problems dealt with in rehabilitation are complex, long term, and frequently multisystem, the only practical solution is to bring together a highly organized group of professionals.

Therapeutic Approach

The therapeutic emphasis in the medical model is on treatment, while in rehabilitation, it is on management. Treatment is defined as effecting a relief or cure of the disease and relies heavily on medication, surgery, and the skills of modern technology. It is often episodic and symptom oriented. Management is defined as effecting relief from illness or disability and enhancing function, using the full resources of the health care system. It implies long-term involvement that actively includes the patient and family.

Objectives

In terms of outcome, the medical model is characterized by concern with curing and enhancing physiological function, while the rehabilitation model is characterized by concern with healing and enhancing functional performance.

Curing is defined as removing, reversing, or retarding a disease process, while healing is defined as decreasing discomfort and enhancing a sense of physical and psychological well being. For both patient and physician, healing is more active, curing more passive. Healing does not exclude curing, but extends beyond it to include caring.

TEAM CARE

The principal objective of interdisciplinary teams is to maximize functioning of the patient with chronic disability through comprehensive, coordinated care. Comprehensive, coordinated team care is defined as services by various professionals who communicate regularly about their observations and who integrate decisions and actions in relation to their separate goals. Through the coordinating process, the different professions focus on the individual as a whole in terms of the total environment and the total problem, thereby avoiding a fragmented approach to the patient.

Tasks of interdisciplinary rehabilitation teams involve assessment, definition of goals, provision of services, and follow-up to ensure continuity of care responsive to changes in the patient's needs. Team members know that the treatment process is not a single set of actions derived from an inflexible set of goals worked out in a clinic or office. Team treatment is a dynamic process of changing goals and service decisions where changes are based on the feedback of information from the patient's environment and the environmental conditions that influence improvement or lack of improvement.

Hospital-based, most rehabilitation teams can only provide restricted services to the community. Some communities, however, have interdisciplinary teams that do provide ongoing restorative services and treatment in the home. These teams include two or more of the following specialists: physicians, nurses, occupational, physical, and speech therapists, home aides, social workers, and vocational counselors. Although home care programs vary widely in their size, base of operations, and scope, they represent a potential model for establishing a network of community resources capable of providing the kinds of comprehensive care required by patients with long-term problems. In many communities, the Visiting Nurse Association provides the nucleus for the extension of rehabilitation services into the home.

Overall, coordinated team care appears to be more effective than the customary, fragmented care currently received by most persons with long-term illnesses. According to studies of coordinated team care, the patient's function usually improves or is at least maintained and disease activity either improves or deteriorates at a slower rate.

FUTURE DIRECTIONS

Costs and Reimbursement

The cost associated with rehabilitation services is often high, and sometimes when compared with other types of health care services, seems to be inappropriately expensive. There is loss of income, increased outlay for medical care, and the costs of special equipment and physical assistance to compensate for lost function. The provision of early preventive care, however, often helps avoid long-term complications that are even more expensive. Obtaining adequate reimbursement from third party payers has been a problem since the inception of rehabilitation medicine, and the provision of rehabilitation services by state and federal programs has often been inadequate. Interestingly, insurance companies providing workmen's compensation have usually been the most generous in their investment of comprehensive care for injured clients.

Rehabilitation Facilities

Although this book emphasizes the application of rehabilitation medicine to the office, home, hospital, and community practice of primary health care providers, it is sometimes advisable to refer a disabled patient to one of the specialized rehabilitation facilities available in many parts of the country. Also available are regional centers that provide specialized rehabilitation services for different types of disability groups, such as federally funded spinal injury centers. Preliminary data indicate that treating spinal injured patients in these specialized centers is more economical and efficient than in community hospitals. For less complex and less demanding kinds of problems, however, rehabilitation care can be applied in almost any health care setting.

Community Needs and Programs

Over the last decade, there has been an enormous increase in the provision of community rehabilitation services. The legislative act of 1976, known as Public Law 504, helped bring disabled persons into the mainstream by providing equal access to all federally funded programs and projects. A comparable law mandates the provision of rehabilitation services in public schools rather than segregating disabled children in specialized facilities. Another important development in recent years has been the implementation of independent living programs. These programs provide housing and other facilities where disabled persons are able to apply the skills learned in rehabilitation programs to living either independently or in groups that share resources and expenses. Through such programs, disabled persons are able to find more effective ways of living full, productive, useful lives.

CONCLUSIONS

A number of areas distinguish rehabilitation from most other medical specialties. Rehabilitation usually deals with patients having long-term problems and, thus, requires ongoing involvement. Ideally, rehabilitation begins as early as possible after the onset of a disability and often continues for many months or years. There is usually no clear-cut point of resolution at which someone is rehabilitated. Constant adjustments must be made as the patient ages and identifies new goals, priorities, and environmental changes. These problems often result from disease or injury for which there is no cure. Therefore, the emphasis is on restoration of residual function and helping the person adapt and become as independent as possible. Because the disease or injury often affects several organ systems, a comprehensive approach directed at the whole person is required. As a result, there is concern with not only physical well-being but also emotional, social, and vocational issues. In addition, multiple specialties and skills are usually involved in rehabilitation programs, which require team care and maximum use of allied health personnel. Finally, rehabilitation emphasizes patient education and helping patients learn to live with their disability in their own environments.

Many of these principles are fundamental not only to rehabilitation but also to primary health care. The philosophical principles underlying the fields, the approach to the patient, the concern for the whole person, the use of allied health personnel, and the emphasis on patient education give the two fields much in common.

Medical Rehabilitation,
edited by L. S. Halstead et al.
Raven Press, New York © 1985.

CHAPTER 2

Rehabilitation Specialists

*Lauro S. Halstead and **Martin Grabois

*Departments of Rehabilitation, Physical Medicine, and Community Medicine, Baylor College of Medicine, and The Institute for Rehabilitation and Research; **Departments of Physical Medicine and Rehabilitation, Baylor College of Medicine, Houston, Texas 77030*

Rehabilitation medicine, as practiced by physiatrists and allied health professionals, involves the coordinated efforts of a team of specialists, as described in Chapter 1. The physician and other rehabilitation professionals often have the advantage of working together as a team in a hospital, especially in larger communities. By contrast, many primary care physicians in private practice or rural settings may have limited access to other health professionals. For them, forming a team capable of handling the complexities of chronic illness can be a difficult and frustrating experience. Yet even a nucleus of two or three professionals, including the primary care physician, is often enough to make a significant difference in managing long-term disability.

An estimated 5% to 10% of the population is in need of physical medicine and rehabilitation services. As medical advances progressively increase the likelihood of survival from serious injury and chronic illness, primary care physicians will encounter more and more patients in their communities whose activities are severely curtailed by disability. At least three times as many as the 2,200 physiatrists currently in practice will be needed to bridge the gap between the supply of rehabilitation specialists and the demand for their services. Consequently, the burden of care for this growing population will fall on the primary care physician, who will need to understand the roles of the members of

a typical rehabilitation team and know how to use to best advantage one or more of the rehabilitation specialists available in the community.

QUALIFICATIONS AND RESPONSIBILITIES

If rehabilitation specialists are in short supply, you may wonder which ones are available in your community, how to select them, what services can be provided safely in your own office, and which services require hospital supervision. Discussion of the training, roles, responsibilities, strengths, and limitations of the various specialists will help you assemble and reassemble flexible teams from among the available public health or rehabilitation nurses, physiatrists, physical therapists, occupational therapists, speech and language pathologists, social workers, psychologists, and orthotists. Depending on the special needs of each patient, your role on this team will range from evaluator, prescriber, and director to actual provider of the therapeutic intervention.

Table 2–1 summarizes the education, training, and licensure, as well as the primary responsibilities, of rehabilitation specialists. The services typically provided by each specialist should be considered as general guidelines rather than as absolute standards. The types of neuromuscular disease and musculoskeletal injuries treated by

TABLE 2–1. *Qualifications and responsibilities of rehabilitation specialists*

Specialist	Education, training, licensure	Primary responsibilities
Physiatrist	M.D. Certified by Board of Physical Medicine and Rehabilitation	Evaluates muscle function, joint ROM, postural and gait patterns; performs EMG studies Leads team, coordinating and interpreting reports from other health care providers on team Prescribes treatment for disorders of neuromuscular and musculoskeletal function
Rehabilitation nurse	R.N. Optional M.S. in rehabilitation nursing	Writes nursing care plan for each patient Provides preventive and restorative nursing care—positions and turns bedridden patients; takes care of skin, preventing breakdown; trains bowel and bladder; performs passive joint ROM Selects special beds, mattresses, and positioning devices Educates patient and family in self-care techniques Coordinates discharge and follow-up plans with visiting nurse service and family
Physical therapist	B.S. Accredited by American Physical Therapy Association; State license	Evaluates, prevents, and manages disorders of human motion Uses physical modalities in treatment—heat, cold, ultraviolet, massage, exercise, TENS, EMG biofeedback, FES Trains in performing functional activities, especially gait with assistance of orthoses, canes, crutches
Occupational therapist	B.S. National certification Registration with American Occupational Therapy Association	Assesses what muscles need strengthening and coordination to enable ADL and recommends practical activities to improve strength Improves basic self-care skills, such as dressing, eating, and personal hygiene Recommends adaptive equipment and upper extremity orthoses to facilitate ADL and trains patient in use of upper extremity orthoses and prostheses Teaches homemaking skills and determines at what level the patient can participate Teaches energy conservation and work simplification methods to improve work tolerance Improves communication skills, such as reading, writing, and using the telephone Redirects vocational, avocational, recreational interests, and social activities to accommodate disability
Orthotist	B.S. Certified by American Academy of Orthotics and Prosthetics	Evaluates need for orthoses in preventing and correcting deformity and restoring function Designs, fabricates, and fits orthoses to achieve treatment objectives of physiatrist or other referring physician Monitors patient during adjustment to orthosis
Prosthetist	B.S. Certified by American Academy of Orthotics and Prosthetics	Designs, fabricates, and fits functional and cosmetic devices to replace amputated body parts and restore function Suggests prosthetic components that will best accommodate the level of amputation and patient's occupational and recreational needs
Speech-language pathologist	M.S. or Ph.D. in speech pathology or audiology Certified by American Speech and Hearing Association	Evaluates and treats dysfunction in reception, perception, decoding, encoding, motor planning, and production of language Administers psycholinguistic, auditory, and speech-language tests

TABLE 2–1. *(continued)*

Specialist	Education, training, licensure	Primary responsibilities
Social worker	M.A. or M.S.W. Some states require certification with Department of Human Resources	Assesses family support systems Serves as liaison between patient, family, and other community resources Assists family in modifying home environment Advises on management of financial burdens and on disability benefits Leads family or group discussions for patients and families trying to cope with severe physical impairment or disability
Clinical psychologist	Ph.D. Internship Board certified by American Psychological Association	Assesses intellectual dysfunction, psychological impact of disability, motivation Recognizes and treats reactive depression Advises physician on strategies for altering patient's behavior Designs behavioral therapy and social skills training programs Does psychotherapy, marital counseling, sexual counseling, assertiveness training, family therapy Suggests psychiatric consultation when appropriate
Vocational rehabilitation counselor	B.S. or M.S. Certified by the Board for Rehabilitation Certification; licensure required in some states	Performs aptitude and intelligence tests, skill tests, vocational intent tests, attitude tests, and personality tests Observes patient during participation in rehabilitation activities to assess functional suitability for work Coordinates restorative and training services, including work adjustment training and sheltered employment Places disabled patient in new job or adjusts responsibilities of premorbid job to functional capacity

ADL, activities of daily living. FES, functional electrical stimulation. ROM, range of motion. TENS, transcutaneous electrical nerve stimulation.

the physiatrist are indicated in Table 2–2. In most states, only the physician is permitted legally to prescribe treatment. As of 1984, six states permit physical therapists to evaluate and treat patients without physician referral. They are able to evaluate without referral in 22 states but must have a physician's prescription to treat patients.

Not only is there considerable overlap of responsibilities among the various specialists, but their roles also vary with the size and focus of the health facility with which they are affiliated. Furthermore, the facilities vary considerably in the levels of service provided. For example, as an employee of the Visiting Nurse Association, Easter Seal Society, Cerebral Palsy Center, or other community agency, a physical therapist may offer evaluation and referral for treatment, consultation, treatment planning, home care, comprehensive outpatient care, follow-up, or any combination of these services, depending on the facility's capacity. Experience with a broad range of services may be expected from a specialist affiliated with a general hospital, in which services range from long-term care for spinal cord injury, brain injury, and arthritis to management of acute problems such as postsurgical repair of a meniscus, low back strain, and fracture.

TABLE 2–2. *Chief categories of diseases and injuries treated by the physiatrist*

Condition	Sample disorders	Treatment aims and modalities
Acute and chronic musculoskeletal conditions	Muscular and ligamentous strains and contusions, peripheral nerve injuries and neuropathies, tendonitis and tenosynovitis, bursitis, myofascitis, back and neck strains, spondylosis, intervertebral disk disease, arthritis	Recovery or control; requires extensive use of physical modalities supplemented by medications, rest, and controlled mobilization
Acute and chronic neuromuscular conditions	Strokes and brain trauma, spinal cord injuries, cerebral palsy, limb amputations, pain syndromes, peripheral nerve and plexus injuries, postural and gait problems	Train patient to use remaining function in the injured part of his body to achieve maximum functional capacity and to develop compensatory function in other body parts to substitute for losses; determine need for corrective surgery, medications, neuromuscular retraining, assistive devices, lifestyle alterations to adjust to disability
Progressive neuromuscular conditions	Muscular dystrophies and atrophies, multiple sclerosis, and degenerative diseases of the central nervous system	Same as for acute and chronic neuromuscular conditions

INDICATIONS AND CONTRAINDICATIONS FOR REFERRAL

Any patient who has a reasonable chance of recovering lost function is a possible candidate for rehabilitation. The patient should be referred to a rehabilitation specialist or facility as soon as vital functions are stabilized. Early activity helps prevent the deconditioning that results from prolonged bed rest, and training of uninjured body parts can hasten their substitution for handicapped parts. Furthermore, preventing deformities and maintaining range of motion of skeletal joints during recovery accelerates restoration of function later.

Patients should be selected carefully for referral according to their likelihood of benefiting from the therapy. Do not assume that a patient expected to sustain only a mild or moderate handicap does not need rehabilitation; final recovery depends not only on how much residual function remains after the injury but also on how it is used. Patients with a great deal of function remaining may benefit more from rehabilitation than patients with minimal residual function. Proper treatment may be able to double a re-

maining 50% function so that function is restored to a nearly normal 100%, whereas doubling a remaining 10% function will yield only 20% restoration. When patients are responding well to rehabilitation measures, treatment should be continued and even escalated, while the potential of patients who are responding poorly may be so limited that further treatment is not worthwhile.

Certain patients may be poor candidates for referral to a physical, occupational, or related therapist. Because they tend to become overly dependent on the therapist and the treatment, patients with numerous psychosomatic complaints and little insight into the emotional precipitants of their illness rarely benefit from therapy. Obviously, patients who remain semicomatose, confused, and stuporous are not ready to follow instructions and participate actively in a rehabilitation program. Others refuse to cooperate in complying with the prescribed treatment. Similarly, the severely crippled arthritic patient, who requires intervention by a team of physicians and therapists, will benefit more from the comprehensive services of a hospital and rehabilitation center.

PRESCRIBING THERAPY FOR REHABILITATION

When requesting assistance from a rehabilitation service, provide a detailed prescription for treatment that clearly presents the therapeutic objectives. Depending on the nature of the patient's disability, therapy may be short-term, requiring one simple prescription, or prolonged, requiring frequent, complex revisions of the prescription for the severely disabled or chronically ill.

The differences between diagnosing disability and diagnosing disease are discussed in Chapter 3. There are comparable differences between prescribing conventional treatments for disease and prescribing physical and occupational therapy to minimize disability. The following are the essential elements of a prescription for therapy:

1. Brief summary of history
2. Diagnosis
3. Modalities and dosage to use
4. Treatment area of body
5. Dates to start treatments
6. Duration of treatment
7. Number and frequency of treatments
8. Precautions to take
9. Goals to achieve
10. Dates of treatments
11. Date for primary care physician's recheck
12. Order to give home treatment instructions

Following several precautions when prescribing therapy will help improve the treatment outcome. Check the therapists' credentials to ensure their qualifications to perform the prescribed treatment. The therapists available in your community may not offer all of the services mentioned in Table 2–1. The prescription should be sufficiently detailed for the therapists to follow.

Patients should be discouraged from prescribing their own treatment and therapists from giving patients whatever they request. Do make sure, however, that the patients can tolerate the treatment you select, encourage patient feedback, and consider their requests when revising the prescription over the course of the treatment period. Individualize each prescription rather than following a standard therapeutic regimen for every patient with a given disorder. There is no set therapeutic routine that will successfully meet the needs of every patient with degenerative joint disease, for example.

Regardless of the nature of the illness, disappointing results can be expected when the frequency of treatment is inadequate. Beginning treatment is usually most effective if administered at least daily and gradually decreased to two or three times weekly as the patient progresses and learns to perform some procedures at home. Weekly treatments are usually adequate only to update a home treatment program. As the patient progresses and responds to the treatments, frequent changes in your orders may be required. Therefore, prompt and frequent follow-up of the patient is critical to avoid unnecessary delay in recovery.

SUGGESTED READINGS

Colachis, S. C. (1984): New directions in health care. *Arch. Phys. Med. Rehabil.*, 65:291–294.

Halstead, L. S. (1976): Team care in chronic illness; a critical review of the literature of the past 25 years. *Arch. Phys. Med. Rehabil.*, 57:507–511.

Logigian, M. K. (1982): *Adult Rehabilitation: A Team Approach for Therapists*. Little, Brown, Boston.

Martin, G. M. (1982): Prescribing physical and occupational therapy. In: *Krusen's Handbook of Physical Medicine and Rehabilitation*, 3rd edit., edited by F. J. Kottke, G. K. Stillwell, and J. F. Lehmann. W. B. Saunders, Philadelphia.

Ruskin, A. P. (1984): Evolving roles of health professionals in the care of the disabled. In: *Current Therapy in Physiatry: Physical Medicine and Rehabilitation*, edited by A. P. Ruskin. W. B. Saunders, Philadelphia.

Medical Rehabilitation,
edited by L. S. Halstead et al.
Raven Press, New York © 1985.

CHAPTER 3

Evaluation of Disability

Martin Grabois

Departments of Physical Medicine and Rehabilitation, Baylor College of Medicine, Houston, Texas 77030

PRINCIPLES OF DIAGNOSING DISEASE VERSUS DISABILITY

In the medical specialty of physical medicine and rehabilitation, diagnosing the disease is only the first step in evaluating a patient. This diagnosis does not reveal what functions were lost as a result of the disease or injury. The evaluation of lost or compromised physical, psychosocial, vocational, and avocational function over the course of a chronic illness or irreversible pathological process comprises the *disability diagnosis*. There are five principles underlying the evaluation of disability versus disease:[1]

1. The symptoms and signs required for the diagnosis of disability differ from those required for the diagnosis of disease.
2. There is not a one-to-one correlation between a disease and the range of associated disability problems; the disability is dependent on the patient's total daily needs.
3. There is not a one-to-one relationship between a disease and the amount of residual disability; disability can be removed without altering the course of the disease.
4. The ability of the patient and physician to remove disability in the face of chronic disease is dependent on the residual capacity of the patient for physiological and psychological adaptation.

5. Disability means lost function, not only physical but also psychosocial-vocational.

These principles are illustrated in the following hypothetical case:

A 57-year-old woman complains of pain in her calves after walking several blocks. Based on her history, physical examination, and laboratory tests, the diagnosis is peripheral vascular disease. Although you have established a diagnosis of this patient's disease, you have not made a disability diagnosis, that is, you do not know how her disease is affecting her daily functioning. Before prescribing a course of therapy it is necessary to determine the extent of disability caused by the disease. This cannot be assumed from the severity or the chronicity of the medical disorder because functional loss is partly a product of individual lifestyle and responsibilities. This particular patient happens to work in an office, a job requiring little walking. Therefore, her vocational disability from the disease is minimal. Had she been a nurse, however, and her discomfort exacerbated by being on her feet all day, she could have been disabled with "loss of primary vocation," unless she were eligible for a sedentary administrative position.

The range of disability problems produced by a disease thus depends upon the interaction of the patient with the environment. The patient's rehabilitation potential, in turn, reflects *the sum of abilities in all body systems assessed against the sum of disabilities*. Based on the diagnosis and extent of disability, rehabilitation goals must be established within realistic time frames and an appropriate, goal-oriented prescription for

---

[1]Adapted from Stolov, W. C. (1981): Comprehensive rehabilitation: Evaluation and treatment. In: *Handbook of Severe Disability*, edited by W. C. Stolov and M. R. Clowers. Department of Rehabilitation Medicine, University of Washington, Seattle.

rehabilitation therapy written. Frequent re-evaluation of the patient is necessary to establish new goals and update the therapy prescription.

Problem-Oriented Medical Record

The Weed problem-oriented medical record, as modified for rehabilitation medicine, provides a model for the clinical evaluation of the patient's disease and resultant disability. This means of organizing the ongoing management of disabled patients is a useful tool for planning patient care and assessing the patient's rehabilitation potential. The problem-oriented record consists of a medical problem list, a rehabilitation problem list, a medical problem-oriented progress note, and a rehabilitation problem-oriented progress note. The problem lists should include subjective and objective data—physiologic syndromes, symptoms, signs, and laboratory test results. Because abnormalities of undetermined disease diagnosis may contribute to disability, these should be recorded, as well as those abnormalities related to the disease diagnosis. In addition to specific impairments of function in basic physical self-care, include problems in social, vocational, or psychological function. These steps will enable you to formulate an impression of the status of both medical problems and disabilities and, ultimately, a therapeutic plan that can be revised frequently as the patient's condition improves or progresses.

The following case history illustrates the application of the problem-oriented approach to a patient following a cerebral vascular accident. Although the patient's primary medical problem, right hemiparesis, could not be resolved, many of the rehabilitation problems did have solutions that decreased disability.

PROBLEM-ORIENTED APPROACH

Report of a Case

HISTORY. This 69-year-old man was admitted to a local hospital for evaluation of sudden right-sided weakness, and after stabilization, he was referred to a physical medicine service for intensive rehabilita-

TABLE 3–1. *Medical problem list*

No.	Problem	Date of onset	Date resolved
M1	Right hemiparesis	5/5/84	—
M2	Urinary tract infection	5/10/84	5/20/84
M3	Hypertension	1981	—
M4	Diabetes mellitus	1981	—

tion. Acute medical problems were limited to right hemiparesis secondary to occlusion of the left middle cerebral artery and urinary tract infection. Past medical history was noncontributory, except for a history of mild hypertension controlled with hydrochlorothiazide and diabetes mellitus controlled by diet. Social history revealed the patient was retired and living with his wife, who had arthritis. Before the onset of right hemiparesis, he had been independent in all functional activities.

PHYSICAL EXAMINATION. This patient had minimal to moderate receptive and expressive aphasia with a seventh cranial nerve central palsy on the right. Gross sensation was intact. Deep tendon reflexes were hyperactive on the right and normal on the left, with positive Babinski and Hoffman signs on the right side. Range of motion was within normal limits, but there was no voluntary motion in the right upper extremity. Increased muscle tone was noted on the right side. There was fair muscle power in the proximal right lower extremity, but poor muscle power of the distal muscle groups. Muscle strength on the left side was within normal limits.

FUNCTIONAL EXAMINATION. The patient's functional status was evaluated by several rehabilitation team members. A physical therapist examined mobilization; an occupational therapist, activities of daily living; a speech pathologist, communication skills; a social worker, economic assets, family and community support; and a psychologist, mental status and coping skills. He was found to be dependent in most

TABLE 3–2. *Rehabilitation problem list*

No.	Problem	Date of onset	Date resolved
R1	Mobilization	5/5/84	—
R2	Activities of daily living	5/5/84	—
R3	Communication	5/5/84	—
R4	Social interaction	5/5/84	—
R5	Psychological status	5/5/84	—

TABLE 3–3. *Medical problem-oriented progress note*

M1 Right hemiparesis
  No change
M2 Urinary tract infection
  S[a]—No complaints
  O[b]—Urine culture negative after 10-day course on nitrofurantoin (Macrodantin®)
  A[c]—No urinary tract infection
  P[d]—Problem resolved
M3 Hypertension
  S—No complaints
  O—Blood pressure ranges from 140/80 to 145/90 mm Hg
  A—Blood pressure under control
  P—Continue hydrochlorothiazide and monitor blood pressure daily

[a]Subjective data—patient's symptoms and personal impressions.
[b]Objective data—patient's physical signs, laboratory and other test data, and quantified progress.
[c]Assessment of the problem—interpretation of subjective and objective data into an impression of the status of the problem.
[d]Plan—necessary additional consultations, diagnostics, therapeutics, or patient education required.

TABLE 3–4. *Rehabilitation problem-oriented progress note*

R1 Mobilization
  S/O—No active motion in right upper extremity. Fair proximal and poor distal power in right lower extremity. Transfers from bed to wheelchair and stands in parallel bars with assistance
  A—Little improvement in strength. Transfers improved from dependent to assistance level. Standing with support
  P—Improve transfers to supervision level. Start ambulation with temporary short leg orthosis in parallel bars
R2 Activities of daily living
  S/O—Self-feeding. Washing of upper extremities with supervision. Washing of lower extremities dependent. Dressing dependent
  A—Feeding and upper extremity dressing improved
  P—Improve lower extremity washing to supervision level. Start dressing techniques
R3 Communication
  S/O—Decreased receptive and expressive language skills. Difficulty finding words
  A—Moderate receptive and expressive aphasia. No improvement noted
  P—Instruct in alternate means of communication. Start work on single-word responses
R4 Social
  S/O—Wife with nondisabling arthritis. Hospital coverage and resources adequate to hire housekeeper, if necessary
  A—No immediate social problems. No vocational training necessary (patient retired)
  P—Purchase adaptive equipment and hire housekeeper after patient's discharge
R5 Psychological status
  S/O—Appropriate depression being worked out
  A—Transition from depressive phase to adjustment phase of disability. Antidepressant medications not indicated
  P—No formal intervention necessary

activities of daily living, such as bathing, dressing, eating, personal hygiene, wheelchair transfers, and ambulation, but bladder and bowel function were intact. He had some difficulty communicating and was depressed.

Tables 3–1 through 3–4 show the organization of this patient's history, physical examination, and functional examination into problem lists and progress notes.

CLINICAL EXAMINATION

The clinical evaluation consists of the medical history, physical examination, and functional evaluation. Standard techniques for taking a history and performing a physical examination are used but expanded to determine the type and degree of disability.

History

Many of the sections of the medical history designed to identify disabilities contain a different emphasis from the typical disease-oriented medical history. The nature of the chief complaint may imply the existence of disability. The present illness data reveal the extent of lost function in basic self-care skills. The review of systems and past medical history sections provide clues to the physical reserve available for participating in the rehabilitation program. The social and vocational history discloses the personality, response patterns to stress, and environmental factors that may accommodate or exacerbate disability.

Chief Complaint

The patient usually describes the presenting symptoms, anatomical area of dysfunction, and reason for seeking medical care in terms of lost function. For example, the patient described above probably stated, "I had a stroke," "I can't walk," "I'm having problems talking," or "I can't take care of myself."

Present Illness

In addition to the development of the disease, include the patient's premorbid physical functioning, as well as a chronological sequence of events and time course for loss of independence. Determine whether the onset of such symptoms as weakness, speech abnormalities, or bladder dysfunction was sudden or progressive, whether the patient has had similar episodes, and whether he has noted associated symptoms.

Past Medical History

Emphasize medical problems that are related to the development of the present condition and note the patient's response to previous medical stress. Previous trauma, diseases, or surgery may have left the patient with residual impairments that are reactivated or compounded by the present illness. In the case report above, for example, the history of hypertension and diabetes is significant not only in the development of the present illness but also in predicting long-term functional outcome and prognosis, since hypertension makes the patient more vulnerable to cerebral vascular accidents and diabetes to peripheral neuropathy.

Review of Systems

The status of four systems in particular must be evaluated to assess a patient's residual capacity for the training required to minimize disability and restore function: cardiovascular, respiratory, neurological, and musculoskeletal systems. Compromised cardiopulmonary function—chest pain, shortness of breath, or claudication—can limit the duration and strenuousness of exercise periods, as well as

quickly deplete the high energy reserves needed for transfers and walking. Musculoskeletal limitations such as pain, weakness, or limited range of motion may interfere with ambulation and the performance of activities of daily living. Before rehabilitation, for example, the patient described earlier was dependent in all functional activities due to hemiparesis. Neurological symptoms such as diminished sensation may limit the use of most heat modalities, while attention deficits secondary to disorders of the central nervous system may decelerate the learning of self-care techniques.

Psychosocial History

The object is to gather information about the patient's environment to determine the social impact of the illness. If the patient has not been working, inquire about current sources of financial support. Are insurance and personal funds adequate to cover the expensive rehabilitation process? If financial assistance will be needed, refer the patient to agencies that can provide support. Also determine whether family relationships are adequate to provide emotional, physical, and economic support, and whether the physical characteristics of the home enable ease of access. Are the bedroom, bathroom, and kitchen on the first floor or must stairs be negotiated?

Note the patient's previous social adjustment, since earlier patterns of response to stress and change are often helpful predictors of how the patient will cope with the current stress. How self-reliant has the patient been? If there have been previous periods of depression, what brought them on? The patient's level of success, maturity, and responsibility achieved as an adult in school, work, and marriage is often a good indicator of how the patient will handle the current disability and rehabilitation process.

Vocational and Avocational History

What were the patient's vocational and recreational activities before and after illness? Record the history of employment, types of skills, and highest educational level, noting any work adjustment problems. Referral to a state Bureau of Vocational Rehabilitation may be needed if job instability is suspected or the current job seems incompatible with the current disability even after rehabilitation.

Recreational activities are particularly important for the retired patient, as in the patient cited above, or if vocational placement is improbable. Determine whether most of the patient's desired activities are symbol oriented, motor oriented, or interpersonally oriented and how distressed the patient is about losing the ability to perform activities in one of these categories. Paraplegia, for example, is less likely to affect performance of symbol-oriented activities such as reading than motor-oriented activities such as hiking and other sports, while a stroke with aphasia may profoundly impair participation in interpersonal and symbol-oriented activities.

Physical Examination

After you have identified areas of disability from the history, a physical examination of the patient will provide three kinds of information about the nature of disability:

1. Signs of deviations from normal structure and function that contribute to formulating the disease diagnosis.
2. Signs of secondary problems which, although not necessarily a direct consequence of the disease, may lengthen the treatment time needed to remove the disabilities induced by the primary disease process. (Secondary problems result from treatment of the disease or from neglect of appropriate preventive measures.)
3. Residual strengths in the system or parts of systems unaffected by the disease.

The search for secondary problems and residual strengths calls for concentration on virtually all organs (or systems) of the body.

HEENT Evaluation

Examination results of the visual, auditory, and speech apparatus reveal communication defects that may interfere with learning, as well as suggest the patient's most effective mode of communication. Patients with stroke or head injury, for example, may have hearing difficulties and visual field losses. In addition, disorders of the mouth and throat may disrupt chewing and swallowing as well as vocalization.

Cardiopulmonary Reserve

Appropriate exercise levels can be established only if the patient's cardiopulmonary reserve is known. Examination of blood pressure, peripheral and carotid pulses, skin temperature, and peripheral edema, as well as cardiac size, rhythm, and sounds, will identify abnormalities that can be treated to improve cardiovascular reserve. Similarly, examination of respiratory rate and rhythm, chest shape, the facies for cyanosis, and the lungs for congestion and obstruction will identify problems compromising respiratory function (see Chapter 13 for more details). Exercise stress testing shows the response of the cardiopulmonary systems to a measured work load. Through a regular schedule of exercise testing, the adequacy with which the cardiopulmonary system responds to a trial quantity of exercise can be monitored and the exercise program adjusted accordingly (see Chapter 14 for details).

Genitourinary and Rectal Examination

Genitourinary and rectal evaluation is important not only to detect neurogenic bladder and bowel but also to determine whether reflexes are adequate for normal physiological sexual response. Inadequate bowel and bladder control, producing unpredictable episodes of incontinence, can make social situations especially stressful and lead to reclusive behavior. Neurologically impaired erectile dysfunction may threaten the patient's marriage as well as his self concept. Included in the examination are patterns of elimination, perineal sensation, prostate size, sphincter tone, and the bulbocavernosus (BC) reflex. The BC reflex is performed by pinching the glans penis while inserting a finger in the anus. Contraction of the external anal sphincter indicates intact afferent and efferent pathways of the voiding reflex. Pressure on the clitoris or a tug on the catheter if one is present are also tests for afferent pathways. A finger in the anus will detect the efferent response. These examinations are covered more thoroughly in Chapter 25.

Neurological Examination

The neurological examination includes evaluation of cerebellar and coordination functions, deep tendon and pathological reflexes, all 12 cranial nerves, cerebral functions, and sensation. Impaired coordination may interfere with, among other functions, voluntary control of gait and grasp, which are important predictors of functional independence. Rehabilitation may require extensive retraining of individual muscles. Cerebral evaluation should detect possible perceptual involvement and determine the patient's ability to learn and communicate, essential for successful outcome of training in new techniques to replace incapacitation by disability.

Sensory examination concentrates on superficial touch and pain, deep pain, position sense of large and small joints, vibration sense, stereognosis, two-point discrimination, hot and cold perception, and the presence or absence of extinction to bilateral confrontation. Application of certain physical modalities, especially some forms of heat, may be contraindicated in patients with diminished sensation, which prevents accurate dose regulation (see Chapter 4). The patient with deficient proprioception, unable to judge where a body part is in space, may require supervision in walking and other activities to prevent accidents. Inadequate proprioception may also impair coordination training and, in severe cases, dictate confinement to a wheelchair. Without adequate perception of pain, patients may inadvertently injure themselves or ignore warnings of skin sore formation. Detection of diminished sensation will alert the health care providers not only to avoid damaging the skin by inappropriate handling but also to teach the patient new means of self-care to compensate for the loss of former sensory cues.

Musculoskeletal Examination

Musculoskeletal evaluation comprises the joints and associated structures, ligaments, and muscles that cross the joints. While the muscles should be inspected for contour and size, atrophy, masses, and swellings and palpated to distinguish between bony masses, edema, and joint effusions, testing of joint range of motion and muscle strength should have priority.

Measurement of joint motion by the universal goniometer helps in diagnosing the degree of functional loss and provides objective criteria for assessing the patient's progress throughout the treatment program. Goniometric measurement can be performed within 5° of accuracy by a physical therapist, occupational therapist, or physician (Fig. 3–1). This reading is compared to the normal range of motion established for each joint. Table 3–5 shows average range of motion data for some commonly measured joints. A joint may retain full functional capacity for most activities of daily living even if the range of motion is less than full. For example, a patient with 70° of shoulder abduction would be able to perform all activities of daily living even though the full range is 180°. The examiner should indicate whether the range of motion was measured under conditions of pain, active or passive motion, and consider the sex and age of the patient. Measuring all possible joint motions is unnecessary; measure only those joint motions that are pertinent to the patient's medical and functional diagnosis and treatment plan.

Using this system, the examiner can measure excessive laxness of a joint, which permits motion beyond normal extension, recurvatum deformity, or flexion contracture, the inability to move a part to its normal position of extension. Perhaps the most serious detriments to energy conservation, especially for efficient ambulation, are hip flexion contracture and knee flexion contracture, common concomitants of bed rest or prolonged sitting. You can test these joints without a goniometer by using your own normal range of motion as a control or by comparing

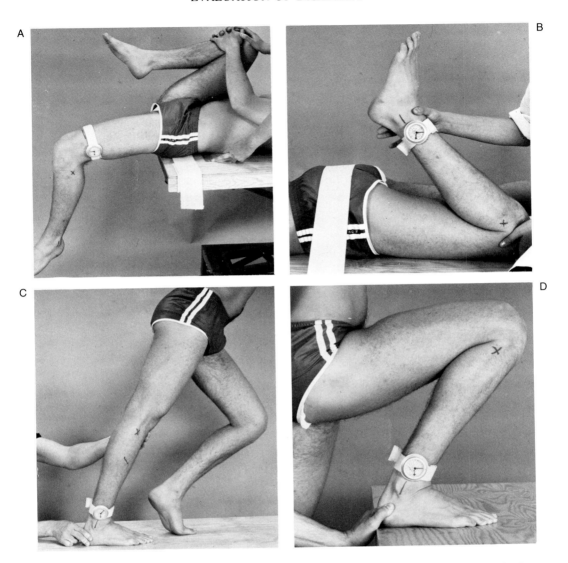

FIG. 3–1. Accuracy of lower extremity goniometer measurements are improved by standardizing the instrument's position in relation to bony anatomic landmarks (x) and the height of the examining bench. **A:** Hip extension is measured with patient supine on bench and flexometer (a type of goniometer) strapped to lateral side of thigh. Placement of plastic ruler under lower back ensures elimination of lumbar lordosis. **B:** Knee flexion is measured with subject lying prone on bench and flexometer strapped to leg above lateral malleolus. Patient's pelvis is immobilized with Velcro band. One examiner passively flexes the knee as the other reads the result at the moment hip flexion begins. **C:** Ankle dorsiflexion is measured as patient stands upright. Patient is asked to lean forward and bring about maximal ankle dorsiflexion, keeping the knee straight and the heel on the floor. Examiner checks knee extension and knee contact against floor. **D:** Standing on the floor with the foot of the leg to be tested on a bench, subject leans forward to produce maximal ankle dorsiflexion. Examiner checks to make sure patient's heel is in contact with the bench. [From Eckstrand, J. (1982): Reliability of goniometric measurements. *Arch. Phys. Med. Rehabil.*, 63:172–175, with permission.]

TABLE 3–5. *Average ranges of joint motion*

Joint	Action	Degrees of motion
Shoulder	Flexion	180
	Extension	45
	Abduction	180
	Adduction	40
	Lateral rotation	90
	Medial rotation	90
Elbow	Flexion	145
Forearm	Pronation	80
	Supination	85
Wrist	Extension	70
	Flexion	80
	Abduction	20
	Adduction	45
Hip	Flexion	125
	Extension	10
	Abduction	45
	Adduction	40
	Medial rotation	45
	Lateral rotation	45
Knee	Flexion	140
Ankle	Flexion	45
	Extension	20
Foot	Inversion	40
	Eversion	20

the patient's abnormal side with the affected side.

In muscle strength testing, a disabled patient's current and potential level of strength has some correlation with functional outcome in activities of daily living. For example, sufficient strength is required to propel a wheelchair over even or uneven terrain, up or down a curb, or across a street that is controlled by a timed traffic light. Similarly, adequate strength is necessary to lift one's body weight on crutches to climb and descend stairs and curbs, to cross a street, or to sit down in and rise from a chair. Therefore, the manual muscle test, which grades the strength of muscles that are under the control of the central nervous system, has become an important part of the objective physical examination for disability. It is most reliable in evaluating lower motor neuron disorders such as Guillain-Barré syndrome and peripheral neuropathy, although it may also be used in upper motor neuron disorders such as stroke or head injury.

Muscle strength is quantitated through a grading system such as the typical one shown in Table

3–6. Regardless of the system selected, the minimal functions evaluated are normal, zero or no contraction, and that strength just adequate to move a body segment or part fully against the resistance of gravity (fair). Strength can be further screened by assigning a plus (+) or minus (−) to each grade, where plus designates that a muscle can be moved two-thirds through the range of motion, and minus indicates that it can be moved one-third through the range of motion. Thus, F − would indicate a muscle that is strong enough to move a body segment two-thirds of its range of motion against gravity but not completely against gravity, whereas P + would indicate a muscle strong enough to move a body segment fully with gravity eliminated but only one-third of the range of motion against gravity.

A skilled therapist or physiatrist is able to differentiate accurately between these fine grades of muscle strength. As a prelude to specific manual muscle testing, you can identify general areas of deficit, which can be more precisely tested by standard techniques later, by performing some simple screening tests. For example, applying resistance over the humerus as the patient holds the arms out to the side will help detect middle or lower trapezius weakness. To detect weakness of the serratus anterior or anterior deltoid muscles, apply downward resistance on the mid-humerus as the patient pushes upward with arms straight out in front. An inability to walk on the

TABLE 3–6. *Muscle strength grading system*

Grade	Muscle activity	Numerical scale
0	No contraction visible or palpable	0
Trace (T)	Contraction seen or palpated but no joint movement	1, or 10%
Poor (P)	Contraction with gravity eliminated	2, or 25%
Fair (F)	Contraction against gravity	3, or 50%
Good (G)	Contraction against minimum to moderate resistance	4, or 75%
Normal (N)	Contraction against maximum resistance	5, or 100%

heels, or walk like a duck, may reveal weak dorsiflexor and evertor muscles of the ankles and toes. Incoordination, deficient afferent senses, or muscle bulk asymmetry may be detected as the patient performs a tandem gait, heel-to-toe and flat-footed. As a general rule, position the patient so that the specific muscle being tested is solely responsible for moving the body part. Strong muscles should be tested against the weight of the patient's body.

FUNCTIONAL EXAMINATION

A functional examination is performed by asking the patient to perform a particular task such as walking, transferring from a wheelchair to a bed, donning a shirt, or reading. Functional skills typically evaluated include eating, dressing, personal hygiene, balance, transfers, ambulation, and mental status. Although an occupational therapist, rehabilitation nurse, physical therapist, or psychologist can test these skills formally using various objective tests, the primary care physician should obtain an estimate of function at the bedside to expedite initiation of an effective rehabilitation program. Note the degree of independence or dependence in performing each of these skills, as well as the need for assistive devices such as special eating utensils, sliding board for transfers, or walkers. Objectivity in assessing these activities can be improved by making motion pictures or video tapes as the patient performs each task, having specific functions, signs, and symptoms scored by multiple judges, and performing factor analysis on their results.

The levels of dependence are as follows:

1. Independent: Patient can perform activities without verbal or physical assistance.
2. Supervision needed: Patient may require verbal instruction or standby assistance to perform functional activity.
3. Assistance needed: Patient requires assistance of another person at minimal, moderate, or maximal level to perform the functional activity.
4. Dependent: Patient cannot perform the activity even with the assistance of adaptive equipment or another person and the functional activity must be performed totally by someone other than the patient.

Activities of Daily Living

To acquire objective evidence of the patient's functional capacity, ask him or her to demonstrate activities such as dressing, feeding, and attending to personal hygiene. Record any assistance required, the ability to perform the task independently, or the necessity for another person to perform the activity. Also record any adaptive equipment and assistive devices needed and the time required to complete the task.

Balance

Test balance in both the sitting and the standing positions. The normal person is able to remain stationary in the sitting and standing positions unsupported and does not fall when nudged from side to side. Record any deviations from normal balance, as these may impair ambulation.

Transfers

Also a prerequisite for ambulation, transfer ability involves turning in bed, sitting up, and standing up. If the patient can perform these maneuvers, evaluate the ability to move to a chair or mat. Specific transfer techniques are described in Chapters 5 and 15.

Ambulation

Evaluation of ambulation consists of the ability to propel a wheelchair or walk using a functional and efficient gait pattern. As the patient ambulates, observe coordination and speed and record any deviations from a smooth, rhythmic pattern. Changes in muscle strength or the skeletal structure produce abnormal shifts in the center of gravity, leading to abnormal gait patterns and additional energy requirements.

You can make a preliminary assessment of a disabled patient's gait as he or she walks into the examination room by noting any lurches or limps that should undergo more extensive evaluation. Observe the patient walking with and without orthoses, crutches, or other supportive devices. Note the motion of the trunk, head, upper extremities, and each joint of the lower extremities as the patient walks at various speeds. Limping is often more exaggerated during fast than slow walking. Referral to a physiatrist for a more thorough gait analysis is recommended before taking any of these actions:

1. Exercise and training to correct gait.
2. Recommending an orthosis for support or correction.
3. Assessing the fit and function of a prosthesis or lower extremity orthosis.
4. Modifying a supportive device, such as crutches, a cane, orthosis, or prosthesis, to improve its fit and function.

Accurate assessment of gait pattern necessitates understanding the normal gait cycle, which consists of two phases—stance and swing (Fig. 3–2)—and requires optimal stride length and timing. Gait is ordinarily an automatic function. Injury to the neuromusculoskeletal system partially replaces this automatic sequencing with a slower, less coordinated, less rhythmic, and asymmetric translation of the body from one position to another. Normal motion is a smooth, sinusoidal pathway of the center of gravity; this center shifts toward the stance leg, alternating as each limb becomes a stance leg and then a swing leg, and rises and falls from the unilateral to the double stance. Maintenance of this smooth progression requires normal range of motion of the hip, knee, and ankle, symmetry of limb length, and an intact neuromuscular system. Abnormalities causing jerky or abrupt movements expend considerably more energy.

Common causes of gait abnormalities are unequal leg lengths, ankylosis or limitation of joint range, equinus deformity of the foot, and joint instability. In addition, pain often leads to avoidance of weight bearing on the painful side and shortening of the stance phase. Extensive discussion of all possible gait deviations is beyond the scope of this chapter, but some typical gait deviations are described in Table 3–7.

These deviations may be combined to form gait disorders that are readily discernible to the observer. The combined gluteus maximus and gluteus medius gait of the patient with Duchenne-type muscular dystrophy, for example, results in a waddling gait composed of a compensated gluteus medius limp or a trunk lurch over the affected side with each step. Exaggerated lordosis also occurs, due to hip extensor weakness.

Another easily recognized gait is the ataxic or unbalanced gait, characterized by impaired width of the gait base, uneven stride length and unequal stride times, and flailing about to retain balance. A typical retropulsion and festinating gait with small, shuffling steps progressing in speed is seen in Parkinson's disease. The steppage gait is commonly observed in weakness of the peroneal innervated musculature, producing drop foot, exaggerated hip and knee flexion, and toe strike prior to heel strike. Orthoses and supportive devices that are useful for correcting these specific gait abnormalities are suggested in the chapters on specific disorders (e.g., Chapters 15 and 19).

Functional Profile

A useful profile for evaluating independence in self-care and mobility is PULSES:

P—Physical condition, including visceral, cardiovascular, gastrointestinal, urological, endocrinological, and neurological disorders.

U—Self-care activities depending mainly on upper limb function, such as drinking, feeding, dressing, applying braces and/or prostheses, grooming, bathing, perineal care.

L—Mobility activities depending mainly on lower limb function, such as transferring between chair and toilet or tub or shower, walking, negotiating stairs, transferring to and from wheelchair.

S—Sensory components relating to communication—speech, hearing, and vision.

E—Excretory functions of the bladder and bowel.

S—Intellectual and emotional adaptability, support from family, and financial capability.

Each of the six functions is scored on a scale from 1 to 4, where 1 represents the least dependence and 4 the greatest dependence. Using such

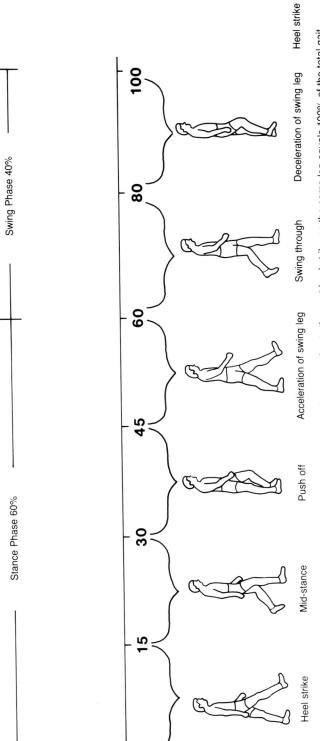

Stance Phase 60%   Swing Phase 40%

| 0 | 15 | 30 | 45 | 60 | 80 | 100 |

Heel strike   Mid-stance   Push off   Acceleration of swing leg   Swing through   Deceleration of swing leg   Heel strike

FIG. 3–2. Phases of the normal gait cycle. The cycle from heel strike on one leg to the next heel strike on the same leg equals 100% of the total gait cycle. The walker spends 60% of the cycle in the stance phase, then proceeds to the swing phase and returns again to the stance phase. (Illustration by Charlotte Holden.)

TABLE 3–7. *Selected gait deviations*

Deviation	Definition	Usual causes
Stance phase		
Trendelenburg sign	Abnormal drop of pelvis on the contralateral limb that is in swing	Weakness of gluteus medius on stance leg
Gluteus maximus gait	Backward lurching of trunk; hyperextension of the hip to achieve stability in stance, also producing lordosis and shortened step length	Weakness of gluteus maximus on stance leg
Genu recurvatum	Hyperextension of knee on stance leg, sometimes accompanied by forward lurch of trunk, decreased stance time, or external rotation of leg	Weakness of hamstrings, quadriceps, or gastrocnemius, quadriceps spasticity, or contracture of Achilles tendon
Swing phase		
Circumduction	Limb moves laterally in wide arc during swing phase but returns to normal orientation at end of swing	Inability to shorten leg in swing because of hip weakness, knee and dorsiflexor or extensor spasticity of swing leg, or shortening of stance leg
Abducted gait	Continuous positioning of swing leg in abduction, with leg held laterally away from normal frontal alignment at all times during gait cycle	Contracture of gluteus medius
Foot drop and steppage gait	As limb begins swing, foot hangs downward, lacking dorsiflexion; patient compensates by increasing hip and knee flexion; foot hits toe first	Paralysis of anterior tibialis, deficient proprioception, abnormal motor control or footdrop

profiles, many rehabilitation centers have developed patient status forms to evaluate function and goals from admission through 1 year after hospital discharge (Table 3–8). These forms can be used with or without the problem-oriented medical record described earlier in this chapter.

Quantitative Methods

Clinicians, biomedical engineers, biostatisticians, psychologists, and computer programmers have been collaborating to develop quantitative methods for objectively assessing pathological sensory and motor function, comparing the relative efficacy of therapeutic drugs, such as for spasticity, and performing activities of daily living. The severity of specific signs and symptoms—involuntary movements, abdominal pain, bladder dysfunction, paresthesias, motor weakness, gait disturbance, loss of associated movements, rigidity, cogwheeling, and bradykinesia—can be rated on an ordinal scale. Sensory tests have been developed to measure touch, pressure, two-point discrimination, vibration, temperature, and pain in the evaluation of some peripheral and central neuropathies. Disability rating scales are available for diseases such as multiple sclerosis and Parkinson's disease in which individual numerical ratings can be summed or weighted based on clinical judgment to obtain an overall index of neurological function. An alternative to rating signs and symptoms is the use of functional categories—pyramidal, cerebellar, sensory, brain stem, bowel and bladder, visual, mental, personal hygiene, upper extremity and lower extremity functions—with each function graded on an ordinal scale. Instrumental sensory-motor test batteries also enable a patient's progress to be followed routinely over many years.

Potvin, Tourtellotte, and colleagues have developed a neurofunction laboratory that administers a broad battery of instrumented tests consisting of a clinical quantitative neurological examination (Fig. 3–3) and complementary simulated activities of daily living tests. When the former tests show altered capacity, the latter tests are given to delineate which basic functions are compromised and disrupting performance of daily activities. The video tape preserves a record of changes in movement impairment over time as the patient performs simple tasks. An asymptomatic technician performs the same tasks at maximum speed to encourage the patient's maximum performance. Since these tests have been automated with microcomputer-controlled patient console stations, several rehabilitation centers have been using them to monitor the effectiveness of therapeutic exercise programs, as well as in drug trials in Parkinson's disease, multiple sclerosis, stroke, cerebellar ataxia, and dementia. Other instruments have been developed to record distance traveled daily by wheelchair or time out of bed each day. Use of some quantitative measures may not be practical if not enough health care providers are available to keep accurate records or supervise the testing.

Mental Status

Review of the medical history and general observation of the patient during the physical examination often provide many clues to the mental status of the patient. The psychological factors that are the most predictive of success in rehabilitating the disabled patient are intellectual functions—judgment, perception, and recent memory—and affect.

Judgment

Stroke or cortical insults often produce defective impulse control and reasoning. Difficulty in monitoring one's own behavior may account for unkempt appearance or family reports of inappropriate behavior, although apathy or physical inability to perform the task should not be ruled out as alternative explanations. Whether a patient's judgment is sufficiently impaired to

create danger to him- or herself or to others often can be determined by reviewing the hospital reports of the patient's daily activities in response to the health care providers. Since most patients with serious disability will initially show periods of confusion, disorientation, and poor judgment that do not portend lingering disorganization, you should determine whether such problems reported in early records were transient. Periodic reassessment of judgment is necessary to prevent prolonged overprotection of the patient that could adversely affect rehabilitation. A family member may have to provide standby assistance as the patient performs functional activities if judgment is sufficiently impaired.

Perception

Brain damage, especially to the right cerebral hemisphere, may result in visual misinterpretation of form, space, and distance. Perceptual difficulties may interfere with the accurate performance of transfers, dressing and personal hygiene, and communication. You can test perception by asking the patient to put on a shirt that has one sleeve inside out, draw a clock face from memory, or copy figures such as a square or triangle. If there are perceptual deficits, alert the other members of the health care team to teach basic self-care skills by verbal instruction rather than by demonstrations that the patient will be unable to follow.

Memory

Short-term memory deficits must be recognized because successful rehabilitation requires the ability to retain newly learned information such as how to transfer from a bed to a wheelchair. Such deficits are the single most likely adverse consequence of brain damage; all brain-damaged patients exhibit some memory impairment. Left-brain injury tends to result in more impairment of memory for language and symbolic material, while right-brain injury tends to impair memory of spatial material. Recent memory can be tested by asking the patient to remember an address or a simple new motor task, then having him or her repeat it later during

TABLE 3-8. *Moss Rehabilitation Hospital status form*

NAME K. R. AGE 60 SEX M ADM. DATE 4-4-73 DISCH. DATE 5-15-73

ADDRESS SERVICE DIAGNOSIS Rt. Hemiparesis

	PRE-MORBID	ADMISSION	DISCHARGE	1 MO. POST DISCHARGE	3 MOS. POST DISCHARGE	6 MOS. POST DISCHARGE	1 YEAR POST DISCHARGE
		Date 4-4-73	Date 5-15-73	Date No visit	Date 8-12-73	Date	Date
A.D.L.							
Dressing	1	31	21		1		
Feeding	1	21	1		1		
Personal Hygiene	1	31	1		1		
Bowel/Bladder	1/1	1/21	1/1	—	1/1	—	
MOBILITY							
Ambulatory	1	31	21		1		
Non-Ambulatory	N/A	21	1		N/A		
Transfers	1	31	21		1		
SPEECH	1	32	22		22		
PSYCHOLOGICAL	1	21	21		22		
VOCATIONAL							
Employment	1	43	43		31		
Homemaker	1	41	21		1		
Avocational	1	31	1		1		
TRANSPORTATION							
Public	1	42	31		21		
Driving	1	43	43		32		

NOTE: LEFT DIGIT REFERS TO PRESENT FUNCTIONAL STATUS. RIGHT DIGIT REFERS TO GOAL. *AN ASTERISK DENOTES STATUS WITH THE USE OF ASSISTIVE DEVICES.

ACTIVITIES OF DAILY LIVING (ADL)	MOBILITY	SPEECH	VOCATIONAL	TRANSPORTATION
Dressing: 1. Independent 2. With supervision 3. With assistance 4. Dependent **Feeding:** 1. Independent 2. With supervision 3. With assistance 4. Dependent **Personal Hygiene:** 1. Independent 2. With supervision 3. With assistance 4. Dependent **Bowel/Bladder:** 1. Continent/Reflex controlled 2. Occasional incontinence 3. Needs assistance 4. Incontinent	**Ambulatory:** 1. Independent ambulation 2. Ambulates with supervision 3. Ambulates with assistance 4. Dependent **Non-Ambulatory:** 1. Independent W/C level 2. W/C level with supervision 3. W/C level with assistance 4. Dependent **Transfers:** 1. Independent 2. With supervision 3. With assistance 4. Dependent	1. Normal communication 2. Some speech with gestures, good comprehension 3. Gestural communication, some speech, some comprehension 4. No communication **PSYCHOLOGICAL** 1. Rational/Well integrated 2. Needs limited support 3. Needs active support 4. Irrational/Disordered	**Employment:** 1. Competitively employed/ Sheltered/ Homebound 2. Awaiting placement 3. Participating work evaluation 4. Not feasible vocationally **Homemaker:** 1. Independent homemaker 2. With supervision 3. With assistance 4. Not feasible **Avocational:** 1. Active participation 2. Limited participation 3. Readiness for involvement 4. Not feasible	**Public:** 1. Travels independent 2. With supervision 3. Readiness for transportation training 4. Not feasible **Driving:** 1. Can drive/ Relicense 2. Participating driver training 3. Readiness for driver training 4. Not feasible

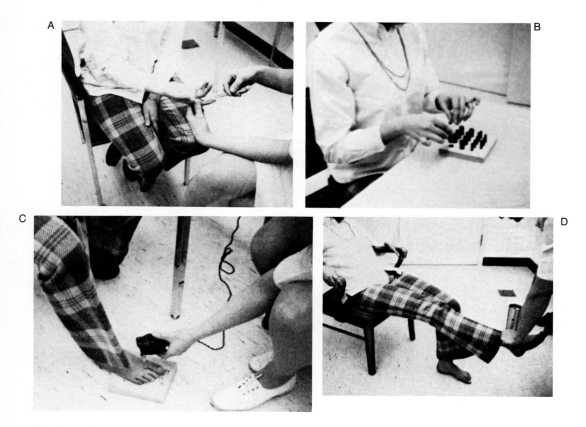

FIG. 3–3. Quantitative measures of neurological function. **A:** Compass is used to measure two-point discrimination sense. **B:** Patient is timed as she grasps, rotates, and reinserts eight pegs. **C:** Biothesiometer is applied to toe to measure vibration sense. **D:** Modified Newman myometer is used to measure flexion strength of extended leg. [From Potvin, A. R., and Tourtellotte, W. W. (1975): The neurological examination: Advancements in its quantification. *Arch. Phys. Med. Rehabil.*, 56:425–437, with permission.]

the examination. Asking the patient to recall what was eaten for lunch is not an accurate test, as this does not represent the learning of totally new information. If memory is impaired, alert all health care providers to repeat instructions frequently during rehabilitation training.

Affect

Affective responses to disability typically include anxiety, anger, and depression. Anxiety not only serves as a cue that stress needs to be alleviated but also often accompanies change; the disabled patient experiences numerous changes in functional capacity. At low to moderate levels, anxiety can enhance adaptation by making the patient more receptive to environmental stimuli; at extreme levels, however, it produces disorientation and inhibits goal-directed behavior. Anger is often expressed in verbal attacks, temper outbursts, destructive behavior, noncooperation with treatment, or escape behaviors designed to avoid perceived punishment. Depression, unless prolonged, should be recognized as a normal stage in coping with disability in which the patient recognizes the full impact of medical and social problems and associated losses. It may be expressed as self-denigration, lethargy, withdrawal from social contact, disregard for self-care, or denial of disability. Lability of mood is probably organic if pseudobulbar neurological signs are also present or if tears are easily interrupted by changing the topic of conversation or simply snapping your fingers.

This mental status examination should be considered a preliminary evaluation. Referral to a psychologist or other mental health professional is necessary for the administration of psychometric tests of intellectual function and affect.

ELECTRODIAGNOSTIC STUDIES

By recording the intrinsic electrical properties of muscles and nerves, electromyography (EMG) and nerve conduction velocity (NCV) studies indicate the pathophysiological status of a motor unit, which consists of the anterior horn cell, axon and terminal branchings, and the muscle fibers it innervates. The major indication for EMG/NCV examination is disease of the lower motor neuron type, as indicated in Fig. 3–4. This examination will determine which segment, or neuroanatomical level, of the motor unit is involved in the disease process, as well as the extent of involvement. Prognosis also can be inferred from the level and completeness of the lesion; EMG findings of reinnervation often precede functional recovery from peripheral nerve and similar injuries. Accurate results from electrodiagnostic examinations are optimized by waiting 14 to 21 days after injury to the nerve or muscle before performing an EMG and 72 hr for the NCV because these techniques may not be able to detect any abnormalities immediately after injury.

Electromyography

Electromyography consists of recording the electrical activity of muscle fibers near a needle inserted into the muscle belly. This technique is useful primarily for identifying denervated muscle, localizing lesions, and following the progress of reinnervation of previously injured or

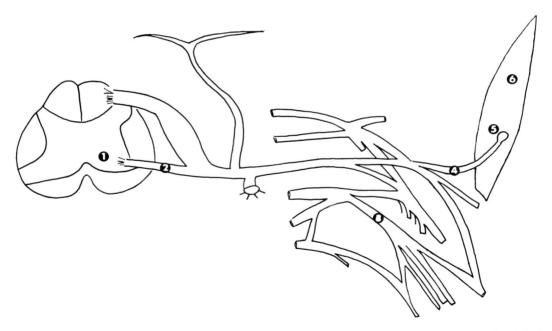

FIG. 3–4. Anatomical levels of neuromuscular disease or injury explored by clinical electromyography. Spinal Cord—Nerve—Muscle Complex. 1, Anterior horn cell (amyotrophic lateral sclerosis, spinal tumors, poliomyelitis, hemorrhage, trauma, cysts); 2, Spinal nerve root (radiculopathy to herniated nucleus pulposus, intervertebral disk protrusion or rupture, extramedullary space-occupying lesions); 3, Plexus (Erb's palsy, dislocations, fractures, wounds, trauma to brachial plexus); 4, Nerve trunk (crutch paralysis, contusions, fractures, cicatrix, wounds, cubital tunnel syndrome, peripheral neuropathy); 5, Myoneural junction (myasthenia gravis, myotonia); 6, Muscular fiber (muscular dystrophy, dermatomyositis, endocrine myopathies).

destroyed nerves. Preparation for the EMG examination includes determining which muscles and nerves will be examined based on the differential diagnosis derived from the history and neurological examination. The five major steps in an EMG examination, along with what they measure, are as follows:

1. Observe the muscle at rest for fasciculation and fibrillation potentials.
2. Compare insertional activity to potentials observed after pin movement stops for fasciculations, fibrillations, and positive waves.
3. Observe minimal motor unit activity for motor unit action potentials (MUAPs) as patient voluntarily produces minimal muscle contractions.
4. Observe maximal motor unit activity for the MUAP firing rate and the number of MUAPs as patient maximally contracts muscle.
5. Assess the distribution or pattern of EMG abnormalities found in the light of the history and physical examination.

Common EMG abnormalities that may indicate disease or disorder are increased or decreased insertional activity, fasciculation potentials, fibrillation potentials, positive sharp waves, polyphasic potentials, myotonic discharges, and neurogenic blocking. Each fasciculation represents the spontaneous firing of all or part of a *single motor unit*. Since fasciculations are often found in normal persons, their pathological significance must be determined on the basis of the other EMG and neurological findings. Anterior horn cell diseases in particular are likely to produce clinically significant fasciculation potentials.

Fibrillation potentials refer to the electrical imprint produced by the spontaneous firing of a *single muscle fiber*. A denervated muscle shows fibrillations, but they are also commonly seen in some myopathic disorders without denervation, such as polymyositis, and in upper motor neuron disorders such as stroke. Fibrillations merely indicate abnormal muscle membrane irritability.

Positive waves have the same diagnostic significance as fibrillation potentials. They are evoked by the mechanical irritation of the muscle fiber as the pin electrode is inserted. In pathological states, additional positive sharp waves may continue after pin movement stops, whereas in normal muscle, these insertional potentials immediately cease when the electromyographer stops moving the pin.

The duration, amplitude, and number of phases of the muscle MUAP are observed as the patient voluntarily contracts the muscle. Neuropathic disorders typically cause polyphasicity of the voluntary MUAPs, as well as an *increase* in their duration and amplitude. By contrast, myopathic disorders typically produce polyphasicity, but show a *decrease* in the amplitude and duration of the MUAPs. Patients with hysterical weakness, malingering, upper motor neuron weakness, or other conditions show a reduction in rate of firing of the MUAPs, rather than an actual reduction in the number of MUAPs that are firing. The specific cause of a reduced rate of firing must then be determined clinically.

Nerve Conduction Studies

The most helpful part of the examination for diagnosing peripheral nerve problems, nerve conduction studies may be used to determine the conduction velocity of either motor or sensory fibers. Nerve conduction velocity determinations can be made for most peripheral nerves that are accessible to stimulation at two or more points. Normal NCV is usually greater than 40 m/sec in the lower extremities and greater than 45 m/sec in the upper extremities. If the myelin sheath is not intact, conduction velocity will be abnormal. Only injury to the myelin sheath of most of the fast-conducting fibers or total destruction of these fibers results in decreased conduction velocity. Nerve conduction study also helps localize the site of injury to the nerve. Interpretation of conduction velocity must consider the normal decrease occurring before ages 4 to 8 and after age 40, as well as variations in core body temperature. Limbs with substantial muscle atrophy or vascular insufficiency may be abnormally cool, thereby also slowing nerve conduction. Defects of the neuromuscular junction, occurring in myoneural joint disease, can be identified through repetitive nerve stimulation before and after exercise periods.

Because EMG/NCV results often must be interpreted during the examination, a physician rather than a technician should be selected to perform the examination. You can find a physician who is qualified to perform electrodiagnostic studies by consulting the American Association of Electrodiagnosis and Electromyography (AAEE).

SUGGESTED READINGS

Goodgold, J. and Eberstein, A. (1983): *Electrodiagnosis of neuromuscular diseases*, 3rd ed. Williams and Wilkins, Baltimore.

Grabois, M. (1977): The problem-oriented medical record: Modification and simplification for rehabilitation medicine. *South. Med. J.*, 70:1383–1385.

Granger, C., Albrecht, G. L., and Hamilton, B. B. (1979): Outcome of comprehensive medical rehabilitation: Measurement by PULSES Profile and Barthel index. *Arch. Phys. Med. Rehabil.*, 60:145–154.

Granger, C. and Greishem, G. (1984): *Functional Assessment in Rehabilitation Medicine*. Williams and Wilkins, Baltimore.

Halstead, L. and Hartley, R. B. (1975): Time care profile: An evaluation of a new method of assessing ADL dependence. *Arch. Phys. Med. Rehabil.*, 56:110–115.

Halstead, L. (1976): Longitudinal unobtrusive measurements in rehabilitation. *Arch. Phys. Med. Rehabil.*, 57:189–193.

Johnson, E. W., editor. (1980): *Practical Electromyography.* Williams and Wilkins, Baltimore.

Kottke, F. J., Stillwell, G. K., and Lehmann, J. F., editors. (1982): *Krusen's Handbook of Physical Medicine and Rehabilitation*, 3rd ed. W. B. Saunders, Philadelphia.

Materson, R. S. (1978): Physical medicine and rehabilitation for the medical practitioner. In *Practice of Medicine.* Harper and Row, Hagerstown, Maryland.

O'Sullivan, S. B., Cullen, K. E., and Schmitz, T. J. (1981): *Physical Rehabilitation: Evaluation and Treatment Procedures.* F. A. Davis, Philadelphia.

Potvin, A. R., Tourtellotte, W. W., Kyndulko, K., and Potvin, J. (1981): Quantitative methods in assessment of neurologic function. *CRC Critical Reviews in Bioengineering*, (Oct):177–224.

Stolov, W. C. and Clowers, M. R., editors. (1981): *Handbook of Severe Disability.* U.S. Government Printing Office, Washington, D.C.

Tovian, S. M. (1982): Psychologic evaluation and treatment. In *The Practice of Rehabilitation Medicine.* Kaplan, P. E. and Materson, R. S., editors. Charles C Thomas, Springfield, Massachusetts.

Medical Rehabilitation,
edited by L. S. Halstead et al.
Raven Press, New York © 1985.

CHAPTER 4

Physical Modalities of Treatment

*Martin Grabois and †Lauro S. Halstead

*Departments of *†Physical Medicine *†Rehabilitation, †and Community Medicine Baylor College of Medicine; †The Institute for Rehabilitation and Research, Houston, Texas 77030*

Rehabilitation specialists are qualified to perform numerous physical and psychosocial therapeutic strategies to prevent secondary disability, maintain existing capability, and restore the disabled patient's ability to function independently. Discussion of the indications and contraindications, as well as the physiological and psychological effects of these treatments, will help you select and prescribe the most appropriate interventions for an individual patient over the course of a neuromuscular or musculoskeletal disease or injury. Many of these therapeutic strategies are adaptable to the facilities in the primary care physician's office. Judgment as to what can be expected of a patient with long-term disability and whether the patient is making adequate progress will be enhanced by sensitivity to the potential and limitations of given treatments.

Physical treatments—exercise, heat, cold, ultraviolet, electrotherapy, traction, and massage—may be prescribed singly, but are effective more often as part of a comprehensive treatment plan in which each modality used potentiates the others. For example, heat application before exercise enhances performance by reducing pain and joint stiffness; exercise, in turn, prepares the patient for transfers and gait training.

THERMOTHERAPY

Guidelines for Prescribing

A prescription for thermotherapy should include the source of heat, the duration and number of daily applications, and the intensity in terms of output or temperature. Specify the body part to be treated, the local area of the part, and the position of the patient.

Whether you decide to prescribe the heat treatment for a physical therapist to carry out, instruct the patient in home application, or apply the heat in your own office, the physician retains responsibility for the order and its outcome. Following ten general guidelines when prescribing or performing thermotherapy will enhance the probability of successful outcome:

1. Prescribe the simplest modality that will work.
2. Select a modality that can be safely used at home over one that requires office or hospital visits.
3. Use wooden, not metal, work tables.
4. Remove clothing, drape for privacy, and eliminate metals near the treatment field.
5. Always place the heat element *on* the patient; placing the patient on the heat element alters the patient's perception of heat change and compresses arterial blood supply so that local temperature rises more rapidly.
6. Follow thermotherapy with massage or exercise.
7. Do not apply heat over areas with arterial insufficiency.
8. Do not use heat over anesthetic or hyperesthetic areas, because the patient's awareness of temperature change is a critical guide to dosimetry.
9. Do not heat an extremity in a dependent position, and follow heat application with

elevation of the limb and exercise to discourage edema.

10. Do not prescribe thermotherapy for infants and elderly patients; they cannot tolerate thermal changes well.

Note that the last four guidelines are not absolute contraindications; however, they should be violated with caution and while closely supervising the patient for untoward effects.

Physical Properties

The physiological effects of thermotherapy include a rise in temperature, increased local metabolic rate, arteriolar dilation, and increased capillary blood flow and capillary hydrostatic pressure. Blood flowing through the heated area dissipates heat from the area being treated. This helps prevent burning, unless the patient's vascular system is unresponsive, as seen in severe arteriosclerosis. Reflex vasodilation and sweating, as well as increased cardiac output and respiratory rate, occur in an attempt to maintain temperature homeostasis. More oxygen, nutrients, antibodies, and leukocytes are available and phagocytosis increases. These physiological changes account for the therapeutic effects of heat, which are both objective and subjective. Objectively, heat relieves muscle spasm, increases the blood flow and the extensibility of collagen tissue, and promotes the resolution of inflammatory infiltrate, edema, and exudates. Subjectively, it produces sedation and relaxation, relieves pain, and decreases joint stiffness.

Four major factors determine the number and intensity of physiological reactions to heat:

1. The level of tissue temperature, the therapeutic range extending from 40 to 45.5°C.
2. The duration of exposure to heat, within a therapeutic range of 3 to 35 min.
3. The rate of temperature rise.
4. The size of the area heated.

The therapeutic effects of heat treatment depend not only on the physiological effects of heat in general but also on the depth of heating attained by specific modalities. Superficial heat modalities include hot pack, paraffin bath, hy-drocollator pack, infrared, hydrotherapy, and moist air cabinet. Deep heat modalities include short-wave diathermy, microwaves, and ultrasound.

Superficial Heat Modalities

Conductive

Conductive modalities transfer their heat directly to the cooler body, the rate of this exchange depending on the specific temperatures of the agent and the body part. The advantages of such devices as the paraffin wax bath are their relative simplicity, safety, home applicability, and affordability. They share the disadvantages, however, of obstructing the observer's view of the body part during treatment and endangering open wounds.

Hot packs can be made at home by heating towels with hot water and wringing them out before application. Temperatures up to 43.3°C can be tolerated. Hydrocollator packs are sized for application to the back, limbs, or neck. These silicate gel packs are immersed in a thermostatically controlled water bath unit and heated to 160°F, then encased in layers of Turkish toweling. The steam released heats the body part, causing the pack to begin cooling in 15 min. Heat dosage can be regulated by removing towels. Recommended treatment time is 20 to 30 min.

The paraffin bath consists of seven parts of paraffin added to one part of mineral oil. This mixture is applied to the skin at 52.2°C by immersion for 20 to 30 min, intervals of dipping, or painting it onto the hands, arms, or feet. As a vigorous form of heating, paraffin produces a significant rise of temperature in small joints, which are covered with very thin tissue.

Radiant

Radiant, usually infrared energy, causes thermal agitation in the tissues in which it is absorbed. The benefits of radiant heat are its drying effect and suitability for home use. However, safety may be compromised by self-use or by the breakage of the hot glass light bulbs. You should train a family member or other attendant in use of the radiation device at home and caution the patient to avoid using it alone. An inexpensive home heating device is a 250-watt bulb with a built-in reflector, which can be clamped onto chairs or other furniture. Only a very small area can be heated evenly, however. The reflective cradle, or baker, is more useful for heating larger areas. Regulate dosage by altering the distance of the infrared lamp from the skin, within a range of 15 to 26 inches. The patient's subjective feeling of warmth is a reliable guide to dosage. Limit treatment time to between 30 and 45 min.

Convective

Convective heating is the exchange of heat between a solid and a fluid or gas moving past the surface of the solid. Modes of hydrotherapy, for example, heat by convection.

The agitated-water bath or whirlpool can be used to heat and massage the extremities or the entire body. The Low-Boy tank, ideal for treating the lower back and lower extremities, enables the patient to sit comfortably with his or her knees and hips either partially flexed or fully extended in the agitated water. The Hubbard tank is a large tub that can accommodate the entire body. Because the tank requires 30 min of cleaning and refilling for each patient in order to prevent cross-contamination and infection, treatments usually can be scheduled no more than once per hour. Treatment in the tub lasts 30 min at a temperature of 37.8 to 42.8°C.

Vapor-saturated air at 40 to 45°C circulated by a blower surrounds the body part in the moist air cabinet. Expensive, bulky, and requiring maintenance, this mode of hydrotherapy is not used as widely as the Hubbard tank.

The therapeutic pool provides comfortable heat for relaxation and easy movement. Water temperature is controlled between 92 and 96°F.

In fluidotherapy, thermostatically controlled hot air is blown through a pad of finely divided solids such as glass beads. The dry, warm semifluid mixture into which the body part is immersed enables the skin to stay dry.

The summary of the advantages, indications, and contraindications of these common superficial heat modalities provided in Table 4–1 will help you choose the most appropriate modality for selective patient problems.

Deep-heating Conversive Modalities

Deep-heating agents, which heat by conversion of electrical, electromagnetic, or sound energy to thermal energy, are indicated when the deeper tissues cannot be heated without burning the surface tissues. Conversive heating is supplied, in order of increasing depth of penetration, by short-wave, microwave, or ultrasonic diathermy (Table 4-2).

Short-Wave Diathermy

Short-wave diathermy is the therapeutic application of a high-frequency oscillating current through the patient. Conduction is greatest through tissue high in water content; muscle is therefore often selectively heated. Knees, elbows, and shoulders, sparsely covered by superficial subcutaneous tissue, are the areas that are the most effectively treated by short-wave diathermy.

Dosimetry depends entirely on the patient's subjective feeling of warmth, which will vary with the amount of body fat in the area being heated. The most efficacious duration of heating is 20 min. Do not expect to attain more therapeutic benefits by extending this heating time; increasing this time even slightly produces a paradoxical effect. Its high cost, bulkiness, and complexity make diathermy impractical for home use. Cautious, continuous monitoring is essential during the application of diathermy.

Microwaves

Like short waves, microwaves are electromagnetic waves that can be reflected, refracted,

TABLE 4–1. *Comparison of common superficial heat modalities*

Modality	Applications	Advantages	Precautions
Hubbard tank or whirlpool	Open wounds—burns, pressure sores; rheumatoid arthritis—repaired cartilage, tendon repair or transfer, hip or knee joint replacement; healed or healing fracture	Body can be immersed fully; active, passive, or resistive exercises can be performed in water; burn wounds can be debrided and bandages removed; water agitation thoroughly cleanses open wounds	Unstable blood pressure; severe debilitation; sensory deficit of skin; respiratory problems; thrombophlebitis; edema persisting after treatment
Therapeutic pool	Arthritis; Guillain-Barré syndrome; stroke; spinal cord injury	Patients of all ages with wide variety of disorders can be treated safely; 90% reduction of body weight enables patients with weakened musculature or painful joints to ambulate or exercise; pool allows freedom of movement, especially for very weak patients; easy movement in water produces positive psychological effects; open wound can be treated	Bowel or bladder incontinence; open wounds; respiratory difficulty; unstable blood pressure
Moist air cabinet	Rheumatoid arthritis; pressure sores and other open wounds	Enables treatment of open wounds	Same as for other types of hydrotherapy
Hydrocollator pack	Pain; muscle spasm; limited motion	Pack can be molded around body part; patient can either sit or lie down; pack can be used at home	Temperature high enough to produce burn or blister; diminished sensation; impaired peripheral circulation; open wounds
Paraffin bath	Painful joints, especially in the hand, prior to exercise for mobilization	Paraffin and oil can be mixed and used by patient at home	Open lesions; diminished or no skin sensation; rash; persistent edema or pain
Infrared	Strains; sprains; open sores; tenosynovitis; arthritis	Lamp or cradle is easy to move about and may be used at bedside; patient has some freedom of movement during heat application	Debility; old age; impaired peripheral circulation; limited cardiovascular or respiratory reserves; dermatitis; diminished or lost sensation; over a scar

or absorbed in tissue. They are selectively absorbed in fluid, subcutaneous fat, and tissues with high water content, such as muscle. Because bone is not a good absorber of microwaves, microwaves should be applied from different directions to ensure effective heating on all sides of a target bone. The highest temperatures are produced at the interfaces between fat and muscle. Microwaves are not very effective for heating the shoulder and are unable to reach the hip. You can control dosimetry by the meter available on the instrument and the distance from the unit to the body part being heated. The recommended treatment time is about 20 min. Microwave is easily applied by following the manufacturer's instructions for the appropriate warm-up period and using the proper director.

Ultrasound

If you plan to purchase only one diathermy instrument, ultrasound is recommended over the others because it offers the greatest deep heating capacity combined with little temperature elevation in the superficial tissues. Joints covered by heavy masses of soft tissue can be heated to tolerance levels without any deleterious effects elsewhere in the tissues. Reflected and absorbed at tissue interfaces, ultrasound can even heat the joint capsules and synovia. A disadvantage of ultrasound, however, is its tendency to potentiate the cavitation of gases in tissue. The destructive effects of cavitation can be minimized with the use of proper equipment, proper technique, and therapeutic dosages. Use a dosage that is lower than the standard therapeutic intensity and frequency when treating joints with effusions, the eyes, and the pregnant uterus. As a general rule, apply 5 to 10 min of ultrasound at a dosage between 0.5 and 2.75 W/cm^2 through the anterior, posterior, and lateral port of each joint site. Give thin patients higher doses for shorter periods and heavy patients with thick

TABLE 4–2. *Comparison of common diathermies*

Modality	Applications	Advantages	Contraindications and precautions
Short wave	Pain in joints from bursitis or tendonitis; back pain	Enables selective heating of muscle and other dense tissue; effectively deep heats tissue with minimal superficial subcutaneous covering such as knees, elbows, or shoulders; enables deep heating of internal tissues such as prostate	Metal implants; diminished or absent sensation; malignancy; tuberculosis; hemorrhage; vascular disease; pregnancy; tuberculosis
Microwave	Same as for short wave	Heat interface between fat and muscle; applied easily; heats deep tissue without heating skin as much as with short waves; patient is free to move within limited range without disturbing treatment	Same as short wave; cardiac pacemaker; early trauma; use over eyes, ischemic areas, male gonads, growing bone in children, anesthetic areas, wet bandages, or adhesive tape; extremes of age; obesity
Ultrasound	Dupuytren's contracture; joint contractures resulting from tightness or periarticular structures or from scarring or capsular tissues; calcific bursitis; pain of tendonitis in shoulder joints; pain from fibromas, especially those embedded in scar tissue	Dosage can be controlled better than in other forms of diathermy; reduces scarring; may be used in areas of body where metal implants are located; more efficient than microwaves in heating shoulder and hip joints; can be used over anesthetic areas; has capacity to specifically heat periosteum and tissues surrounding joint; enables greater stretching of collagen tissues than other heat modalities	Use over eyes, gravid uterus, ischemic areas, or heart; acutely inflamed joints or bursa; malignancy; hemorrhage

subcutaneous fat tissue lower doses for longer periods.

Therapeutic Cold

Cryotherapy reduces edema, decreases extravasation of blood cells and substances across the vascular membrane, slows enzymatic reactions within the area, and decreases nerve conduction velocity. Skin temperature drops rapidly, while muscle temperature will take 10 min to drop in a thin person and 30 min in an obese person. These physiological reactions produce the following therapeutic effects:

1. Decrease muscle spasm and spasticity.
2. Reduce swelling, bleeding, and edema resulting from mechanical trauma such as sprains.
3. Reduce tissue damage from burns when applied soon after the thermal trauma.
4. Relieve pain directly or, by acting as a counterirritant, increasing the pain threshold.
5. Reduce edema and destructive enzyme activity of inflamed joints.
6. Decrease local metabolic activity, enabling the preservation of a limb with threatened arterial supply.

Cold and simultaneous compression should be applied for 4 to 6 hrs, immediately after trauma, to prevent substantial swelling and hemorrhage. Otherwise, treatments usually last about 20 min and are administered once or twice a day. Avoid excessive cooling, which may increase joint stiffness and retard healing. Methods of application include ice bags, cold packs, ice baths, ice towels, and ice massage. With minimal instruction, all of these methods are easily applied at home. Another effective cooling agent is ethyl chloride sprayed on the patient's skin; the cooling spray relieves pain by acting as a counterirritant as it evaporates.

Under certain conditions, cold is a more efficacious treatment than heat, and vice versa. Some of the therapeutic effects of heat and cold are similar, as indicated in Table 4–3. The therapeutic effects of cold tend to last longer, however, making it more efficient than heat. Cold

TABLE 4–3. *Comparison of the effects of therapeutic heat and cold*

Condition	Heat	Cold
Muscle spasm	Decreased	Decreased
Pain	Decreased	Decreased
Bleeding	Increased	Decreased
Edema (trauma-related)	Increased	Decreased
Swelling	Increased	Decreased
Tissue damage from burns	Increased	Decreased
Joint stiffness	Decreased	Increased

and heat have many more opposite effects, also shown in Table 4–3, which should be considered when selecting a treatment modality to best meet the special needs of each patient.

ULTRAVIOLET THERAPY

The therapeutic effects of ultraviolet waves include the production of vitamin D, sterilization of the skin, pigmentation and erythema of the skin, and exfoliation of the skin. These effects help heal acne vulgaris, psoriasis, pressure sores, indolent ulcers, herpes zoster, lupus vulgaris, and carbuncles. Ultraviolet therapy is contraindicated in other skin disorders, including lupus erythematosus, herpes simplex, and acute eczema.

Ultraviolet therapy is often more effective when used in conjunction with another therapeutic modality. The Goeckerman technique, for example, involves the application of a crude coal tar ointment to a psoriatic patch of skin the evening before ultraviolet exposure. An effective alternative is the simultaneous ingestion of a photosensitizing drug such as methoxsalen.

Dosage is measured in MED, the minimum efficacious dose producing slight erythema in average Caucasian skin. This dosage not only varies considerably from one individual to another but also decreases as the lamp ages. For a new hot quartz lamp, the average MED is 15 sec at a distance of 30 inches. The physical effects on average skin at increasing dosage levels, as well as therapeutic ranges for various skin disorders, are given in Fig. 4–1. To avoid epi-

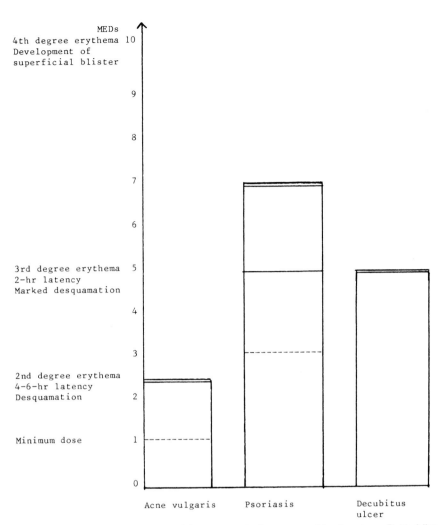

FIG. 4–1. Average dosage ranges for ultraviolet treatment of common skin disorders. *Dotted line*, minimum efficacious dosage; *solid line*, moderate, second treatment dosage; *double line*, maximum dosage.

thelialization and tissue destruction, higher doses should be applied only to the lesion itself, protecting the surrounding tissue. Both you and the patient should wear lenses that block the passage of ultraviolet radiation because of the danger of photoophthalmia.

THERAPEUTIC EXERCISE

Therapeutic exercise is the prescription of bodily movement to correct an impairment, improve musculoskeletal function, or maintain a state of well-being. Its early introduction into a rehabilitation plan is often the critical determinant of speed and extent of functional recovery and independence. The goals of therapeutic exercise, toward the ultimate objective of functional independence, are as follows:

1. Improve coordination.
2. Increase range of motion, flexibility, and endurance.
3. Strengthen musculature weakened by disease, injury, or disuse.

4. Maintain musculoskeletal function.
5. Facilitate relaxation.

A prescription for therapeutic exercise should always be preceded by a thorough evaluation, including manual muscle tests, range of motion, status of bones and joints, and coordination problems, as described in Chapter 3. Based on this evaluation, the prescription should include the essential elements described in Chapter 2. Some indications and contraindications for the major exercise approaches are presented in Table 4–4.

Despite thorough evaluation, selection of suitable patients, custom-designed prescription, prompt initiation of the exercise program, frequent treatments, and progressive neurophysiological training, there is no guarantee that the most carefully prescribed exercise program will succeed. The program may overwhelm a patient if it exceeds his or her capabilities, aggravates pain or other symptoms, exacerbates fatigue, or triggers excessive fear, insecurity, excitement, or other strong emotions. The patient may have been severely weakened by unavoidable periods of inactivity, especially postcoma or postsurgery (see Chapter 22). In addition, the therapist's instructions may bewilder the patient, who may not understand what the therapist wants him or her to do. Any of these factors may inhibit learning, increase incoordination, diminish motivation, and discourage the patient from cooperating fully with the therapist. On the other hand, inadequate supervision by a therapist who is treating too many patients to note the problems of individuals may also lead to failure. In some cases, you will need to refer the patient to a physical therapist who uses a different approach, seek psychosocial consultation, or enlist greater participation by the patient's family.

ELECTRICAL STIMULATION

Guidelines for Prescribing

Manual muscle tests and sensory tests should be done before you select a mode of electrical stimulation to relieve pain, relax spasm, re-

educate muscles, or produce movement in non-functioning muscles. Innervated muscle responds to short-duration, faradic current of 30 to 1,000 Hz, whereas denervated muscle responds only to long-duration, galvanic currents of 25 Hz or less lasting about 100 msec.

To obtain an optimal response from denervated muscle, prescribe three to four daily sessions of 25 to 50 strong contractions, preceded by heat application. If introduced soon after denervation, this regimen sometimes retards the progression of muscle atrophy. A battery-operated stimulator for the patient to use at home is indicated for long-term treatment.

There are several comparable uses for faradic stimulation of innervated muscle. Short-duration electrical stimulation of the quadriceps can retard disuse atrophy after knee injury. In spastic paralysis associated with spinal cord injury, this procedure can help reduce spasticity. If the spinal lesion is above C4, stimulating the phrenic nerve, or diaphragmatic pacing, facilitates respiration. Stimulation of the calf muscles after surgery may help ward off phlebothrombosis. In general, electrical stimulation helps relax and reeducate muscles. Innervated skeletal muscles are most effectively stimulated at the points where the motor nerve penetrates the epimysium.

Transcutaneous Electrical Nerve Stimulation

In transcutaneous electrical nerve stimulation (TENS), electrodes may be placed on the skin surface over afferent nerve paths to relieve pain (Fig. 4–2). Treatment trials will identify the best location and most effective duration, which may range from 30 min of intense stimulation to several hours of low-intensity stimulation. Therefore, your prescription should request an evaluation of the effectiveness of several frequencies and intensities over a 2- or 3-day trial period.

These small, battery-powered units provide a high-frequency electrical current of varying duration and amplitude that excites sensory nerve fibers while modifying the perception of pain

TABLE 4–4. *Approaches to therapeutic exercise*

Approach	Definition	Purpose and indications	Contraindications
Passive range of motion	Body part is completely supported, manually or mechanically, and taken through the available range of a joint	Maintain joint mobility when control of voluntary muscles about a joint is lost or when patient is unconscious or unresponsive	Thrombophlebitis; unsupported fractures; joints lacking sensation
Active exercise	Patient moves the body part through the available range of motion without assistance or resistance	Maintain joint range of motion and minimal strength when activity is limited and stimulate cardiopulmonary systems	Total bed rest
Active assistive exercise	Body part is moved through available range of motion with manual or mechanical assistance	Maintain joint mobility and some strength when patient lacks strength to complete range of motion and when weight of body part being exercised cannot be eliminated by positioning	Total bed rest; need to immobilize joint
Resistive exercise	Manual or mechanical resistance is applied through the available joint range of motion or at the end of joint range of motion	Build strength rapidly in preparation for crutch walking, independent transfers, or wheelchair ambulation or to stabilize joints after fracture has healed	Pain or edema after an exercise session
Isometric exercise	Maximal contraction of muscle or muscle group is elicited without joint movement	Maintain limited strength and muscle bulk when body part is immobilized, e.g., in skeletal traction or cast	Pain or edema after an exercise session
Neurophysiological	Desired motor patterns are repeated frequently while eliminating errors; activities are broken down into simple components	Teach control or inhibition of individual muscles and multimuscular coordination to enable performance of desired activities; develop highest level of coordination in shortest possible time	Total bed rest

and the patient's reaction to it. Helping about 50% of patients, these units may remain efficacious for years or for only a few weeks.

Various musculoskeletal pain syndromes or causalgia may also be indications for TENS (Fig. 4–3). However, it is contraindicated in patients with pacemakers and should not be placed over the uterus during pregnancy. Danger and discomfort are minimized by carefully cleaning and debriding the skin to reduce skin resistance, using well-soaked electrical contact pads or electrode jelly, and setting up the electrode leads unilaterally for cardiac safety.

Functional Electrical Stimulation

Contraction of muscles lacking voluntary nervous control can be elicited by functional electrical stimulation (FES) in order to produce a functionally useful movement. The most com-

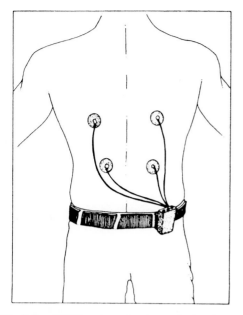

FIG. 4–2. TENS system showing typical surface arrangement of electrodes. [From O'Sullivan, S. B., Cullen, K. E., and Schmitz, T. J. (1981): *Physical Rehabilitation: Evaluation and Treatment Procedures.* F. A. Davis, Philadelphia.]

mon application of FES is in the gait training of patients with damaged upper motor neurons, but it may also be used to retrain the fingers to grasp objects when grasping is inhibited by extensor paralysis. In addition, spasticity can be alleviated in patients with hemiplegia, paraparesis, cerebral palsy, or multiple sclerosis. This modality is usually ineffective, however, when flaccid paralysis originates in the central nervous system or the lower motor neuron pathways are damaged. Contraindications to FES are strong spastic equinovalgus, diminished excitability of the peroneal nerve, and extremely weak hip, knee, or ankle joints. Functional electrical stimulation does not prevent contractures and deformities, nor is it useful in the presence of dyskinesia or hyperkinetic hypertonic syndromes.

Muscle contraction is elicited directly, by stimulating efferent nerve fibers, or indirectly, by stimulating afferent nerve fibers. Efferent FES involves the neuromuscular transmission of electrical impulses to motor nerve fibers. Its success depends on the muscles retaining some capacity

to contract. In afferent FES, spinal reflex mechanisms are excited to indirectly influence muscle contraction.

Despite its efficacy in about 25% to 30% of hemiplegics, the FES unit does pose the disadvantages of being complicated and expensive. Determining the optimal pulse repetition rate to achieve adequate movement, yet minimize pain and skin irritation, may require considerable trial and error. Generally slower for patients with upper motor neuron lesions than for healthier patients, the rate should be increased as function improves. Applying and maintaining the units require extra effort that may inconvenience the patient and family.

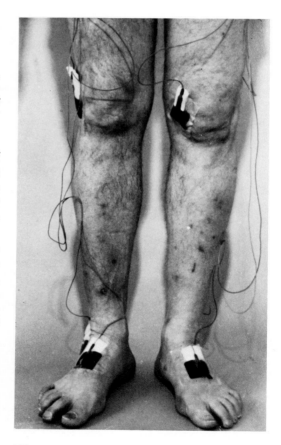

FIG. 4–3. Transcutaneous nerve stimulators arranged over lower extremities of man with intractable foot pain following frostbite. [From Kuman, V. N. (1982): Intractable foot pain following frostbite: Case report. *Arch. Phys. Med. Rehabil.* 63:284.]

Traction

Traction applied to joints relieves pressure or tension on muscles, tendons, or disks. The force may be applied intermittently or continuously through manual or mechanical means, and in conjunction with a program of heat, massage, manipulation, and exercise. The weight of the traction and the duration of application are determined by the nature and severity of the patient's condition, as well as the patient's tolerance. Taking care to align the body properly will increase tolerance and improve the therapeutic results.

In the treatment of spinal disorders, traction is most commonly applied to the cervical or lumbar spine. Traction is indicated in painful conditions caused by irritation or compression of nerve roots from trauma, degenerative processes, or disk protrusion. It is not indicated, however, in all painful conditions of the neck or low back and seems to be more effective in acute rather than chronic pain.

Cervical traction is delivered manually or mechanically by head halter. The manual method, rarely used in the United States, is applied in combination with manipulation of the cervical spine as the patient lies supine. Compared with mechanical traction, it allows greater control of head position. For mechanical traction, the patient may sit or lie on an inclined plane, using the body weight as the tractive force. To prevent dizziness or nausea, the force of traction should begin at about 5 lb and progressively increase in duration and force. Traction is ineffective until it exceeds the weight of the head; good response is usually obtained at 20 to 30 lb. A typical regimen is intermittent sessions of 15 to 20 min daily for 7 to 10 days, tapering off to three times a week, for a total of 3 or 4 weeks. Traction should be discontinued if the patient does not experience relief by the end of this period.

Cervical traction may be continued at home by rigging a spreader bar, pulley, rope, brackets, and head halter in a doorway. Advise the patient that proper head position can be roughly gauged by the patient's ability to read a book comfortably during application.

Lumbar traction may be applied in an upright, horizontal, or inclined position. Usually, the patient hangs from an overhead bar or beam by the arms, using the body as the tractive force, as in cervical traction. Due to the strong forces required to separate the disks of the lumbar spine, manual traction is not feasible. This force must exceed 26% of the patient's body weight to be effective, although using a special table to eliminate friction can reduce the amount of weight needed. Usually, a force of at least 100 lb is used. Lumbar traction is best tolerated if administered intermittently by motorized devices. The patient wears a pelvic corset or harness while a thoracic corset provides countertraction for stabilization.

Massage

Massage consists of four therapeutic techniques: compression, for mobilizing tissue deposits and stretching adhesions; stroking, for removing tissue deposits or edema fluid; friction, for treating very limited areas, particularly nodules; and percussion, for psychological or sedating effects at the end of the treatment session. Through these techniques, massage relieves pain, reduces swelling, and mobilizes contracted tissue. Among the conditions helped by massage are sequelae of fractures, dislocations, joint injuries, sprains, strains, bruises, tendon and nerve injuries, and neuritis. Massage combined with heat therapy for relaxation and pain relief may precede exercise to increase range of motion or flexibility. Massage should not be considered a substitute for exercise, however, because it cannot increase muscle strength.

Because massage may spread infection throughout the tissues, spread tumors beyond their confined limits, or spread contagious skin diseases to the masseur, this modality is contraindicated in the presence of any of these conditions. Massage is likewise contraindicated in patients with thrombophlebitis.

SUGGESTED READINGS

Basmajian, J. V., editor (1978): *Therapeutic Exercise*, 3rd edit. Williams and Wilkins, Baltimore.

Downer, A. H. (1978): *Physical Therapy Procedures: Selected Techniques*, 3rd edit. Charles C Thomas, Springfield, Ill.

Lehmann, J. F., editor (1982): *Therapeutic Heat and Cold*, 3rd edit. Williams and Wilkins, Baltimore.

Rogoff, J. B., editor (1980): *Manipulation, Traction, and Massage*, 2nd edit. Williams and Wilkins, Baltimore.

Stillwell, G. K., editor (1983): *Therapeutic Electricity and Ultraviolet Radiation*, 3rd edit. Williams and Wilkins, Baltimore.

Voss, D. E., Ionta, M. K., and Myers, B. J. (1985): *Proprioceptive Neuromuscular Facilitation: Patterns and Techniques*, 3rd edit. J. B. Lippincott, Hagerstown, Maryland.

Wood, E. C. (1974): *Beard's Massage, Principles and Techniques*, 2nd edit. W. B. Saunders, Philadelphia.

Medical Rehabilitation,
edited by L. S. Halstead et al.
Raven Press, New York © 1985.

CHAPTER 5

Functional Training for Independent Living

*Mary Joyce Newsom and **Martin Grabois

*The Institute for Rehabilitation and Research, and Department of Rehabilitation, Baylor College of Medicine; **Departments of Physical Medicine and Rehabilitation, Baylor College of Medicine, Houston, Texas 77030*

PROGRESSIVE MOBILIZATION

The mobility of many hospitalized patients is limited because of surgery, traction, extensive diagnostic tests, or pain. Mobility is likely to be even more severely curtailed in patients with chronic illness or neuromuscular disorders. Since prolonged immobilization produces adverse effects on virtually all body systems (see Chapter 22), disability resulting from inactivity may be more severe than that caused by the original illness. Therefore, as soon as possible after such patients have become medically stable, preparations should begin for resuming independent self-care and normal activities of daily living in the community. A program of progressive mobilization is necessary ultimately to attain these goals and immediately to counteract the effects of immobilization on the patient's physical and psychological status. There are basically eight steps in progressive mobilization:

1. Positioning and passive range of motion (ROM) exercises in bed.
2. Moving up, down, and sideways and rolling over in bed.
3. Sitting up and balancing.
4. Transfers, sitting, and standing.
5. Wheelchair ambulation.
6. Standing up and balancing.
7. Stair climbing.
8. Walking, with or without crutches or cane.

Bed Positioning

Positioning and turning regimens are aimed at reducing the force of gravity, maintaining alignment, and preventing pressure that leads to skin breakdown. The physician's order should specify any variations to accommodate such problems as edema, spasticity, and contractures. The order should designate equipment (Table 5–1), positions to use, positions to avoid, and frequency of turning. The prone position is favored since it distributes pressure more evenly than the others. Initially, patients are turned every 2 hr. Turning time is then gradually decreased until the patient can tolerate 3 or 4 hr in one position and eventually get through the night without being turned. Special beds that mechanically turn the patient are described in Chapter 23.

Bridging is a simple but effective technique to prevent pressure sores in patients with special problems. In this technique, pillows and wedges are positioned to allow free space between the bed surface and bony prominences (Fig. 5–1). This method is inexpensive and easily taught to family members who position the patient after discharge from the hospital.

Transfers

Since learning most activities of daily living requires sitting upright, the next step in the progressive mobilization program is practicing transfers from bed to wheelchair, and wheel-

TABLE 5–1. *Equipment to facilitate positioning*

Equipment	Physical requirements	Purpose
High-low bed with board	Adjustable, 20–30 in	Wheelchair transfers and crutch walking in low position; nursing care and ROM in high position
Foam rubber mattress	4 in thick, 34-lb compression ratio	Firm support helps prevent hip flexion contracture
Short side rails	33 in long, extending 11 in above mattress level	Improve safety when moving, sitting, or transferring
Positioning frames (Foster, Stryker)	Canvas stretched on anterior and posterior frames that can be rotated along their long axes	Enable easier positioning when spine is immobile
Electrically powered rotating frames	Remote control switch rotates frames along their short axes	Permit more comfortable positioning by patient or family member without assistance of others
Standing bed	Electrically or manually controlled	Enables patient to attain upright position; reduces osteoporosis; preserves morale; shifts weight-bearing to alleviate pressure

ROM, range of motion.

chair to bath. Until the patient can sit upright, a reclining-back wheelchair will provide adequate support. Selection of the most appropriate method of transfer involves matching the physical requirements of the methods with the patient's capabilities (Table 5–2). Most hemiplegics are able to learn standing transfers (see Chapter 15), whereas spinal cord injured patients, or double amputees, are able to learn one of the sitting transfers, with or without the assistance of a sliding board (Fig. 5–2). Sliding board transfers are simple enough to be performed by families who do not have access to a nurse or therapist; many spinal cord injured patients can learn to do this transfer independently.

The ability to get in and out of a bathtub and to transfer from a wheelchair to the toilet is an important step toward independent self-care. These more difficult, potentially dangerous transfers may require assistance or supervision, chiefly due to the need to remove or adjust clothing. Methods of bath and toilet transfer are depicted in Fig. 5–3.

Ambulation

After transfers have been mastered, wheelchair ambulation and pregait training begin. Wheelchair push-ups will help patients strengthen their arms and shift their weight to prevent decubiti from prolonged sitting. Ability to maneuver a wheelchair will greatly extend the patient's scope of activities, enabling independent trips home, as well as to physical and occupational therapy rooms. Pregait training consists of mat exercises, standing up and balancing, and stair climbing. These procedures, most applicable to hemiplegics and other patients with one good leg, are described in Chapter 15.

Walkers, crutches, or canes (in increasing order of progression toward independent ambulation) are used to assist patients who cannot walk without them, or to make the gait more efficient. Select the safest type of gait, which will depend on the patient's diagnosis, as well as strength, coordination, mental status, and age. Providing the most stability, the walker is indicated for generally weak, elderly patients who have problems balancing and a fractured hip, leg or foot but two good arms. Crutches are more suitable for younger patients with good balance and two strong arms.

How to walk with the assistance of crutches is shown in Figs. 5–4 and 5–5. When walking with crutches, a disabled patient may either take a step with one leg and then the other as in normal walking, which would call for a four-

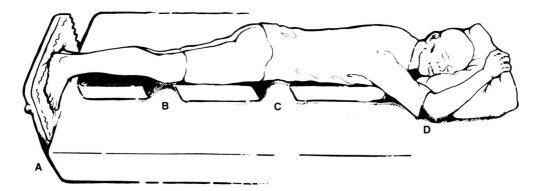

FIG. 5–1. Prone position with bridging. **A,** Footboard. **B,** Knees free to prevent skin breakdown over bony prominence. **C,** Genitals free for easy catheter care and to prevent hip contracture. **D,** Pillow prevents hyper-extension of neck (Used with permission of the Rehabilitation Institute of Chicago).

point or two-point crutch gait, or move both legs simultaneously, as in the tripod or swinging gaits. Regardless of the gait pattern chosen, never allow the patient to line up both crutches with both feet; instead, a triangle should be formed with the crutches and feet. Bearing weight on the crutch tops should also be discouraged because the resulting pressure on the nerves in the armpits could cause paralysis.

A stable gait, the tripod or three-point gait, is indicated for patients who are allowed minimal or no weight bearing in one lower extremity, as with a healing fracture or sprain. To perform the two-point or four-point gaits, patients must be able to move each leg separately and bear significant weight on each leg. Patients who lack strength in the lower extremities are usually able to execute the swing-to gait, which is slow but stable because of the wide base of support provided by the crutches and because the feet are in contact with the floor. The swing-through gait, less stable and faster than the swing-to, requires more strength, trunk flexibility, and coordination. Patients who have enough strength to lift their weight and sufficient endurance to maintain a rhythmic forward pace, but who lack function completely in one or both lower extremities, usually are able to use this gait.

The swing-to and three-point gaits can be easily adapted to a walker. Patients using a wheeled

TABLE 5–2. *Physical requirements of bed to wheelchair transfers*

Type of transfer	Physical requirements of patient
Standing	Hand and wrist function on one side
	Good sitting balance without postural hypotension
	Ability to extend the hip and knee by voluntary muscle contraction, long leg braces, or extensor spasticity
	Reasonably strong shoulder depressors and adductors, elbow flexors and extensors
Lateral sliding with aid of sliding board	Good sitting balance
	Enough strength in arms to lift hip from bed
Anterior-posterior sitting, sliding	Loose hamstrings
	Slightly more strength than required for lateral, especially in elbow extensors
	Better balance than in lateral
Lateral sitting without aid of sliding board	Exceptionally good shoulder depressors and abductors
	Excellent balance
	Ability to lift buttocks off bed and move from bed to wheelchair in single motion

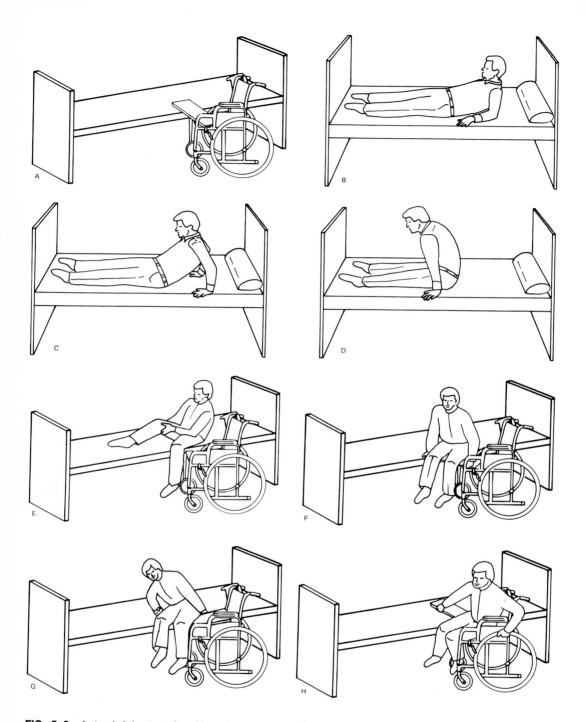

FIG. 5–2. Lateral sitting transfer with assistance of sliding board. **A:** Position of wheelchair and sliding board for lateral sliding transfer. **B:** To sit up, patient raises his shoulders by pushing down on his forearms and gradually moving them backward. **C:** He straightens his elbows, one at a time. **D:** He walks his hands forward one at a time until his trunk is forward and he is sitting upright. **E:** Patient moves his legs over the side of the bed with his arms. **F:** He slides to edge of bed. **G:** Leaning on his right forearm, he places one end of the sliding board under him. **H:** He moves across the sliding board to the wheelchair and leaning over onto his left forearm, removes the sliding board. (Illustrations by Charlotte Holden.)

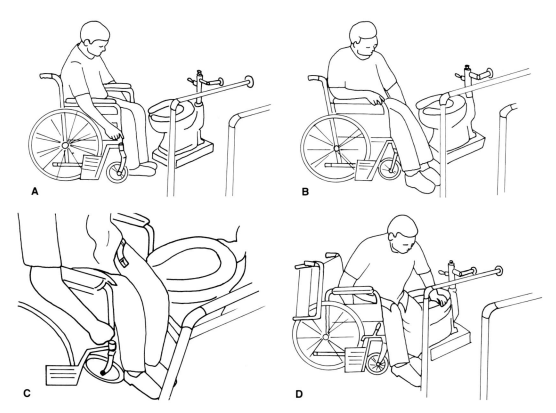

FIG. 5–3. Independent lateral transfer from wheelchair to toilet with raised seat. **A:** Patient swings footrests to the side, moves wheelchair so that his knee is close to the toilet, and locks brakes. **B:** He shifts his hips to sit sideways on chair and moves his knees away from toilet. **C:** He unlocks the brakes and moves wheelchair as close as possible to toilet. Then he relocks the brakes and loosens his trousers, gradually working them down to midthigh by leaning from side to side. **D:** He removes the armrest and places it on the back of the chair within easy reach; then, placing one hand on the opposite side of the toilet seat and the other on the wheelchair seat, he uses his upper extremities to raise his hips and move toward toilet seat (Illustrations by Charlotte Holden.)

walker, however, must use a modified four-point gait, since reciprocal movement of the upper and lower extremities is impossible.

Cane gait, similar to crutch gait, provides lateral support and enables the patient to ambulate more independently. A patient needing the most support would start with a walkcane, which has four legs, then progress to a quad or regular cane as strength improved. As indicated in Fig. 5–6, the various cane gaits are based on forming a triangle with the cane and feet, as with crutches.

ACTIVITIES OF DAILY LIVING

Whereas functional training for mobilization requires conditioning of the lower extremities, most other activities of daily living—eating, dressing, grooming and personal hygiene—are facilitated by attending to function of the upper extremities. To perform these formerly routine tasks, each disabled patient must be instructed in new techniques that accommodate the disability in a progressive sequence of functional training (Table 5–3). Just as otherwise nonambulatory patients can be taught to walk with the assistance of walkers, canes, and crutches, patients otherwise unable to take care of everyday needs often can feed, wash, and dress themselves using special assistive devices and prostheses that compensate for weakness or paralysis.

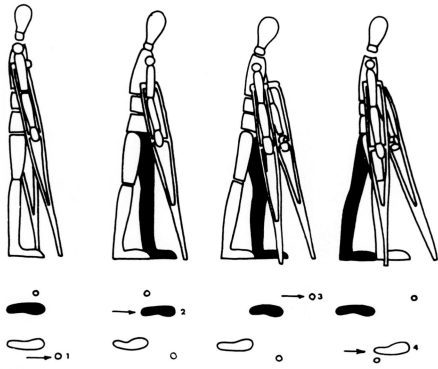

FIG. 5–4. Four-point alternate crutch gait. Crutch sequence: 1, right crutch; 2, left foot; 3, left crutch; 4, right foot. As patient gains strength and balance, crutch and opposite foot may move almost simultaneously [From Wilson, G. (1981): Progressive mobilization. In: *Basic Rehabilitation Techniques: A Self-Instructional Guide*, 2nd edit., edited by R. D. Sine, S. E. Liss, R. E. Roush, and J. D. Holcomb. Aspen Systems, Rockville, MD, with permission.]

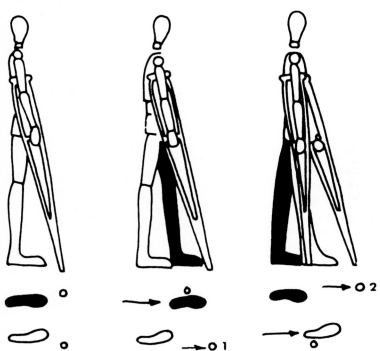

FIG. 5–5. Two-point alternate crutch gait. Crutch-foot sequence: 1, right crutch and left foot together; 2, left crutch and right foot together [From Wilson, G. (1981): Progressive mobilization. In: *Basic Rehabilitation Techniques: A Self-Instructional Guide*, 2nd edit., edited by R. D. Sine, S. E. Liss, R. E. Roush, and J. D. Holcomb. Aspen Systems, Rockville, MD, with permission.]

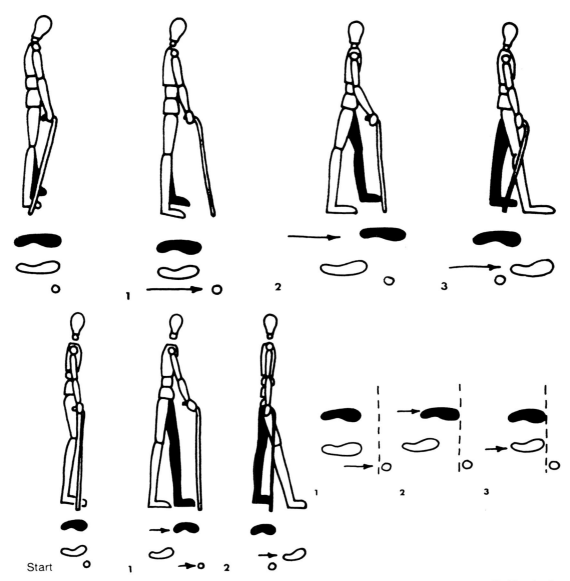

FIG. 5–6. Top: Step-through gait pattern. Move cane forward and out to the side. Shift weight off of involved leg and onto cane. Move involved leg up even with cane. Putting as much weight as possible on the involved leg, step past the cane with the uninvolved leg. **Bottom right:** Step-to cane gait. Indicated when patient can step to, but not past, the cane. Keep the walkcane well ahead of the feet. **Bottom left:** Cane-together gait. Patient moves cane and involved foot forward at same time, then steps past cane with his uninvolved foot [From Wilson, G. (1981): Progressive mobilization. In: *Basic Rehabilitation Techniques: A Self-Instructional Guide*, 2nd edit., edited by R. D. Sine, S. E. Liss, R. E. Roush, and J. D. Holcomb. Aspen Systems, Rockville, MD, with permission.]

TABLE 5–3. *Sequence of functional training from beginning to advanced activities*

Elementary
  A. Self care
    Eating and drinking
    Facial hygiene
    Toothbrushing
    Shaving or applying make-up
    Hair grooming
Intermediate
  B. Communication skills
    Conversing
    Reading
    Writing
    Using the telephone
  C. Dressing techniques
  D. Homemaking
Advanced
  E. Vocational and avocational activities
    Schooling or job training
    Driving a car
    Community social life
    Hobbies and interests

Instruction is usually coordinated by a nurse and occupational therapist. Although, for most activities, the patient is taught to lead with the dominant hand and assist with the nondominant one, performance is usually maximized by switching handedness if the dominant side is partially or totally disabled.

Eating

Disabled patients may have difficulty getting food to the mouth and then chewing and swallowing it. Patients with dysphagia, for example, may be unable to control oral musculature, protect the airway from choking, or swallow. These patients can be instructed in proper positioning, feeding rate, and bite size, as well as shown a method of voluntary swallowing. Special utensils can be purchased, but most patients are more likely to accept adaptations to regular utensils they already have at home than buying special utensils. Handles can be built up with adhesive-backed foam padding, or round foam hair curlers, for instance, to compensate for a weak grasp. Incoordination or lack of pronation/supination is best accommodated by using a spoon instead of a fork. Steak knives are easier to cut with than flatware knives. Patients with very weak hands may use a knife that has a ring where the knife handle joins the blade, to slip over the first finger as the palm of the hand provides leverage. A slice of bread held against the side of the plate enables getting food onto a utensil without pushing it off the plate.

For drinking, mugs with large handles and lightweight thermal cups, which prevent the patient from burning him or herself, can be used. Long straws made from hollow plastic tubing, with a 45° angle at the top, are helpful if the patient cannot pick up a mug.

Electric toothbrushes, or regular toothbrushes with padded handles, will encourage a disabled patient to accomplish routine oral hygiene. Caution patients with diminished sensation to avoid prolonged holding of any electric appliance; they may not notice progressive heat build-up and resulting burns. A universal cuff will help a patient with inadequate grasp hold a toothbrush. Likewise, electric razors facilitate shaving. Elastic straps can be sewn on to the razor and wrapped around the hand to assist in holding the razor. A washcloth can be folded and stitched to make a terrycloth wash mitt with a pocket for storing small pieces of soap. Hair is combed most easily by a rattailed comb with a padded handle.

Dressing

Most disabled patients have difficulty dressing themselves unless they are taught new techniques. Dressing the lower extremities is usually easier in bed, with the patient sitting up or leaning against the headboard, whereas the upper extremities and feet are more easily dressed in a chair. When dressing the upper or lower extremities, the more involved limb should be placed into the garment first and removed last. Pull tabs inside clothing, Velcro closures, button hooks, loops attached to zipper tabs, and various aids enable independent dressing with practice and trial and error to determine the best method.

Homemaking

A disabled patient's ability to function independently in the home often depends on the position of furniture and appliances, as well as the

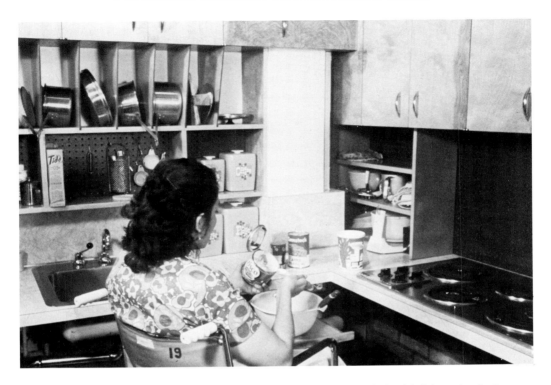

FIG. 5–7. Cooking utensils and supplies kept within easy reach of wheelchair-bound patient.

availability of labor-saving devices. Important considerations in adapting the home, especially the kitchen, for working include the following:

1. Safety.
2. Movement from one place to another, between and within rooms.
3. Energy consumption, with emphasis on economy of motion.
4. Automation of manual activities whenever possible.
5. Range of reach relative to position of objects.

The patient's mental alertness should be considered due to the prevalance of safety hazards in the kitchen. Insulation of the sink and pipes will prevent them from burning the patient's knees and legs. If the patient cannot see the stove top, a mirror should be installed over the stove or a hot plate used on a low table.

An occupational therapist should be consulted for instruction in principles of work simplification and economy of motion. Fixed work stations for each task should be assigned, so that the appropriate supplies can be kept ready at each station for immediate use (Fig. 5–7). Work areas should be laid out within normal reach so that supplies can be arranged in a semicircle. Select equipment that can be adapted to more than one task and appliances that are easy to operate, with controls and switches placed within easy reach. When possible, both hands are used in opposite, symmetric motions while working and any unnecessary motions are eliminated. Energy should not be wasted in holding utensils; instead, they should be secured by suction cups or clamps, freeing the hands for work. Also avoided are lifting and carrying; a table with casters can transport objects from one work area to another. Laundry chutes, refuse chutes, and gravity-feed flour bins enable gravity to replace some manual labor. Removing the cabinet doors in front of the sink, and installing a false base so that the sink will not be too deep, enable dishes to be washed from a wheelchair. The patient should also be encouraged to sit in a comfortable chair whenever working, to adjust the height of the work place to that of the chair, or to use an adjustable chair. Inspect the work environment for adequate light and ventilation.

SUGGESTED READINGS

Cynkin, S. (1979): *Occupational Therapy: Toward Health Through Activities*, 1st edit. Little, Brown, Boston.

Eggers, O. (1983): *Occupational Therapy in the Treatment of Adult Hemiplegia*. Heinemann, London.

Hopkins, H. L., and Smith, H. D. (1983): *Willard and Spackman's Occupational Therapy*, 6th edit. J. B. Lippincott Co., Philadelphia.

Lucci, J. A. (1980): *Occupational Therapy: Case Studies. A Compilation of 41 Case Studies*, 2nd edit. Medical Examination, Garden City, NY.

Martin, N., Holt, N., and Hicks, D. (1981): *Comprehensive Rehabilitation Nursing*. McGraw-Hill, New York.

Murray, R., and Kijek, J. C., editors. (1979): *Current Perspectives in Rehabilitation Nursing*. C. V. Mosby, St. Louis.

Pedretti, L. W. (1981): *Occupational Therapy: Practice Skills for Physical Dysfunction*. C. V. Mosby, St. Louis.

Reed, K. L. (1984): *Models of Practice in Occupational Therapy*. Williams and Wilkins, Baltimore, MD.

Stolov, W. C. (1980): Normal and pathologic ambulation. In: *The Musculoskeletal System in Health and Disease*, edited by C. Rosse and D. K. Clawson. Harper and Row, Hagerstown, MD.

Stryker, R. (1977): *Rehabilitative Aspect of Acute and Chronic Nursing Care*. W. B. Saunders, Philadelphia.

Wilson, G. (1977): Progressive mobilization. In: *Basic Rehabilitation Techniques: A Self-Instructional Guide*, edited by R. D. Sine, S. E. Liss, R. E. Roush, and J. D. Holcomb. Aspen Systems, Rockville, MD.

Medical Rehabilitation,
edited by L. S. Halstead et al.
Raven Press, New York © 1985.

CHAPTER 6

Orthoses and Adaptive Equipment

Thorkild J. Engen

Departments of Physical Medicine and Rehabilitation, Baylor College of Medicine, and Orthotics Department, The Institute of Rehabilitation and Research, Houston, Texas 77030

Orthoses and adaptive equipment support independent functioning by compensating for impairment of the upper and lower extremities, as well as the spine. Also called braces or splints, orthoses support, enhance, or alter the remaining capabilities of body parts disabled by various skeletal, muscular, or neuromuscular dysfunctions. Within the past 15 years, a major revolution has taken place in orthotic patient management. New highly sophisticated synthetic materials such as thermoplastics are enabling the application of new or improved design concepts in meeting the orthotic needs of individual patients. In addition, a properly fitted wheelchair, ambulatory aids, and architectural adaptations of the home often enable an otherwise institutionalized patient to live in the community.

ORTHOSES

Orthoses are designed to prevent or correct deformities or restore function. To encourage compliance with use of a prescribed orthosis, you should ensure that the device selected has the following qualities:

1. Purpose acceptable and accomplishable by patient.
2. Proper fit.
3. Lightweight.
4. Easy to apply and simple to use.
5. Reasonable in cost.
6. Safe to use, not causing deformity or discomfort.

Upper Extremity Braces

Splints or braces for the upper extremities—designed to be static, dynamic, or both—can support the hands, wrists, elbows, shoulders, or entire limb. They range in complexity from simple thermoplastic molds to cable- or motor-driven devices with several lever attachments and extension mechanisms.

Static orthoses, which support and immobilize joints to provide rest and promote healing, are used for acute conditions such as sprains, strains, soft tissue injuries, fractures, and acute arthritis. They may also prevent deformities by maintaining position in burns or paralysis. Examples of static orthoses for the upper extremities are basic hand, short opponens orthoses and wrist hand, long opponens orthoses (Fig. 6–1). To support arthritic or injured wrists, you can purchase kits to make low-temperature, thermoplastic splints in your office or clinic.

Dynamic or functional orthoses allow motion and improve function, strength, and range of motion (Fig. 6–2). The functional orthoses most commonly used for the upper extremity are body-powered orthoses (Fig. 6–3), which use several weaker muscles together to provide effective motion of splinted thumb, index, and long fingers. Static and dynamic function also can be combined on two adjacent segments of an upper limb in a single orthosis, so that, for example, the wrist is immobile and the fingers mobile.

Spinal Orthoses

Spinal orthoses are useful for alleviating pain, protecting against further injury, assisting weak muscles, preventing or correcting deformities, and stabilizing bone. These therapeutic results are gained through the biomechanical effects of trunk support, motion control, and spinal realignment. Some indications for various types of rigid and nonrigid spinal orthoses are described in Tables 6–1 and 6–2.

Application of an orthosis to the cervical spine adds the advantage of partial weight transfer of the head to the trunk when the patient is upright. Cervical orthoses can help alleviate complications of systemic diseases affecting the cervical spine, as well as the adverse effects of trauma on the cervical spine (Table 6–3). The advantages of various types of cervical collars and braces are compared in Table 6–4.

Unlike some upper extremity orthoses and the body jacket used in progressive neuromuscular diseases, most spinal orthoses are considered temporary devices. With unwarranted, prolonged wearing, spinal orthoses can produce contractures in the immobilized area, as well as muscle atrophy and weakness that could interfere with ambulation after removal of the orthosis. In addition, a greater expenditure of energy is required to walk while wearing a

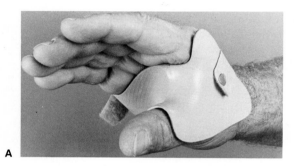

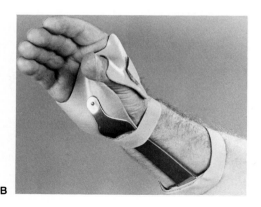

FIG. 6–1. Short opponens (basic hand) orthosis by Engen maintains thumb in opposition with index and middle finger **(A)** and supports palmar arch. Its main indications are impaired function of hand intrinsics secondary to median nerve and ulnar nerve involvement, polio, Guillain-Barré, amyotrophic lateral sclerosis, and spinal cord injury at the C8–T1 level. In addition to these functions, the long opponens orthosis by Engen **(B)** stabilizes and maintains wrist in neutral position. Its main indications are weak intrinsics, wrist extensor weakness, ulnar and radial nerve involvement at elbow, and spinal cord injury at C5–C6 level. (Photos by Gordon Stanley.)

TABLE 6–1. *Nonrigid spinal orthoses for pain and instability*

Type	Description	Indications
Trochanteric belt (Fig. 6–4A)	Belt made of canvas or leather, 2–3 in wide, encircles pelvis between trochanters and iliac crests	Support during healing of pelvic fractures; improve gait of patients with long-standing congenital dislocation of hip; relieve pain in sacroiliac joints or posterior superior spine of ilium in rheumatoid arthritis involving sacroiliac joints
Sacroiliac (SIO) and lumbar (LSO) belts (Fig.6–4B)	Belt made of heavy cotton, 4–6 in wide (SIO) or 8–16 in wide (LSO), reinforced with lightweight stays, worn at level of sacroiliac joint	Low back pain associated with degenerative disk disorders, postural fatigue, acute flexion injuries; other conditions that could benefit from abdominal compression
Sacroiliac, lumbosacral, and thoracolumbar corsets (Figs. 6–4C–E)	Cotton, nylon, or spandex garment that, in addition to compressing abdomen, extends over buttocks and thighs; may lace at back, sides, or front; shoulder straps maintain thoracic extension in thoracolumbar type	Shorter style for degenerative disk disorders, postural fatigue, acute flexion injuries, osteoarthritis, lumbosacral osteoporosis; longer style for pain control in generalized osteoporosis, metastatic malignancy, myeloma, osteoarthritis of mid- and low-thoracic parts of spine; better tolerated by obese patients

spinal orthosis. There is also the possibility of the patient becoming psychologically dependent on the orthosis and unable to function without it.

Lower Extremity Orthoses

There are four functional classes of lower extremity orthoses (Table 6–5), which may overlap to serve more than one purpose in a given patient. The chief indications for lower extremity orthoses are (1) neuromuscular conditions in which weakness impairs ambulation, and (2) bone and joint disease. Ankle-foot orthoses (AFOs), knee-ankle-foot orthoses (KA-FOs), and hip-KAFOs are designed to compensate for weakness in spinal cord injury and neuromuscular diseases, as well as prevent deformities.

Ankle-foot orthoses are by far the most commonly prescribed lower-extremity braces. Proper bracing with an AFO improves functional ambulation safely and with less energy consumption than walking without the brace. Consequently, the patient consumes less oxygen and walks more efficiently. The degree to which the various models accomplish these goals depends mainly on their mechanical design (Fig. 6–8) rather than on their weight or the materials used. The main applications of AFOs are the prevention of ankle twisting during the stance phase, as well as toe dragging, stumbling, and falling during the swing phase, the regulation of gait during pushoff, and some knee stability.

Knee-ankle orthoses are indicated when unstable knees compound foot and ankle weakness. Their most typical use is in spinal cord injuries, which limit gait to swing-through or swing-to patterns. Due to the excessive energy required for functional ambulation, however, few paraplegics at levels above T10 use their knee-ankle orthoses for any activity besides exercise. Paraplegics at L2–L5 levels are the most likely to require the orthosis for ambulation. The older models are being replaced by orthoses of new lightweight materials and modified designs that are easier to put on and take off, yet require little force to stabilize the knee. The addition of pelvic bands is no longer advised because their excessive energy requirement does not warrant the extra support provided.

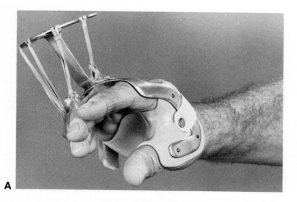

A

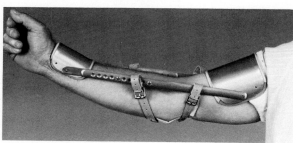

B

FIG. 6–2. Dynamic upper extremity orthoses. **A:** Knuckle bender is used in radial nerve injuries to improve ROM of MP joints and to stretch contractures. **B:** Adjustable elbow extension orthosis is applied to slowly stretch elbow flexion contractures. (Photos by Gordon Stanley.)

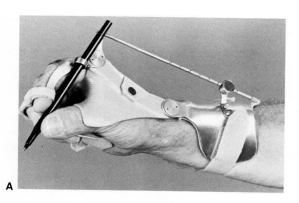

A

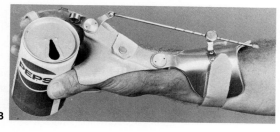

B

FIG. 6–3. Reciprocal wrist extension orthosis by Engen enables closing **(A)** and opening **(B)** of fingers. (Photos by Gordon Stanley.)

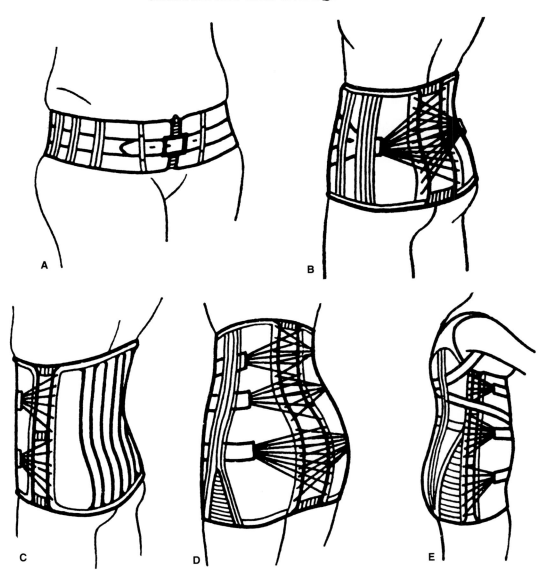

FIG. 6–4. Nonrigid spinal orthoses. **A:** Trochanteric belt. **B:** Sacroiliac belt. **C:** Lumbosacral belt. **D:** Lumbosacral corset. **E:** Thoracolumbar corset. [From Lucas, D. B. (1980): Spinal orthoses for pain and instability. In: *Orthotics Etcetera*, 2nd edit., edited by J. B. Redford. Williams & Wilkins, Baltimore.]

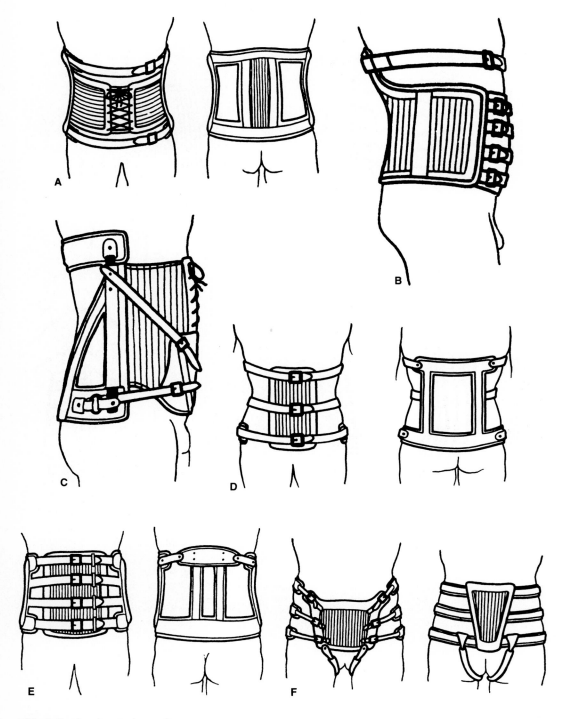

FIG. 6–5. Lumbar and sacroiliac rigid spinal orthoses. **A:** Knight brace. **B:** Brackett brace. **C:** Williams brace. **D:** MacAusland brace. **E:** Wilcox, or Lipscomb, brace. **F:** Osgood, or Goldthwait, brace. [From Lucas, D. B. (1980): Spinal orthoses for pain and instability. In: *Orthotics Etcetera*, 2nd edit., edited by J. B. Redford. Williams & Wilkins, Baltimore.]

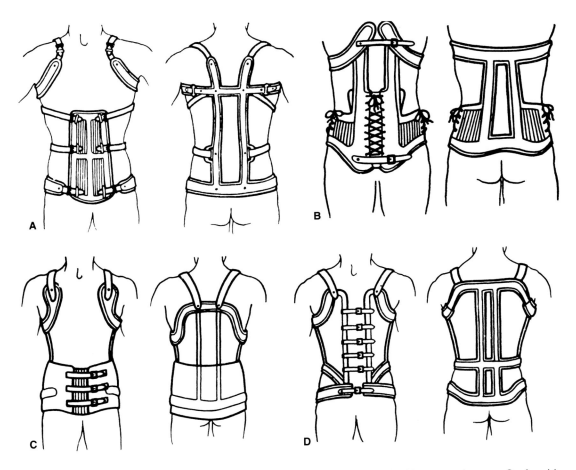

FIG. 6–6. Thoracolumbar rigid spinal orthoses. **A:** Taylor brace. **B:** Magnuson brace. **C:** Arnold brace. **D:** Steindler brace. [From Lucas, D. B. (1980): Spinal orthoses for pain and instability. In: *Orthotics Etcetera*, 2nd edit., edited by J. B. Redford. Williams & Wilkins, Baltimore.]

Orthoses for disorders of the bones and joints are designed to limit weight bearing and maintain correct joint and bone alignment. They are either patellar tendon bearing or ischial weight bearing and, in addition, may have a fracture cast design constructed of plaster of Paris or heat-forming plastic. Ischial weight bearing orthoses transmit force from the ischium to the orthosis, then through the orthosis to the ground. To compensate for specific structural problems, they may have locked or free knee joints, fixed or free ankle joints, a sole plate, and an optional rocker or patten bottom. Their function is significantly improved by the addition of a rigid quadrilateral cuff. Since these orthoses do not

protect the hip joint, a cane or crutches must also be used for successful ambulation. The Thomas ring, formerly the ischial brace of choice, is no longer recommended because it causes more discomfort than the newer models.

Patellar tendon bearing orthoses transmit force from the knee through the patellar tendon, then into the cuff through the upright and from the shoe to the ground. Weight bearing may be enhanced by a locked or free knee joint, fixed or free ankle, sole plate, and optional rocker or patten bottom.

Fracture cast braces (Fig. 6–9), unlike traditional plaster casts, also provide ischial or patellar tendon weight bearing. By maintaining

TABLE 6–2. *Rigid spinal orthoses for pain and instability*

Type	Description	Indications
Lumbar (LSO) or chairback (Fig. 6–5): Brackett, Williams, Wilcox, MacAusland, Knight	Short brace surrounds and compresses entire abdomen, pelvis, and lower back	Progressively straightening paraspinal uprights gradually reduces lordosis; Williams allows free flexion but limits extension and uses lever action to additionally flatten lumbar spine; movable joint in Wilcox permits more mobility and comfort; MacAusland has no lateral uprights to inhibit flexibility but still compresses abdomen
Sacroiliac (SIO) (Fig. 6–5): Osgood or Goldthwait	Very short orthosis provides lower abdominal pressure and pelvic arch support without significantly limiting lumbar motion	Treatment of pelvic fractures and immobilization of sacroiliac joints; lumbosacral arthralgia
Thorocolumbar (TLSO) (Fig. 6–6): Taylor, Bennett, Magnuson, Steindler, Arnold	Fixes lumbar spine to pelvis to provide a base and hold the thoracic part to rigid paraspinal uprights in varying degrees of extension; models differ in amount of rigidity and immobilization provided	Assists maintenance of extension; Arnold model is used in osteoporosis, degenerative joint disease, rheumatoid spondylitis, moderate muscle weakness; Taylor is used after vertebral body compression fractures, treatment of patients with severely rounded back caused by epiphysitis, spondylitis, or marked weakness of trunk; Steindler is reserved for maximum immobilization in limiting axial rotation
Anterior hyperextension	Modified rectangular metal frame exerts pressure over pubis and manubrium while counterpressure is maintained over midback with straps; lightweight construction	Permits ambulation during treatment of compression fractures of vertebral bodies
Molded jackets (see Fig. 17–3)	Plaster of Paris, leather, plastic, or polyethylene foam fits body contours accurately to distribute pressure evenly over widest possible area of body surface; can immobilize entire spine for 6–12 months, yet be removed for comfortable bed rest	Spinal support of elderly, chronically ill, or debilitated patient; advanced metastatic tumor involvement of spine; multiple myeloma; severe osteoporosis; patients with severe deformities; spinal cord injury

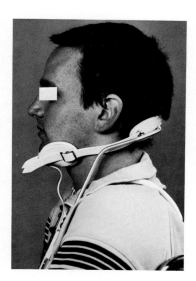

FIG. 6–7. SOMI collar, lateral view.

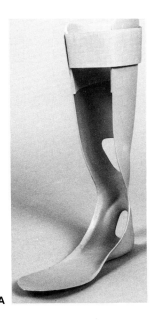

A

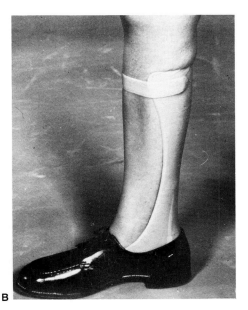

B

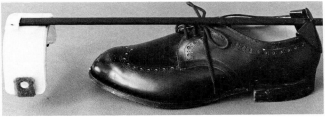

C

FIG. 6–8. Some current designs for ankle-foot orthoses. **A:** TIRR orthosis by Engen provides toe pick-up for patients with flaccid paralysis or mild spasticity. **B:** Seattle orthosis provides maximal mediolateral stability. A similar, but less expensive version, has been made from polypropylene by Rancho Los Amigos orthotists. **C:** Veterans Administration Prosthetics Center Shoe-Clasp is easily attached to any shoe, but collapses readily into maximal dorsiflexion. [From Lehmann, J. F. (1979): Biomechanics of ankle-foot orthoses: Prescription and design. *Arch. Phys. Med. Rehabil.*, 60:203,206.]

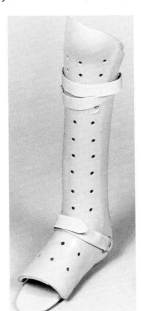

FIG. 6–9. Fracture cast brace constructed of thermoplastic for weight bearing.

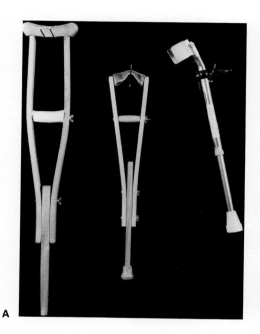

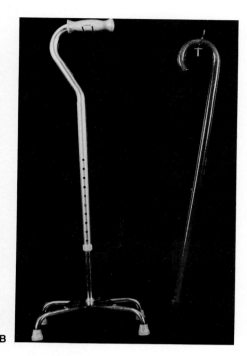

FIG. 6–10. Commonly used crutches and canes. **A:** Axillary crutch *(left)*, forearm crutch with leather cuff *(middle)*, forearm aluminum crutch *(right)*. **B:** Quad cane *(left)*, standard cane *(right)*.

bony alignment while limiting weight bearing through the fracture site, these casts reduce the period of immobilization. Because the bone heals faster, the patient can resume normal ambulation much earlier than with a plaster cast alone.

WALKING AIDS

The most important considerations when selecting walkers, canes, crutches, and other assistive devices for ambulation are the patient's

TABLE 6–3. *Complications of disease and trauma affecting the cervical spine*

Disease or traumatic stress	Complication
Rheumatoid arthritis	Decreased ligamentous stability and odontoid pathology, particularly at atlantoaxial joints
Rheumatoid spondylitis	Spinal rigidity and ankylosis caused by connective tissue autoimmune disease
Duchenne muscular dystrophy	Lack of muscle support and head control against gravitational forces
Parkinson's disease	Neck rigidity and postural changes produced by lack of synergistic neurological control
Cerebral palsy	Lack of volitional fine motor coordination with need to position head to help control tonic neck reflexes
Congenital cervical anomalies	Fusion or partial absence of vertebrae alters stress pattern of breakdown, build-up, and replacement
Repetitive stresses	Adverse effects of abnormal posturing and occupational stresses
Acceleration forces	Hyperextension injury mainly at C4 vertebral area
Deceleration forces	Hyperflexion injury at C5–C6 vertebral area

TABLE 6–4. *Comparison of cervical orthoses for pain and instability*

Type	Advantages
Skin Contact	
Soft collar	Serves as reminder to restrict motion of head and neck; slightly restricts cervical flexion-extension; comfortable; apply to cervical strain for 4–5 days following injury
Hard collar: Thomas, Mayo, wire-frame	Significantly restricts cervical flexion-extension, lateral bending, and rotation; apply to cervical strain, sprain, or whiplash
Head cervical orthosis (HCO): Chin piece collar, Queen Anne collar, Camp collar (double support), molded collar with chin and occipital support, Philadelphia or Plastiazote collar (custom-molded), four-poster	Firm plastic provides more neck control by further restricting head motion, but not totally restricting forward movement of head; apply chin piece for greater limitation of flexion without limiting extension; apply Queen Anne for limiting cervical extension but not atlantoaxial extension; apply Camp for best sagittal immobilization of C1 and C2; polyethylene foam, two-piece Philadelphia collar restricts gross flexion and extension of cervical spine, but is less effective than four-poster in controlling rotation and side-bending, easily applied to and removed from bedridden patient; four-poster restricts lateral bending the least of all HCOs, but is more effective for restricting extension of cervical spine compared with SOMI
Head cervical thoracic orthosis (HCTO): SOMI[a] (Fig. 6–7), Wilson, Guilford, rigid APRO[b]	SOMI is easily fitted on supine patient and can be mounted onto bivalved TLSO; others are modifications of SOMI; Wilson frees chin for talking and chewing, with no undesirable force over temporomandibular joints; rigid APRO combines SOMI chest plate and four-poster superstructure with posterior SOMI chest plate; HCTOs are lightweight and less cumbersome than halo orthoses, but are not good inhibitors of lateral bending
Head cervical thoracic lumbar orthosis (HCTLO): Florida two-poster, Jewett brace with cervical attachment, Dennison-Boldrey	Provides nearly total restriction of flexion, extension, lateral bending, and rotation; Florida type provides good trunk stabilization, but occipital and mandibular portions are connected only by leather straps, not rigidly; Dennison-Boldrey decreases flexion-extension by holding head firmly against cup attached by ear
Head cervical thoracic lumbar sacral orthosis (HCTLSO): Stryker	Provides secure immobilization with traction up to 30 lb; enables easy transportation of patient; permits cervical spine X-ray while brace is worn; permits lumbar puncture and myelogram; adjusts to any adult body shape; applied and removed with ease
Bony Contact	
Halo: Halo bed, SCTO halo vest[c], SCTLO halo body jacket[d], SCTLPO halo hoop[e], Halo femoral pin traction	Rigid fixation improves rate of fracture union; increases application force without causing skin necrosis; countertraction allows early mobility out of bed; quadriplegics usually wear halo for about 8 weeks, then switch to Dennison brace for additional 4–6 weeks

[a]Sternal-occipital-mandibular immobilizer.
[b]Anterior-posterior-rotational orthosis.
[c]Skull cervical thoracic orthosis.
[d]Skull cervical thoracic lumbar orthosis.
[e]Skull cervical thoracic lumbar pelvic orthosis.

height, weight, age, and diagnosis, as well as the cost. Before prescribing nonadjustable equipment, take accurate measurements of the patient while he or she is standing and wearing walking shoes with a broad, flat heel. The patient is likely to avoid using uncomfortable equipment that functions poorly due to imprecise fitting.

Walkers

More stable than crutches or canes, walkers may be adjustable, and crutch pieces, a seat,

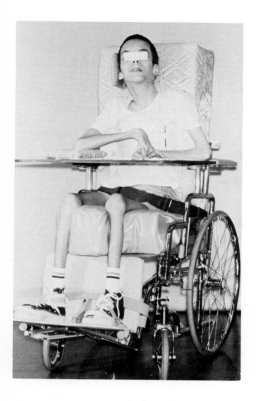

FIG. 6–11. Severely disabled patient travels safely using wheelchair with adaptive items: head positioner, safety belt with chest straps, legs and feet positioners, and hip belt.

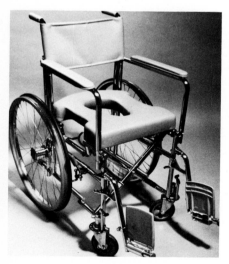

FIG. 6–12. Wheelchair for commode and shower use.

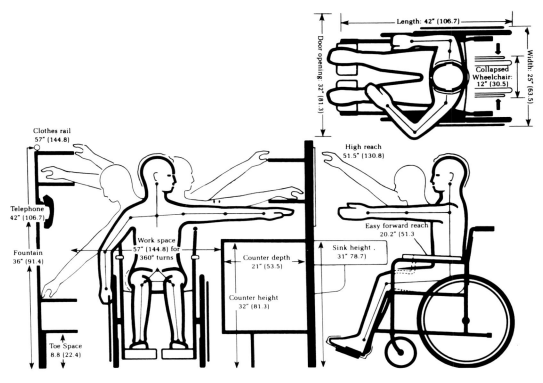

FIG. 6–13. Basic measurements and proportions for modifying home to accommodate wheelchairs. [From Hopkins, H. L., and Smith, H. D. (1978): *Willard and Spackman's Occupational Therapy*. J. B. Lippincott, Philadelphia.]

TABLE 6–5. *Functional classes of lower extremity orthosis*

Class	Purpose	Clinical application
Stabilizing or supportive	Permit patient to control otherwise uncontrollable segment or entire limb; stabilize joints by preventing unwanted motion and stabilize limbs for weight bearing	Spastic paralysis, flaccid paralysis, painful joints, structural inadequacies produced by variety of diseases, post-trauma, congenital abnormalities
Motorized or functional	Provide active function to otherwise paralyzed or paretic limb segment by replacing lost muscle power	Flaccid paralysis
Corrective	Correct or realign parts of a limb by applying intermittent, strong force in desired direction	Congenital club foot, congenital metatarsus varus, developmental flat foot, congenital dislocation of hip, tibial torsion
Protective	Protect or maintain alignment of diseased or injured limb; relieve weight on femur or tibia	Fractures, hip disorders, especially aseptic necrosis

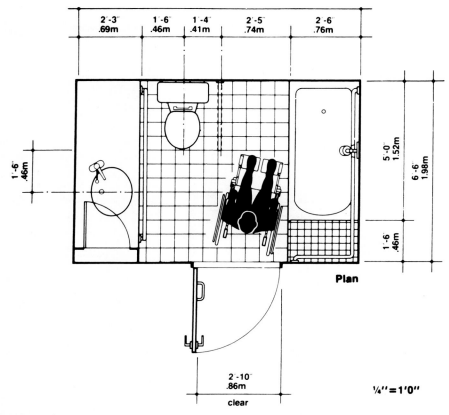

FIG. 6–14. Bathroom that will accommodate disabled person in wheelchair. [From Hopkins, H. L., and Smith, H. D. (1978): *Willard and Spackman's Occupational Therapy.* J. B. Lippincott, Philadelphia.]

and casters may be added. A typical candidate for a walker is a debilitated elderly patient who has had a hip fracture. Walkers also offer safer ambulation for disoriented patients than do canes.

Crutches

Axillary crutches provide more stability than either canes or forearm crutches (Fig. 6–10) because motion of the hip and trunk can be controlled more easily. Another advantage is their capacity to transfer some of the patient's body weight to the shoulders and upper extremities, if necessary, to relieve weight bearing on a lower extremity. Very thin patients, however, may be unable to use them comfortably if they cannot tolerate the pressure or friction of the axillary crossbar against the rib cage. Although similar to a cane, the forearm crutch provides

more stability by supporting the forearm and providing some control of hip motion.

Canes

Standard canes (Fig. 6–10), available in wood or metal, provide the least support in ambulation, but are ideal for patients who are almost fully weight bearing yet need assistance with balance. Metal canes are usually adjustable, whereas wooden canes are not. The quad cane, a broad-based metal cane with four feet (Fig. 6–10), offers additional stability. It is indicated for elderly patients whose weakness, incoordination, spasticity, or imbalance make ambulation unstable. The cane is held in the hand opposite to that of the involved leg. If a patient requires minimal support for balance while walking, you may prefer to prescribe two canes instead of two crutches.

WHEELCHAIR SELECTION

The mandatory requirements for any wheelchair are brakes, leg rests, handrims for easy propulsion, durability, easy folding, and 8-inch front casters. The most important considerations when prescribing a wheelchair include safety, cost, and mode of propulsion, as well as the patient's size, body weight, diagnosis, prognosis, preferred transfer technique, and lifestyle. Available in several standard sizes for adults and children, wheelchairs should be properly fitted for:

1. Seat width—hip measurement across, plus 2 inches.
2. Seat depth—from back of hip to 2 inches from bend of knee.
3. Back height—from seat rail to top of scapulae; add height for trunk weakness and head support for neck weakness.
4. Arm heights—from seat rail, supports arm and shoulder with elbow flexed to a 90° angle; add removable arms for sitting transfers, or adjustable height arms for growing children.
5. Footrests—support foot with femur parallel to floor, heel loops to prevent feet from sliding off.

All measurements should be made as the patient sits on the cushion he or she will be using.

To suit special needs, many adaptive items, such as a safety belt with chest straps, can be ordered from a wheelchair catalogue. Even severely disabled patients can travel independently by operating a motorized wheelchair, which may have hand, chin, or puff-and-suck control. Side or head positioners are available for patients who cannot maintain trunk balance. Positioners can also hold the legs and feet, or hyperflex the hips to minimize extension spasticity (Fig. 6–11). Special wheelchairs are also available for shower and commode use (Fig. 6–12).

Cushions should also be custom selected. Polymer foam cushions, 2 inches thick for patients with sensation and 3 inches thick for patients lacking sensation, are usually chosen for their good support, light weight, and low cost.

Overrated, gel cushions are not recommended. However, some patients may benefit from the superior pressure distribution provided by air-filled cushions.

HOME ADAPTATION

The goal of adapting a home for a wheelchair-bound or other disabled individual is to enable free movement between and within rooms with maximal convenience and minimal effort. The disabled person must be able to use the facilities in every room, not just in the kitchen. Appliances and furniture should be selected for ease of maintenance and serviceability. Since certain disorders are exacerbated by cold, the house must have an adequate heating system. Each addition to the home also should be selected for its cost effectiveness. Optimal measurements and proportions for the efficient functioning of a wheelchair-bound patient at home are given in Figs. 6–13 and 6–14.

SUGGESTED READINGS

American Academy of Orthopaedic Surgeons (1975): *Atlas of Orthotics: Biomechanical Principles and Application.* C. V. Mosby, St. Louis.

Engen, T. (1971): *Research Developments of Lower Extremity Orthotic Systems for Patients with Various Functional Deficits: Final Report.* The Institute for Rehabilitation and Research, Houston.

Engen, T., and Spencer, W. (1969): *Development of Externally Powered Upper Extremity Orthotics: Final Report.* The Institute for Rehabilitation and Research, Houston.

Hopkins, H. L., and Smith H. D. (1983): *Willard and Spackman's Occupational Therapy,* 6th edit. J. B. Lippincott Co., Philadelphia.

Lal, S., and Kaplan, P. E. (1982): Orthotics. In: *The Practice of Rehabilitation Medicine,* edited by P. E. Kaplan and R. S. Materson. Charles C Thomas, Springfield, Ill.

Lehmann, J. F. (1979): Biomechanics of ankle-foot orthoses: Prescription and design. *Arch. Phys. Med. Rehabil.,* 60:200–207.

Malick, M., and Meyer, C. (1978): *Manual of Management of the Quadriplegic Upper Extremity.* Harmarville Rehabilitation Center, Pittsburgh.

Mastro, B. A., and Mastro, R. T. (1980): *Selected Reading: A Review of Orthotics and Prosthetics.* American Orthotic and Prosthetic Association, Washington, D.C.

Prosthetics and Orthotics Department, New York University Post-Graduate Medical School (1983): *Spinal Orthotics.* New York University, New York.

Prosthetics and Orthotics Department, New York University Post-Graduate Medical School (1981): *Lower-Limb Orthotics.* New York University, New York.

Redford, J. B., editor (1980): *Orthotics Etcetera,* 2nd edit. Williams & Wilkins, Baltimore.

Medical Rehabilitation,
edited by L. S. Halstead et al.
Raven Press, New York © 1985.

CHAPTER 7

Psychological, Social, and Vocational Adjustment to Physical Disability

Roberta B. Trieschmann

Private Practice, Scottsdale, Arizona 85261

The onset of any physical disability will have an impact on the behavior of the person. Generally, the greater the number of compromised behaviors that, before disability, were prized by the patient or necessary for independent function, the greater the change in lifestyle after disability and, accordingly, the greater the psychosocial adjustment required. An exception is severe disfigurement, which, while not impairing function, may require significant psychosocial adjustment. Disfigurement from burns or accidents usually has a great impact on the person's social value, resulting in many changes in lifestyle.

The patient's ability to cope will also depend partly on the family's acceptance and adjustment. The family is likely to be anxious about the patient's prognosis regarding deterioration of health and longevity, as well as their own ability to make the changes that may be required of them. Financial worries are often considerable as medical expenses mount, insurance plans must be interpreted, and concerns regarding future sources of income become nagging doubts.

If the disabled person has a job that is no longer appropriate, changes in self-image will be required, which can be particularly threatening to those whose main source of self-identification is through their work. Thus, vocational evaluation and retraining may be necessary. The disabled person occasionally cannot return to the world of work, however, and either the non-disabled spouse must work outside the home for the first time or the entire burden of family income falls on one person's shoulders instead of two.

Thus, most physical impairments will influence the person's lifestyle in some fashion and require changes and adjustments by the disabled person and the family. Assessing the impact of a disability requires a thorough knowledge of the individual's premorbid lifestyle, as well as a complete evaluation of current functioning and environmental resources.

REACTIONS TO DISABILITY

Sudden Versus Gradual Onset

If disability is of sudden onset, and there is no obtundation from associated cerebral trauma, patients may appear unresponsive if they are heavily medicated, have had a disrupted sleep pattern, or are suffering from sensory deprivation. If these conditions are not present, or when they remit, the average person would benefit from information about the disability in general terms and about future rehabilitation plans. Information should be given within the context of hope, that the patient will get better, without giving unrealistic expectations of total recovery. Do not provide too much detail about the patient's condition soon after the injury or acute illness unless the patient specifically requests it.

If disability is of gradual onset, share information with the patient as requested and present the prognosis for the future factually. Emphasize what improvements the patient can expect by complying with the rehabilitation program.

Congenital or Early Childhood Disability

Disabilities acquired early in life will require that the physician deal with the parents more than with the disabled child regarding psychosocial issues. The attitude of the parents toward the disabled child has a critical influence on the child's attitude about himself or herself that will become obvious at adulthood. The primary concern for the disabled child is that he or she participate as much as possible in the normal play and interactions with childhood and teenage peers. Overly protective parents can unintentionally cripple the child's social development, which can lead to profound emotional immaturity by the time adulthood is reached. Therefore, if you observe significant overprotection by the parents, refer the family to a clinical psychologist for assessment of the child's behavioral status and the family interaction pattern.

Static Versus Progressive Disabilities

Reactions to static disability are likely to differ from reactions to progressive disability. Patients experiencing a static disability will typically react with anxiety, depression, and anger. They may ruminate about why the accident happened to them, what they had done to deserve the misfortune. As they find new sources of reward and satisfaction, however, they are better able to resolve these emotional reactions and adjust to disability than patients with progressive disability, whose anxiety about the future can never be fully resolved. The progressively disabled patient therefore often succumbs to chronic depression.

Whether disability is static or progressive, a clinical psychologist is the best qualified specialist to organize a behavioral therapy program emphasizing the activities the patients can do to replace their worries about what they can no longer do.

Emotional Reactions

Emotional reactions to disability often manifest as the patterns of behavior discussed in Table 7–1. Depression is often related to loss of valued independence, social roles, and daily activities, engendering feelings of helplessness, as well as hopelessness about the future. The immediate world seems to contain few rewarding experiences. Behavioral strategies that introduce a graduated series of rewarding accomplishments in an accepting environment are recommended. Antidepressant drugs are indicated only when clinically relevant somatic symptoms, such as loss of appetite, insomnia, and psychomotor retardation, are present.

Irritability and anger, considered normal reactions to the frustrations of disability, should not be treated unless they interfere significantly with daily life. Reassure the patient's family and the health care staff that these emotional reactions will decrease as function improves. The patient can be encouraged to channel this emotional energy into some physical activity.

Active intervention is required to alleviate apathy and passivity, since the resulting inertia can greatly retard recovery. An external structure that *specifies* goals and behavioral quotas, *sequences* activities from easy to difficult, *focuses* on small, easy segments of tasks, and *rewards* accomplishments may motivate a patient who feels overwhelmed by the amount of work required in rehabilitation. Providing an external structure, identifying those rewards and goals for which the person will work, is especially helpful for motivating people who are not self-starters. Behavior therapy techniques, in which a reward is contingent on a specified behavior, can transform the behavior of unmotivated persons into behavior similar to that of self-motivated persons.

Social Implications of Disability

Devaluation

Disabled people may expect to be devalued and treated as inferiors by others because our society tends to reject people who are different,

TABLE 7–1. *Five patterns of behavior often observed in disabled patients*

Behavior	Causes	Therapeutic strategies
Depression	Decreased participation in activities and social interaction; overwhelming novelty and change; loss of control and choices; loss of independence; perceived loss of identity	Listen to the patient; structure environment to encourage participation in pleasurable activities; encourage activities that will result in positive feedback; recognize and call attention to patient's assets and progress; allow as many choices as possible; initiate counseling; prescribe antidepressant medication
Anxiety	Lack of understanding about medical status; lack of predictability; novel roles, situations, and people; social isolation; anticipation of pain and discomfort; fear of the future; discomfort with institutions and authority figures	Listen to the patient; provide reassurance and support; offer information; structure a predictable environment and set clear expectations; plan and reward activities incompatible with anxiety, chiefly requiring active participation; teach and encourage relaxation; initiate counseling; prescribe anxiolytic medication
Excessive demands and complaints	Fear and anxiety; need for contact, social interaction, attention, personal care; emotional distress; premorbid behavior pattern	Establish rapport; identify what the patient wants; try to satisfy the patient's wants without reinforcing complaining; identify and treat underlying emotional distress; respond nondefensively and politely
Lack of motivation	Goal conflicts between patient and caretakers; unclear relationship between goals and prescribed behaviors; cognitive and psychological limitations; practical obstacles to compliance with rehabilitation regimens; countertherapeutic reinforcement, in which cooperative behaviors are implicitly punished and uncooperative behaviors rewarded; interpersonal conflicts expressed as oppositional or uncooperative behavior	Establish rapport; agree on goals and the ways to achieve them; make cooperation easy
Disorientation and confusion	Organic disorders; overwhelming anxiety and fear; excessive emotional excitement or stimulation in patient with marginal neurological or psychological functioning; unfamiliar surroundings and people; lack of routine that differentiates days; little variety of stimulation; minimal need for problem solving or critical thinking; positive reinforcement of confused behavior	Give orienting information frequently, such as names, places, and dates; provide an environment that stimulates orientation—clock, window, radio, TV, familiar objects; arrange highly structured predictable environment; talk simply and repeat important communications; ignore confused talk and respond to sensible talk; give corrective feedback; ease anxieties; treat the patient respectfully, showing respect for privacy, independence, and control

deformed, or disabled. This concept of difference is learned at an early age along with an appreciation for physical attractiveness. Thus, people who are different or less physically attractive are often less preferred as companions and occasionally rejected. The person with the disability has learned these standards, now applies them to himself or herself, and expects others to apply them towards him or her also. As a result, there usually is a significant change in the disabled person's interpersonal relationships, since he or she will be treated as "less than" before disability. Withdrawal from social situations typically occurs. They may benefit from social skills training programs that teach assertiveness and how to combat prejudice. A psychologist, social worker, or vocational counselor should be consulted to implement such an intervention strategy.

Impact on the Family

The onset of a disability can instigate a family crisis. Disability changes the nature of the marital relationship between husband and wife. The spouse of a disabled mate will feel the strain of assuming more family and household obligations. The range of sexual activities may be limited, as discussed in Chapter 26. If a child becomes disabled, the parents may become overprotective, not allowing the child to grow up and live independently. The parents' shift in attention to the disabled child may make the siblings feel neglected. Sorting out these problems may require counseling to improve communication and determine appropriate expectations and roles for each family member. The quality of a disabled patient's relationship with his or her family and other supportive people often has a marked influence on rate and extent of recovery and adaptation.

Sociocultural Influences

In certain cultures, physical ability is necessary for acceptance as a man by the community. Furthermore, in lower socioeconomic groups, physical ability may be required to earn an income. Therefore, the disabled man may no longer be accepted as an equal by his peers. In other socioeconomic groups where intellectual abilities are prized, the physically disabled man may be able to compete successfully with his peers in a profession or business. In certain ethnic groups, women are valued for their physical attractiveness and homemaking skills. Disability may eliminate these women from the dating game and minimize the opportunity to get married and have a family. Thus, sociocultural issues should be evaluated carefully and considered when planning rehabilitation goals.

Financial Concerns

Rehabilitation is expensive. Not only are there hospital and treatment bills, but special assistive devices and equipment used to restore function, compounded by the increased costs of living, will require a higher income than prior to the onset of disability or a significant reduction in the standard of living. If the primary income producer becomes disabled, these concerns become particularly acute. Social workers can help evaluate sources of income and provide assistance in seeking disability benefits.

Productivity

Our society puts pressure on every man to be employed, and employment is often a criterion for acceptance in the community. Many men obtain their primary sources of satisfaction through their work, while others consider work to be a tedious and demeaning experience forced on them to earn money for survival. Following a disability, the person's predisability attitudes toward employment will be a critical factor in rehabilitation planning. Whether or not vocational retraining or further education is appropriate depends on the person, the nature of the disability, and financial circumstances. Unfortunately, welfare legislation of the early 1980s contains many financial disincentives to productivity; most benefits are lost upon earning a small amount of money that in itself would not be sufficient for survival. These financial disincentives to productivity often prevent eager and capable disabled persons from accepting employment because they cannot earn enough to make up for the lost benefits. For this reason, the broader aspects of disability should be considered, such as family participation, community activities, group memberships, education, and volunteerism, in addition to employment.

Every person needs a reason to get out of bed in the morning, and a disabled person particularly needs a reason to endure the hardships imposed by disability. Involvement in productive activities of some kind is often the key to the person's health and rehabilitation efforts.

Sexuality

The onset of disability need not interfere with a desire for a satisfying sexual relationship, regardless of age. Advise the disabled person and partner about the range of sexual activities available to them and about any precautionary measures that should be taken. The physician should be aware of the impotence-producing side effects of certain therapeutic agents for treating hypertension. In addition, impotence may be associated with peripheral vascular disease and diabetes. When sexual intercourse is not possible or advisable, the couple should be counseled on the varieties of sexual satisfaction available. Take care, however, to assess the cultural and religious attitudes toward sexuality before recommending any particular course of action. Rather than focusing on sexual techniques, emphasize the variety of communication and loving behaviors between two people, sexual acts being only one form of communication. Sexual alternatives for the disabled are discussed in more detail in Chapter 26.

INTELLECTUAL DYSFUNCTIONS

Definitions of Intellectual Skills

Human intellectual functioning consists of verbal, perceptual, memory, and quality control skills, as well as emotional appropriateness, and alertness. Verbal skill is the ability to receive verbal inputs accurately and to transmit verbal outputs that are appropriate to the given situation. Perceptual skill is the ability to evaluate one's position in space in relation to other objects and to navigate through space accurately. Another type of perceptual skill is the ability to receive visual, nonverbal auditory, tactual, and kinesthetic information correctly and to use this information to accomplish tasks appropriately. Memory skill is the ability to receive verbal and perceptual information, retain it, and later recall it. Information about the present or very recent past comprises recent memory, while information obtained long ago, usually prior to disability and often used in everyday life, comprises remote memory.

Quality control skill is the ability to monitor one's own behavior for inaccuracies or inappropriateness, to determine what other behavior would be more accurate or appropriate, and to correct the behavior. Given cues as to the appropriateness of emotional displays on particular occasions, individuals should be able to control their emotions, or exhibit emotional appropriateness. Influencing overall intellectual efficiency in all of the above areas, alertness is the continuum from somnolence or unconsciousness to full wakefulness and cognizance of one's surroundings. Alertness also includes orientation to person, place, and time.

Characteristic Intellectual Dysfunctions

Intellectual deficits are typically found in patients following cerebral vascular accidents with hemiplegia or cerebral trauma. They are also associated with multiple sclerosis, cerebral neoplasm, arteriosclerosis, and presenile dementias such as Pick's and Alzheimer's disease. Specific deficits in right and left cerebral vascular accidents are compared in Chapter 15. Intellectual impairment associated with other disorders is discussed in Chapters 12, 16, and 19.

Preliminary Screening Techniques

There are several easy and short screening procedures you can perform in your office to determine whether a patient has some intellectual deficits. These tests will reveal gross deficits, but subtle deficits may remain hidden. Therefore, when the patient has sustained one of the disorders mentioned in the preceding section, refer him or her to a clinical psychologist for further evaluation. Figure 7–1 shows the many kinds of errors that may occur when the patient is asked to draw and identify geometric figures. In addition to the ability to identify person, place, and time factors, some tests for orientation and alertness are having the person recite the letters of the alphabet and count backwards from 20 to 1. Considering the complexity and range of intellectual function, these screening procedures are quite primitive. Anyone who has difficulty with any of these tests should be re-

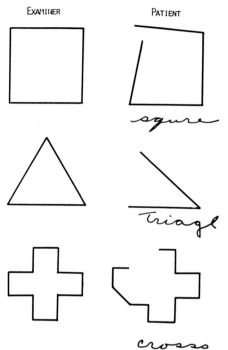

EXAMINER   PATIENT

Fig. 7–1. Examples of patient errors on intellectual screening test. **Left column:** Draw each of the geometric figures on a plain, white, unlined sheet of paper without lifting your pencil from the paper. After drawing each figure, instruct the patient, "Draw this without lifting your pencil from the paper." Do not say the name of the geometric figure (square, triangle, cross). After the patient has completed the three drawings, say, "Now write on the paper what this is, " pointing first to the square, then to the triangle, then to the cross. Do not identify the name of the figure. **Right column:** Similar distortions in any one of the geometric figures suggests the possibility of right hemispheric damage. Errors in writing or identifying the geometric figure suggest left hemispheric involvement. The reproduction of the triangle is an example of left neglect, a perceptual problem. Any patient who exhibited all of the types of problems shown would have bilateral damage or a diffuse deficit.

ferred to a clinical psychologist for further evaluation. When no difficulties appear on these tests, use your judgment and seek further evaluation if you sense problems that may be more subtle.

MANAGEMENT AND REFERRAL

Psychosocial issues may, in certain cases, hold the key to the disabled person's future function; thus, the primary care physician will want to work with the patient and family to solve some of these problems. However, the physician may benefit from input from other professionals who have expertise in evaluating and treating such issues.

For example, the clinical psychologist will be helpful in evaluating cerebral dysfunctions and the psychosocial impact of the disability on the patient and family. The psychologist's report will delineate those intellectual skills that are intact and those that are impaired, and recommendations will be given regarding management of the intellectual and psychosocial issues. Table 7–2 lists the psychological tests that may

be used in an evaluation process. The psychologist can be most helpful in planning a behavioral program for the patient and family, in conjunction with the primary care physician, aimed at returning the person to as normal a life as possible.

The psychologist or social worker can be helpful in family counseling since the disability has an impact on all family members. Sexual counseling can be accomplished most effectively by a team of the primary care physician and psychologist or social worker, if feasible. Counseling sessions should include the patient and partner.

Advice regarding financial concerns and assistance in obtaining disability benefits can be obtained from a social worker, and referral should be made soon after onset of a severe disability so that the disabled person does not feel so overwhelmed by the uncertainties of the future.

Referral to a behaviorally oriented clinical psychologist or social worker may be advisable for social skills training and assertiveness training. Organizations such as the local Easter Seal Society or independent living centers run by

TABLE 7–2. *Objective assessment of intellectual function*

Instrument	Description	Advantages
Wechsler Adult Intelligence Scale (WAIS) and WISC-R for children	Standardized measure of intelligence by age group, measures verbal and perceptual skills, recent and remote memory, general problem solving, judgment, abstract reasoning, and quality control	Results influenced by severe primary sensory or motor deficits, such as aphasia, paralysis, and blindness; identifies specific areas of strength and weakness that would influence the learning of new skills
Wechsler Memory Scale	Brief memory battery assessing personal and current information, orientation to time and place, mental control, and logical memory	Useful for periodic reassessment during crisis and recovery to determine when patient is ready for active participation in rehabilitation program
Halstead-Reitan Battery	Includes tests of verbal and nonverbal intelligence, concept formation, expressive and receptive language, auditory perception, time perception, memory, perceptual motor speed, tactile performance, spatial relations	Provides comprehensive view of intellectual and communicative deficits sustained by brain injury; helps localize suspected neoplasm or cerebral trauma
Progressive Matrices Test	Progressively more difficult matrices for assessment of nonverbal intelligence, with responses made verbally or nonverbally	Adaptable for patients with motor or language deficits; can be used to measure right hemispheric function
Strong-Campbell Interest Inventory	Measures vocational interest patterns based on norms of individuals who are satisfied with and successful in a particular field	Provides guide when disability requires change in chief occupation

disabled persons may provide social outlets initially and advice on daily problems of living with disability.

Advice regarding educational and vocational planning can be obtained from a rehabilitation counselor, usually associated with the state Department of Rehabilitation. Each state has such a department with branch offices in most cities.

Thus, there are a variety of professionals who can assist the primary care physician when any of his or her patients sustain a physical disability. The key to management in such cases is the recognition that all physical disabilities have psychosocial consequences that must be treated to ensure maximal return of physical function and satisfactory return to the world of living.

THERAPEUTIC APPROACHES

Rehabilitation is the process of learning to live with a disability in one's own environment. To help the patient accomplish this, the health care providers must know as much as possible about the person's predisability lifestyle and the resources available to him or her (family, financial, and community). All stages of the treatment plan should be formulated with the disabled person and family rather than presented to the person by the physician. Goals should be specified in concrete behavioral terms so that everyone involved will know when success has been achieved. The more the disabled person is incorporated into the goal-setting process, the greater the probability of accomplishing the goal. The decisions should actually be the disabled person's decisions based on the counsel and advice of the primary care physician.

The family of the disabled person may benefit from counseling that attempts to identify areas of stress and methods of coping with the stress. Marital counseling may help the nondisabled partner establish open communication with the disabled partner so that difficulties and conflicts can be discussed and solutions identified. Financial worry is often a critical issue between partners following a disability.

In cases of intellectual dysfunction, communication patterns may be established that circumvent the deficit. In cases of perceptual deficit, for example, give all instructions verbally. To aid the patient, write out instructions for future reference and as a memory device. When verbal skills have been impaired, give instructions through pantomime, gesture, demonstration, or drawn out on paper using pictures rather than words. Following a cerebral insult, patients will benefit from a well-planned routine that is not changed frequently. Structure and routine assist the person to anticipate the next move and will lead to less confusion. Quality control problems cannot be completely solved, but monitoring of the impaired individual by another person is the key to preventing accidents. This, however, can become a hardship for family members, and practical guidelines should be worked out through discussions between the family and physician.

The decision as to when an older disabled person requires nursing home placement is a difficult one, especially when there is a chance that the person may be able to function at home. But as a rule, a person should be allowed to try to live at home, even if alone, until the person's safety from accidents is truly at risk, because many older persons lose all will to live once placed in a nursing home.

For younger persons, educational and vocational counseling may be appropriate if the disabled person is unable to resume his or her previous vocational endeavor. In some cases,

such counseling may be appropriate for the non-disabled spouse.

Because many physical disabilities change a person's lifestyle to some degree, the disabled person should be assisted in resuming a social life. Therefore, specific training in social skills and assertiveness should be planned in order to counteract the social withdrawal that so frequently occurs.

SUGGESTED READINGS

Browne, J. A., Kirlin, B. A., and Watt, S. (1981): *Rehabilitation Services and the Social Work Role: Challenge for Change*. Williams and Wilkins, Baltimore.

Greif, E., and Matarazzo, R. G. (1982): *Behavioral Approaches to Rehabilitation: Coping with Change*. Springer Series on Rehabilitation, Vol. 3. Springer, New York.

Griffith, E., and Trieschmann, R. (1976): Sexual functioning in patients with physical disorders. In: *Clinical Management of Sexual Disorders*, edited by J. Meyer. Williams and Wilkins, Baltimore.

Krueger, D. W. (1984): *Rehabilitation Psychology: A Comprehensive Textbook*. Aspen Systems, Rockville, MD.

Marinelli, R. P., and Dell Orto, A. E., editors (1984): *The Psychological and Social Impact of Physical Disability*. Springer, New York.

Romano, M. (1976): Social skills training with the newly handicapped. *Arch. Phys. Med. Rehabil.*, 57:302–303.

Trieschmann, R. (1976): Coping with disability: A sliding scale of goals. *Arch. Phys. Med. Rehabil.*, 55:556–560.

Trieschmann, R. (1978): The role of the psychologist in the treatment of spinal cord injury. *Paraplegia*, 16:212–219.

Trieschmann, R. (1980): *Spinal Cord Injuries: The Psychological, Social, and Vocational Adjustment*. Pergamon Press, Elmsford, NY.

Medical Rehabilitation,
edited by L. S. Halstead et al.
Raven Press, New York © 1985.

CHAPTER 8

Adjustment to Disturbed Communication

Kris M. Halstead

Private Practice, Houston, Texas 77025

Confusion and disorientation, hearing loss, visual loss, aphasia, dysarthria, loss of voice, and respiratory insufficiency are among the many conditions that can interfere with communication. The most frequent cause of communication dysfunction in adults is atherosclerosis and its effects, primarily cerebrovascular accident (CVA). Other causes include hearing problems and neuromuscular disorders such as multiple sclerosis and brain injury. Disturbance at any level of the communication process—at the reception, perception, decoding, encoding, motor planning, or production level—upsets the dynamic balance of all other levels (Table 8–1). The evaluation of communication disturbance involves identifying which level of the process is disturbed then determining the specific disorder associated with that level.

RECEPTIVE DISORDER: HEARING LOSS

Evaluation

The anatomical source of the inability to receive an auditory signal can range from the outer ear structures to the peripheral nervous system. Extraneural losses, occurring outside of the nervous system, are called conductive losses, while dysfunction of the auditory nerve is a sensorineural loss. Patients with conductive loss have difficulty hearing any sound, regardless of the frequency, whereas patients with sensorineural loss have difficulty discriminating one speech sound from another, regardless of the loudness of speech. Table 8–2 lists the symptoms and tests you can perform in your office for conductive and senso-

rineural hearing losses. Once you determine, through preliminary screening, the onset, type, and severity of hearing loss, refer the patient to an audiologist. Referrals should never be made directly to a hearing aid dealer until a sufficient audiological evaluation has been done by a certified audiologist; the audiologist, not the dealer, is certified to prescribe a treatment plan.

Management

Treatments available to correct hearing impairments include surgical-medical, corrective amplification, and education. Surgery and medication are the first line of treatment for conductive hearing loss. Provide a hearing aid only if these treatments are ineffective or the patient refuses surgery.

Sensorineural hearing loss is usually untreatable by surgery or medication, unless it is due to acoustic neuroma or Menière's disease. The latter condition responds somewhat to a hearing aid, but sound will be distorted. If the patient has no residual hearing, a cochlear implant can provide electrical stimulation of the auditory nerve to enable the recognition of familiar environmental sounds, but speech will not be intelligible. Training is available, however, to aid patients with sensorineural loss in hearing discrimination. Be alert for background noise that may mask speech when talking to the person with a hearing aid, since this noise is also amplified indiscriminately. Other assistive aids include telephone adaptation devices, which convert auditory signals to a visible form, captioned television, alarm clocks that turn on room lights, and home appliances with light signals replacing auditory signals.

TABLE 8–1. *Steps in the communication process*

Process	Definition	Sample disorder
Reception	Impingement of auditory stimuli on the brain through the ear and auditory nerve, visual stimuli on the brain through the eye and optic nerve, and tactual stimuli through the skin and sensory nervous system	Hearing loss
Perception	Awareness that one has received auditory, visual, or tactual stimuli and that those stimuli differ in intensity, duration, and frequency	Auditory-verbal agnosia
Decoding	Understanding the meaning of spoken sounds, words, and multiword messages, as well as the movement symbols of gestures	Receptive aphasia
Encoding	Retrieving from memory the sounds or manual symbols needed to prepare a message	Expressive aphasia
Motor planning	Nervous system plans how the prepared message will be executed and projected into the environment	Verbal apraxia
Production	Actual projection of the message orally, graphically, or gesturally into the environment	Voice and articulation problem

If the patient did not become deaf until after learning how to speak, provide feedback to maintain good quality in voice melody, rhythm, articulation, and loudness. Speechreading—by watching lip movements and other situational and contextual cues—is also easier for adults whose hearing was once normal. Language deficits, on the average maintained at the fourth grade level among the prelingually deaf, will require special education, using visual means of instruction to overcome them.

PERCEPTION DISORDER: AUDITORY-VERBAL AGNOSIAS

Evaluation

Auditory-verbal agnosias result from the nervous system's inability to integrate, sequence, and remember phonemes, the basic units or sounds of the native language system. Patients with these perceptual disorders are unable to recognize and differentiate incoming signals that give informa-

TABLE 8–2. *Tests for hearing loss*

Dysfunction	Symptoms	Instrument	Test
Conductive hearing loss	Difficulty hearing all sounds regardless of frequency; itching, pain, burning, fullness of the ear	Tuning fork	Patient has difficulty hearing the sound through air conduction, but can hear it when the vibrating fork is placed on the mastoid bone
		Pure tone audiometer	Vary the frequency and intensity of the signals
		Impedance audiometer or tymphanometry	Electronically measures the change in a pure tone signal when there is resistance to its transmission through the middle ear
Sensorineural hearing loss	Difficulty discriminating speech sounds; omission or distortion in speech of some high frequency consonant sounds (f,s,k,t,); tinnitus	Pure tone audiometer	Discriminates the pitch and intensity of pure tone signals
		Speech audiometer	Discriminates speech sounds, words, and sentences
		Galvanic skin response	Electrodermal response to functional or nonorganic hearing problem

tion about the size, color, and shape of objects, and the pitch, loudness, and duration of sounds. Agnosias are usually seen in children, and they are associated with any number of the following behaviors:

1. The inability to pay attention, sometimes appearing as a hearing disorder.
2. Fine and gross motor coordination problems, clumsiness.
3. Left-right confusion.
4. Dyslexia, a developmental reading problem relating more to decoding than to comprehension of reading material.
5. Articulatory dyscoordination, the inability to orally sequence and produce a series of phonemes.
6. Other learning disabilities, such as inability to recognize musical or numerical concepts.
7. Hyperactivity.

Evaluation includes neurological examination for the locus, extent, and nature of the lesion, if present, and tomographic studies to determine the size of the cerebral hemispheres in relation to handedness and perceptual function. In patients with developmental perceptual deficits, the dominant hemisphere, which is normally larger than the nondominant hemisphere, tends to be smaller than the nondominant hemisphere. Diagnosis is through standardized tests. A simple office test for visual, auditory, and tactile agnosias is to ask the client to listen to, observe, or touch objects and identify them. Matching rather than naming objects is the best way to test for agnosias.

Management

Any environment that intensifies the perceptual problem must be altered, whether at home, school, or work. These situations can be identified through interviewing the client, any other physicians involved, teacher or employer, and family. In addition to medical and educational interventions, counseling of the client and family is essential.

DECODING AND ENCODING DISORDER: APHASIA

Evaluation

Aphasia, the brain's inability to process one's native language code, affects the visual and auditory systems. The language deficit may be expressive, with disturbed speaking or writing abilities, receptive, with disturbed listening or reading abilities, or global, with some deficit in all language functions. Aphasia can manifest as incorrect grammar (syntactical), stereotyped or unintelligible communication (jargon), disrupted associations between words and ideas (semantic), or the inability to process words at all (global). The type of aphasia is often associated with the locus of the lesion in the dominant hemisphere of the cerebral cortex (Table 8–3).

Evaluation includes neurological examination of the cranial nerves, motor and sensory systems, and reflexes, tests for apraxias (Table 8–4), tests for agnosias, and application of speech-language measuring instruments.

Common medical conditions that should alert you to the possibility of associated aphasia include the following:

1. Occlusion of the internal carotid artery, resulting in decreased blood supply to the dominant side of the brain.
2. Direct injury to the brain, caused by a bullet wound, surgery, or blow to the head.
3. Skull injury, producing hemorrhage, inflammation, or compression in the language area.
4. Brain disease.

By far the most common cause of aphasia is CVA affecting the left hemisphere (85%).

Prognosis for Rehabilitation

Recovery rates of speech-language abilities differ according to the cause of aphasia combined with the extent of damage to the brain. Deficits caused by cerebral hemorrhage may improve steadily over 6 months and then stabilize, whereas aphasia resulting from a thrombosis or embolism may improve rapidly for a few months but halt within 6 months. Occasionally, an old CVA with

TABLE 8–3. *Aphasia classification system*

Classification	Locus of lesion	Symptoms
Broca's, expressive anterior, nonfluent	Third frontal convolution; Broca's area	Hemiparesis, usually on right side; apraxia (inability to carry out preplanned, purposeful sequence of movements in absence of muscle weakness); telegraphic speech; agrammatic speech; client appears to comprehend
Wernicke's receptive, posterior, fluent, sensory	Left temporal lobe, Wernicke's area	Fluent speech, good prosody; articulation intact, poor auditory comprehension; speech may lack content (empty speech); use of jargon; circumlocution; inability to follow verbal directions; usually no hemiparesis
Conduction aphasia	Arcuate fasciculus (fibers that form connection between Broca's and Wernicke's areas)	Good auditory comprehension but inability to repeat what is heard
Transcortical motor aphasia	Areas anterior to Broca's area and extending into it	Same symptoms as Broca's aphasia, but with ability to repeat what is heard
Transcortical sensory aphasia	Areas surrounding Wernicke's area	Fluent, empty speech; echolalia (automatically repeats everything heard)

associated untreated aphasia is discovered in a patient who is admitted to the hospital for an unrelated medical problem. Do not automatically assume that this patient could not benefit from reevaluation and treatment of the communication problem merely because family members report no improvement in communication for months or years, or because a brief bedside examination suggests the patient is beyond the recovery phase. The patient who is suffering from disuse of speech-language abilities or lack of adequate stimulation may significantly improve when enrolled in an aggressive treatment program with massive stimulation and encouragement. Discontinue treatment only if the patient fails to respond to intensive stimulation in 2 to 4 weeks.

Recovery from aphasia associated with massive trauma or brain surgery is less predictable. Successful treatment mandates continuous adjustment within the hospital, family, or other system in which the patient is functioning.

Hospital Management Program

Stimulation of communication ability should be introduced at the beginning of the patient's recovery period and scheduled once or twice daily for the first few months. Withholding sensory input because the patient is unable to complain about discomfort or understand instructions will only encourage the patient to withdraw and become apathetic to future rehabilitation attempts. Some

TABLE 8–4. *Simple clinical tests for apraxis*

Type of apraxia	Test
Buccofacial	Ask patient to perform sequenced movements of tongue, lips, jaws (la-la-la, ma-ma-ma) Ask patient to blow, whistle, and suck
Limb	Ask patient to wave goodbye, pantomime use of telephone, snap fingers Check left and right limbs
Ideational	Ask patient to tie shoe

patients will become irritable, angry, and depressed when unable to answer questions they understand. Avoid talking to such patients as though they have no faculties, allow extra time for them to make choices and decisions, and do not give sudden, rapid instructions or requests. Consistency in using the same wording each time you give an instruction or ask a question will also facilitate comprehension, as will telling the patient you are changing tasks before giving new instructions, thereby discouraging a previous response to the new subject. Since the patient may be unable to screen out small movements and sounds that are unrelated to the task at hand, try to reduce or eliminate all distractions during the communication period. Help the patient find the right word when necessary. In response to unintelligible speech, nod or make neutral statements, watching the patient's gestures for clues about his or her topic, then shift the conversation to the topic of your choice. Frequent standardized tests of speech, writing, or gesture ability will help quantify the extent of improvement from one session to the next. When addressing the patient, simplify your speech when needed, but do not markedly change your usual speaking habits or raise the pitch and loudness of your voice.

Telling the patients not to worry about their communication problems without providing an explanation of what they are experiencing will only raise their anxiety level. Explaining the problem and appearing relaxed and unhurried throughout the training sessions will help reduce anxiety and tension.

Home Management Program

After aphasic patients have been discharged into the care of their families, they may appear to relapse and become more impaired. This is the result of replacing the consistent hospital schedule they have memorized with a relatively unstructured situation. The family needs to provide the patients with new activities and consistent verbal instructions. The patients' progress may be further impaired by well-meaning relatives, who anticipate their needs and speak to them less often so response is unnecessary, or speak for them

when there are visitors. Thus, the patients are discouraged from improving through practice. Others may overwhelm the patients with too many, too difficult, or irrelevant speaking tasks. These patients become too frustrated to improve. Instruct the family to guard against overprotecting the patients and excluding them from family activities and conversations.

A family member may initiate daily structured lessons in speech, writing, reading, and listening. To avoid overfatiguing the patient, he or she should not be asked to apply the lessons throughout the day; instead, rest periods should be allowed between lessons. Improvement from lessons will be the most dramatic in the first 2 or 3 months, then become less obvious.

The daily lessons should have a consistent format and begin with easy tasks at which the patient can succeed. Then review the material covered in the previous lesson and introduce new material related to the patient's needs and interests. Do not proceed to new material until the patient has mastered all previous material. The instructor should present a relaxed and friendly attitude, using humor whenever appropriate and commenting on successful attempts rather than errors. The family member should stop before the patient becomes too tired and tell him or her what time the next lesson will be presented.

In summary, both the hospital and home programs should embody the following principles of management:

1. Speak slowly and distinctly in a normal voice.
2. Use short, simple phrases to compensate for reduced memory span.
3. Ask direct questions that can be answered with a simple yes or no.
4. Give one instruction at a time, and wait for a response before continuing.
5. Repeat questions and instructions, rephrasing to clarify meaning.
6. Supplement speech with gestures and demonstrations if the patient does not seem to understand.
7. Stand in good light and make sure the patient can see your face to enable lip reading.

8. Give instructions to hemiplegic patients from the nonaffected side.
9. Write and draw pictures when speech is not effective.
10. Allow plenty of time for the patient to respond, encouraging nodding, pointing, and pantomime if these improve the patient's response.

SPEECH PRODUCTION DISORDERS

Evaluation

Disorders of speech production may involve phonation—vocal pitch, intensity, and vocal qualities such as hoarseness; or resonation and articulation. Phonatory dysfunction is the inability of the facial skeletal bones, tongue, teeth, palate, nasal bones, or lips to modify sound into intelligible speech.

Evaluation of phonatory dysfunction considers symptoms in vocal intensity, pitch, and quality. Intensity may be too loud or too soft, loudness may trail off or be inappropriate due to an inability to monitor loudness. A patient may have a very limited pitch range, be unable to monitor pitch, or consistently use a pitch that is uncomfortably high or low. Voice quality may be breathy, harsh and scratchy, too nasal or too dense, or continuously hoarse. Phonatory disorders can result from vocal abuse, cord thickening, nodules, polyps or papillomas, endocrine changes, contact ulcers, tension of the tongue, pharynx, and oral cavity, or improper use of the respiratory mechanism. Voice evaluation includes indirect laryngoscopy and a careful history of the onset and duration of the disorder, as well as the patient's general health and voice habits.

Symptoms of the most common articulatory disorders include:

1. "Baby talk," "sloppy speech," "lisps," and "mumbling."
2. Misarticulation of a specific phoneme, as when a child substitutes w for r.
3. Muscle weakness, or dysarthria, which results in a slurring of all speech sounds and difficulty with swallowing, chewing, and whistling.

The articulation disorder seen most frequently in rehabilitation centers is dysarthria, muscle weakness resulting in a slurring of all speech accompanied by difficulty swallowing and chewing. Common causes of dysarthria are stroke, cerebral palsy, mental retardation, and head injury.

Management

Treatment of articulatory disorders involves muscle strengthening and control exercises necessary for the production of single sounds, then single words, phrases, and finally, functional speech for communication of daily needs. Patients can compensate for muscle weakness by speaking more carefully and deliberately to give slow-moving muscles time to reach the correct positions for production of intelligible words. Schedule short training sessions daily, preferably in the morning before fatigue sets in. Patients whose articulation remains poor despite training can use gestures to supplement speech. Patients may be fitted with palatal lifts to reduce hypernasality, use an alphabet board, or use communication augmentation systems, such as the Canon communicator (Fig. 8–1), in cases of severe dysfunction. The athetoid patient, for example, may be able to type using a stick attached to a headband, or use head motions to activate an alarm or call light.

COMMUNICATION AIDS

Contact the telephone company for recommended equipment, such as a phone amplifier, to accommodate the patient's disability. A dialing stick or the eraser end of a pencil can facilitate dialing. In writing, felt tip pens that are built up to keep the fingers from sliding down the pen can compensate for inadequate strength. Typewriters with key guards are indicated for severe disability and incoordination. Book holders, rubber bands placed lengthwise to keep pages flat, and rubber finger caps for turning pages will facilitate reading. The expense of electric page turners, however, makes them impractical except for severely

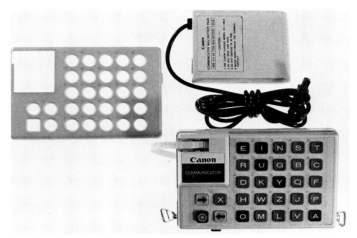

FIG. 8–1. Canon communicator, a small portable tape typewriter, provides displacement keys that are directly selected by the user and a strip printer that produces permanent visual output. [From Beukelman, D. R., and Yorkston, K. M. (1982): Speech and language disorders. In: *Krusen's Handbook of Physical Medicine and Rehabilitation*, edited by F. J. Kottke, G. K. Stillwell, and J. F. Lehmann. W. B. Saunders, Philadelphia.]

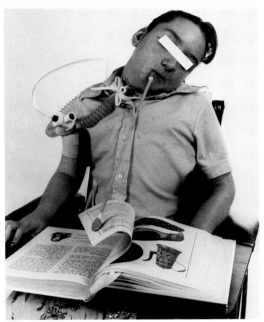

FIG. 8–2. Patient uses mouth stick to turn pages of book.

disabled patients who must wield a stick held between the teeth (Fig. 8–2) in lieu of all upper body motion.

SUGGESTED READINGS

Chase, J. B. (1977): Techniques to facilitate communication. In: *Basic Rehabilitation Techniques: A Self-Instructional Guide*, edited by R. D. Sine, S. E. Liss, R. E. Roush, and J. D. Holcomb. Aspen Systems, Germantown, MD.

Darley, F. L., editor (1979): *Evaluation of Appraisal Techniques in Speech and Language Pathology*. Addison-Wesley, Reading, MA.

Hintgen, T. L., and Mueller, P. B. (1983): *Communicating with Aphasic Adults: A Guide for Families and Caregivers*. Charles C Thomas, Springfield, IL.

Holland, A., editor (1984): *Language Disorders in Adults: Recent Advances*. College-Hill Press, San Diego.

Jerger, J. (1984): *Hearing Disorders in Adults*. College-Hill Press, San Diego.

Mohr, J. P. (1981): The evaluation of aphasia. *Curr. Concepts Cerebrovasc. Dis. Stroke*, 16:29–32.

Musselwhite, C. R. (1982): *Communication Programming for the Severely Handicapped: Vocal and Nonvocal Strategies*. College-Hill Press, Houston.

Peterson, H. A., and Marquardt, T. P. (1981): *Appraisal and Diagnosis of Speech and Language Disorders*. Prentice-Hall, Englewood Cliffs, NJ.

Porch, B. E. (1976): Communication. In: *Rehabilitation: A Manual for the Care of the Disabled and Elderly*, 2nd edit., edited by G. G. Hirschberg, L. Lewis, and P. Vaughan. J. B. Lippincott, Philadelphia.

Rieber, R. W., editor (1981): *Communication Disorders*. Plenum Press, New York.

Sarno, M. T. (1981): *Acquired Aphasia*. Academic Press, New York.

Shames, G. H., and Wiig, E. H. (1982): *Human Communication Disorders: An Introduction*. Merrill, Columbus, OH.

Medical Rehabilitation,
edited by L. S. Halstead et al.
Raven Press, New York © 1985.

CHAPTER 9

Musculoskeletal Pain

Ralph M. Mancini

Rosewood Rehabilitation Center, and Department of Physical Medicine, Baylor College of Medicine, Houston, Texas 77030

DISTINGUISHING MUSCULOSKELETAL PAIN FROM VISCERAL PAIN

Pain in its myriad forms is by far the most common complaint of patients to physicians. In evaluating these complaints, the physician must consider the vast array of painful stimuli, including visceral sources, that could cause pain in a particular area, as well as the functional anatomy and kinesiology of the region involved. Musculoskeletal pain most commonly originates in the low back, neck, or shoulder, but may radiate to adjacent areas such as a leg or arm. The history should provide answers to several questions concerning the nature of the complaint:

1. Is the pain elicited by motion or other stress of a structure either remote or proximal to the area in which pain is perceived?
2. Is there a history of symmetry or bilaterality that could suggest a systemic or otherwise diffuse process?
3. Are the symptoms produced only by activities of certain body parts or by any exertion?

Answering these questions may help determine whether the problem is visceral or musculoskeletal in origin.

The physical examination begins when the patient first walks into the office, when he or she is less aware of being examined, and ease of movement, smoothness of gait, and facial expression are readily observed. Active and passive motion of the potentially defective body part and palpation of soft tissue and bony struc-

tures are as important as a thorough neurological examination. Using this approach to differentiate musculoskeletal pain syndromes from other more serious disorders can avoid delay in making an accurate diagnosis.

In some cases, diagnosis can be confirmed only by ruling out more serious conditions. X-rays, electromyography, nerve conduction studies, myelography, CT scan, bone scan, blood chemistry, and other appropriate laboratory tests may then be important sources of differential diagnosis.

KEY ANATOMY AND BIOMECHANICS OF THE SPINE AND THE SHOULDER

The spine is composed of superincumbent functional units supported in equilibrium on the sacral base. A functional unit consists of any two neighboring vertebrae and their connections. The vertebral column contains seven cervical vertebrae, 12 thoracic vertebrae, five lumbar vertebrae, the sacrum, and the coccyx. Holding the upright position is possible with minimal muscular effort only because the line of the center of gravity falls through the major weight-bearing joints, which are the first thoracic, twelfth thoracic, and fifth lumbar vertebrae, in front of the knees, and through the hip joints.

With reinforcement by ligaments, the functional units of the vertebral column enable erect posture and the various movements needed to perform daily activities. In the abnormal state, they produce pain and disability. Tissues that can cause localized or radiating pain if they are irritated, injured, or inflamed include the posterior longitudinal ligament, the outer layers of the annulus fibrosis, the spinal nerve passing through the intervertebral foramen, the posterior synovial joints and capsules, the interspinous ligaments, and the back muscles (Fig. 9–1). The vertebral body and ligamenta flava, however, are not pain sensitive. The components of each individual functional unit—enabling weight bearing, protection of neural tissues, movement or inhibition of movement, and muscular attachment—are shown in Figs. 9–2 and 9–3.

Lumbosacral Vulnerability

The lumbosacral spine is more susceptible to injury and instability than the cervical spine. The anatomical differences that account for this increased vulnerability include the orientation of the facet joint planes, the architecture of the longitudinal ligaments, and the much greater leverage forces encountered in the lumbosacral region.

The facet joints between L1 and L5 permit flexion and extension but only minimal rotation and side bending. Normal, relative alignment between superior and inferior facets enables pain-free, unobstructed motion. The posterior longitudinal ligament is narrower than in the upper spinal regions but more centrally located, leaving the posterolateral arcs of the intervertebral disks without protective reinforcement (Fig. 9–4). Lateral disk herniations, therefore, are much more prevalent in the lumbosacral region.

The usual lumbar lordosis that develops in early childhood enables erect stance. However, it in turn allows gravity to impose shear forces along the inclined planes of the vertebral bodies,

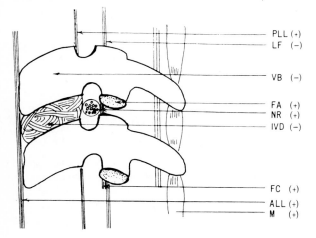

PLL (+)
LF (−)

VB (−)

FA (+)
NR (+)
IVD (−)

FC (+)
ALL (+)
M (+)

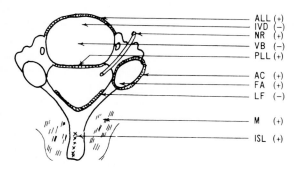

ALL (+)
IVD (−)
NR (+)
VB (−)
PLL (+)

AC (+)
FA (+)
LF (−)

M (+)

ISL (+)

FIG. 9–1. Tissue sites of pain production. PLL, Posterior longitudinal ligament. LF, Ligamentum flavum. VB, Vertebral body. FA, Facet articulation. NR, Nerve root. IVD, Intervertebral disk. FC, Facet capsule. ALL, Anterior longitudinal ligament. M, Muscle. ISL, Interspinous ligament. +, Pain sensitive. −, Not pain sensitive. [From Cailliet, R. (1981): *Neck and Arm Pain*, 2nd edit. F. A. Davis, Philadelphia.]

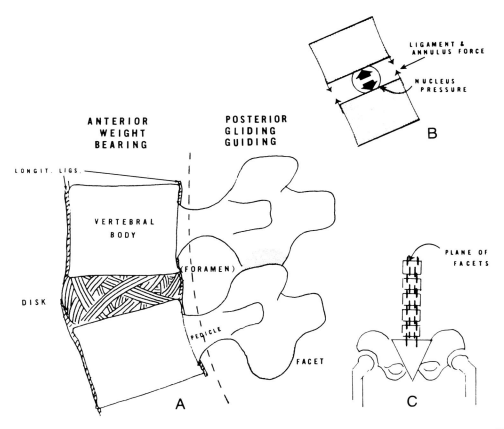

FIG. 9–2. Functional unit. The anterior weight-bearing portion consists of two adjacent vertebrae separated by the disk. This portion is reinforced by longitudinal ligaments. The posterior portion contains the facets, or articulations that oppose each other in the sagittal plane. The spinal nerves emerge through the foramina. The intradiskal pressure within the nucleus separates the vertebrae. The annulus and longitudinal ligaments oppose this pressure. [From Cailliet, R. (1981): *Low Back Pain Syndrome*, 3rd edit. F. A. Davis, Philadelphia.]

particularly at L4–L5 and L5–S1. The only junction where these shear forces have good bony opposition is at L5–S1. During everyday activities, even without lifting heavy objects, leverage forces averaging several hundred pounds per square inch are commonplace. Intervertebral foramina are somewhat larger here than in the cervical region except at L5–S1. Since the spinal cord ends approximately at the L2–L3 junction, the nerves that exit in the lumbar and sacral region originate above. Consequently, there is less opportunity for selective irritation of sensory, as compared to motor, components.

The greatest motion in flexion and extension takes place at levels L4–L5 and L5–S1. Con-

sidering that these levels also bear the greatest shear forces, it is no wonder that these are the most common areas of derangement. During full flexion, stress is placed on the posterior longitudinal ligament, as well as on those ligaments bridging the posterior arches. In hyperextension, there is less ligamentous stress, but impaction of facet joints is a potential problem.

Supportive abdominal and spinal musculature is crucial for reducing some of the leverage forces borne by the skeletal structures. The abdominal cavity directly anterior to the spinal column is potentially a semirigid, semihydraulic cylinder that can buttress stresses on the spinal column. The oblique and transverse muscles of the ab-

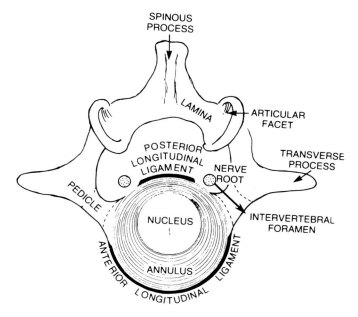

FIG. 9–3. Lumbar vertebral functional unit viewed from above, dorsal view. [From Cailliet, R. (1981): *Low Back Pain Syndrome*, 3rd edit. F. A. Davis, Philadelphia.]

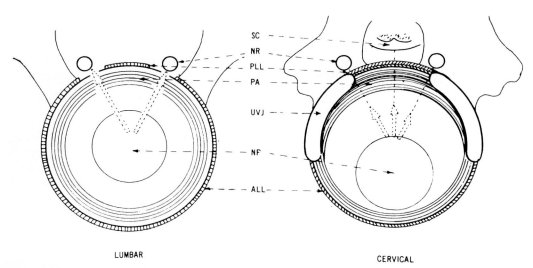

LUMBAR   CERVICAL

FIG. 9–4. Comparison of lumbar and cervical disk containers. The lumbar region has an incomplete posterior longitudinal ligament (PLL), a thin layer posterior to the annulus fibrosus (PA), and thus a relatively exposed nerve root (NR). Arrows show the routes by which herniation of the nucleus can approach the nerve roots. The nucleus pulposus (NP) is centrally located. In the cervical region, a posterior longitudinal ligament (PLL) spans the entire posterior portion of the vertebral body, a double-layered ligament. The posterior portion of the annulus (PA) is broader and firmer. The nerve root (NR) is partially protected by the interposed uncovertebral joints of von Luschka (UVJ), and the anterior position of the nucleus (NP) places it far from the nerve roots and the spinal cord. All these factors protect the nerve roots and the spinal cord (SC) from the protruding disk material. [From Cailliet, R. (1981): *Neck and Arm Pain*, 2nd edit. F. A. Davis, Philadelphia.]

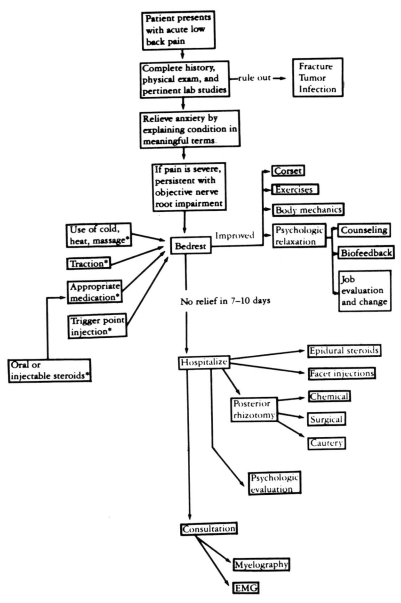

FIG. 9–9. Decision steps in evaluating and treating the patient who presents with acute low back pain. [From Cailliet, R. (1977): *Soft Tissue Pain and Disability.* F. A. Davis, Philadelphia.]

some helpful guidelines for instructing your patients in preventing exacerbations of lumbosacral injury:

1. Never bend from the waist only; bend the hips and knees.

2. Never lift a heavy object higher than your waist.

3. Always turn and face the object you wish to lift.

4. Avoid carrying unbalanced loads; hold heavy objects close to your body.

TABLE 9-3. *Evaluation and treatment of cervical injuries*

Type of injury	Description and causes	Findings, history, and physical examination	Findings, X-ray, and laboratory tests	Treatment
Cervical sprain, acceleration-deceleration injury ("whiplash" syndrome)	Partial disruption or tear of soft tissue, resulting in weakening, edema or microhemorrhage and inflammation; may be transient subluxation of spine; caused by exceeding normal limits of distensibility or tensile strength; abrupt, unanticipated passive movement or action of muscles against overpowering, sudden resistance; symptoms worsen 24–48 hr after injury; cervical subluxation may involve spinal cord or nerve roots	Upper or lower motor neuron findings in severe cases; pain may extend distal to shoulders down upper extremities and to interscapular region and back of head; dizziness, nausea, blurred vision; asymmetry in texture and coolness of skin in upper extremities, sometimes with Horner's syndrome	On X-ray, change in cervical lordosis, enhanced soft tissue shadows suggesting edema or hemorrhage, usually retropharyngeal; spondylosis; segmental subluxation different from fracture or ligamentous rupture; EMG—radiculopathy or anterior horn cell injury; long wave studies confirm root injury	If spine is stable, intermittent cervical traction, to tolerance or up to 35 lb; soft or rigid cervical collar worn longer than for strain; nonsteroidal anti-inflammatory agents; short course of steroids
Cervical nerve root compression syndrome	Injury to specialized components of nerve root, its covering, or related structures, beginning from where dorsal or ventral rootlets leave spinal cord or recesses of neural foramina; caused by traction, compression, or contusion of cervical nerve root; herniated nucleus pulposus, spondylosis secondary to	Pain usually originates in neck, but may radiate inferiorly to interscapular region, shoulder, variable distances into upper extremity, occipital region of head; flexion or extension aggravates symptoms; hypesthesia or dysesthesia; segmental reflex changes; segmental muscle weakness on shoulder abduction, elbow	On X-ray, disk space narrowing and foraminal encroachment; excessive motion between any two segments indicating level of involvement; myelography for potential surgery; EMG—diagnostic when few physical findings, may show reduced motor unit recruitment, increased polyphasic activity, or	Same as for whiplash with radiculopathy; also pillow of sufficient height to maintain alignment of neck with rest of spine; discourage sleeping on stomach; muscle relaxers for patient with spasm or induration; avoid positioning neck in any unnatural position

	Etiology	Clinical features	Laboratory findings	Treatment
	degenerative disk disease, nerve root or brachial plexus traction injury, fracture or dislocation, subluxation, neoplastic disorders	flexion and extension, forearm pronation, wrist extension, grip strength, abduction of fingers, and thumb apposition; asymmetry of reflexes at biceps, triceps, and brachioradialis	evidence of ongoing denervation	
Cervical strain	Prolonged, extreme positioning in any direction; awkward sleeping position; abrupt change of direction; minor trauma; predisposing factors of prolonged disuse, general fatigue, cervical spondylosis and reduction of free motion	Pain on lateral rotation, extension, or flexion, with flexion the most uncomfortable; pain pattern contralateral with lateral bending and to side of rotation; tenderness on palpation; negative Sperling maneuver	Often noncontributory; may be normal or show spondylosis of any degree; may show loss of cervical lordosis; normal EMG	Support with soft or semirigid collar 48–60 hr; hot moist heat with hydrocollator packs; ultrasound; deep or sedative massage; in subacute stage, exercise to regain normal excursion and distensibility of ligaments and muscles; spray-stretch technique using fluoromethane; rhythmic stabilization exercises; routine schedule of nonsteroidal anti-inflammatory drugs; narcotics 1–2 weeks only; muscle relaxers; supervise patient's activities; avoid heavy labor
Tension myalgia	Somatic response to stress, exacerbated by poor posture; prolonged muscle contraction increases intramuscular pressure, interfering with nutrient supply and export of metabolites; insertion of muscle on periosteum	Depression; poor posture with increased cervical lordosis and round shoulders; compulsive personality with perfectionistic tendencies; state chronic anxiety with tendency to somatize; pain does not radiate to upper extremities	Same as for cervical strain	Postural exercises; relaxation training by instructional tape recordings or biofeedback; nonaddictive pain medications; minor tranquilizers; antidepressants; psychiatric counseling for difficult cases

5. Never carry anything heavier than you can manage with ease.
6. If physically unconditioned, do not lift or move heavy furniture; allow someone who knows the principles of leverage to do it.
7. Avoid sudden movements, sudden overloading of muscles; practice moving deliberately, swinging the legs from the hips.
8. Keep the head in line with the spine when standing, sitting, or lying in bed.
9. Avoid sitting on soft chairs and deep couches; during prolonged sitting, cross your legs to rest your back.
10. Wear shoes with moderate heels, all about the same height; avoid changing from low to high heels.
11. Get a rocking chair; rocking rests the back by changing the muscle groups used.
12. Use your abdominal muscles to flatten your lower abdomen.

NECK PAIN

Cervical injury is the second most common cause of musculoskeletal pain. The great flexibility and range of movement of the cervical spine and adjacent soft tissues increase the susceptibility of this functional unit to considerable stress and strain. Less absolute force is required for cervical injury than for thoracic and lumbar injury, since cervical structures are less stable and less well protected. Pain may arise primarily from soft tissue, nerve compression, or skeletal derangement. Table 9–3 describes the evaluation and treatment of cervical strain, tension myalgia, cervical sprain "whiplash" syndrome, and cervical nerve root compression syndrome.

Pathogenesis of Cervical Nerve Root Compression

As in lumbosacral nerve root compression, the two most common causes of cervical nerve root compression are herniated nucleus pulposus and degenerative disk disease with spondylosis. When the central nucleus pulposus of the intervertebral disk loses flexibility, undergoes hyaline degeneration, and shrinks in volume, the disk space narrows, and the annulus bulges and

tears. As a result, nuclear material is more likely to protrude with abrupt force. The bulging annulus may also dissect or cause avulsion of the posterior longitudinal ligament and periosteum from the underlying vertebral body. New bone forms in the space created by the bulging disk and in the adjacent vertebral margin, eventually reducing mobility and degenerating the articular cartilage. Consequently, the joint capsules and ligaments hypertrophy, making the neck more susceptible to injury.

Differential Diagnosis

When injury is limited to cervical soft tissue, signs of fracture, dislocation, and nerve root entrapment are absent. In some instances of cervical nerve root compression syndrome, usually C6 or C7 irritation, the pain may involve the anterolateral portion of the chest and can be confused with coronary insufficiency. This syndrome may be primarily motor in one case and sensory in another because, in contrast to nerve roots in the caudal regions, nerve roots in the cervical region are formed from a combination of dorsal and ventral rootlets at or near the site of exit from the spinal column. In some patients, the pain is dull and vague, not dermatomal, and is accompanied by muscle weakness, while in other patients, sensory aberrations fit a dermatomal pattern and are accompanied by little or no muscle weakness.

Both soft tissue and nerve root injuries can produce pain on either extension or flexion, but flexion tends to be more uncomfortable. Pain tends to radiate into the upper extremities in both cervical sprain and nerve root compression, but rarely in strain or tension myalgia. Movement is more restricted in sprain than in other cervical injuries.

Treatment

The treatment of soft tissue cervical injuries should emphasize physical modalities, medications, and close supervision of daily activities. Goals are to avoid additional injury and the complications of disuse, minimize inflammation, and reduce pain. In addition, correct faulty posture,

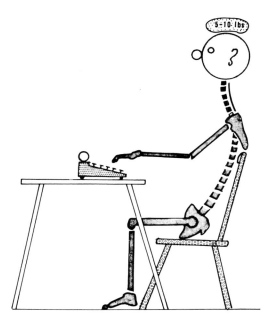

FIG. 9–10. Distraction exercise for posture training. Sandbag weighing 5 to 10 lb placed on head maintains erect posture and minimizes cervical lordosis. Proprioceptive concept of posture learned with no effort. [From Cailliet, R. (1981): *Neck and Arm Pain*, 2nd edit. F. A. Davis, Philadelphia.]

teach relaxation techniques, and identify aspects of the personality or environment that aggravate tension myalgia.

Useful physical modalities include superficial and deep heating, massage, active exercise, and a soft or semirigid cervical collar. A therapeutic level of aspirin, ibuprophen, sulindac, tolmetin, indomethacin, naproxen, oxyphenbutazone, or phenylbutazone should be maintained for best results. Excessive sedation should be avoided because reducing distracting stimuli may draw attention to the pain. Bed rest should be kept to a minimum to prevent adoption of the "sick role."

Distraction exercise is particularly effective for instilling a proprioceptive concept of proper posture (Fig. 9–10). Intermittent cervical traction, the mainstay of treatment for cervical sprain, may also help relieve cervical strain. Effective and ineffective cervical traction for home use are shown in Fig. 9–11. These and other treatments are applied to the primary types of cervical injury listed in Table 9–3.

THORACIC OUTLET SYNDROME

Pathogenesis

The group of conditions known as thoracic outlet or cervical dorsal outlet syndrome involve mechanical compression of extradural cervical roots along their course as they combine to form the brachial plexus. En route this bundle of nerves passes behind, in front of, or through certain anatomical structures that are potential points of compression [accompanied by the subclavian (and later, brachial) artery] (Fig. 9–5). Symptoms are related to the combined neurovascular compromise.

Differential Diagnosis

Cervical rib, anterior scalene, costoclavicular, and pectoralis minor syndromes should be considered as possible diagnoses whenever there is upper extremity pain and neurovascular compromise is suspected. Patients present with various qualities of pain, dysesthesia, and hyperesthesia of the upper extremity. Notably lacking is neck pain, which so often accompanies cervical radiculopathy and cervical strain. Occurrence of the syndrome is relatively rare when compared with that of cervical radiculopathy or entrapment neuropathy distally in the upper extremity.

Evaluation and Treatment

The evaluation and treatment of common thoracic outlet syndromes are outlined in Table 9–4. In general, the neurological examination may be negative because the vascular component of these syndromes may supersede neurological involvement. Neurological compromise may be transient enough to resist detection by electromyography. Although nerve conduction studies are often negative, they can demonstrate proximal slowing across the thoracic outlet, particularly when stimulation is proximal to all of the potentially offending structures such as percutaneous stimulation of C8 that exits the spine.

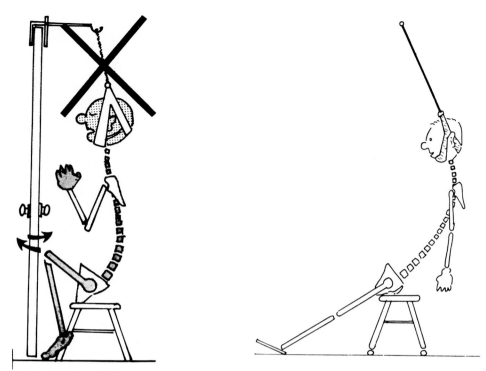

FIG. 9–11. Ineffective vs. effective cervical traction for home use. **Left:** Ineffective door traction. Patient is too close to door to get correct neck flexion angle. Door freely opens and closes, not permitting constant traction. Patient cannot extend legs or assume comfortable position. **Right:** Effective overhead traction. With rope securely fastened overhead and slightly in front of seated patient, traction is applied on flexed neck. Patient should be seated in fully relaxed position with low back flexed, legs extended, and arms dangling at side. This position enables maximum relaxation. [From Cailliet, R. (1981): *Neck and Arm Pain*, 2nd edit. F. A. Davis, Philadelphia.]

Noninvasive treatment is directed toward alleviating the faulty biomechanics and improving posture. Surgical treatment is indicated only after medical management has failed; the results of surgery have been disappointing.

SHOULDER PAIN

Differential Diagnosis

Since shoulder pain may be referred from the cervical spine, or reflect any of several shoulder conditions (Table 9–5), differential diagnosis may be difficult. Understanding the functional anatomy and biomechanics of the shoulder discussed earlier in this chapter will help differentiate pain caused by shoulder impairment from disorders actually arising in the cervical region. Early,

accurate diagnosis and treatment are crucial for preventing further disuse leading to functional disability. The end result is the total loss of shoulder motion characterized by adhesive capsulitis.

During the physical examination, palpable "trigger points" for pain reveal the site of the disorder, corroborate the history, and indicate what types of therapy will alleviate the condition (Fig. 9–12). Tenderness in the deltoid bursa may be difficult to distinguish from tenderness at the supraspinatus insertion, but soft tissue compression may reveal that the pain is originating superficially at the tendon insertion. Careful attention to local tenderness discourages the common practice of concluding that any patient who complains of shoulder pain has bursitis. This term tends to be overused, yet bursitis is rare compared to biceps tendonitis and supraspinatus tendonitis; the latter is the most

TABLE 9–4. *Evaluation and treatment of thoracic outlet syndrome*

Syndrome	Causes	Evaluation	Treatment
Cervical rib	Extradural complex of cervical roots is elevated and stretched by cervical rib, without affecting subclavian artery	Neurological symptoms but usually no vascular symptoms; X-ray shows cervical ribs that may look like spondylosis; differentiate from radiculopathy; possible vascular signs are arm and hand pain or numbness	Alleviate faulty biomechanics and improve posture; exercises to strengthen shoulder girdle muscles, particularly elevators such as trapezii and levator scapulae; surgical resection of cervical rib if noninvasive methods are ineffective
Anterior scalene	Compression of neurovascular bundle between anterior scalene muscle and first rib	Reproduce neurological symptoms by having patient rotate head toward symptomatic side for prolonged period, providing some downward traction to shoulder and palpating radial pulse for weakening; venography or angiography	Exercise to improve flexibility of cervical spine, stretch scalene muscles, and reduce round-shouldered posture and cervical lordosis; myotomy of scalene muscle if all else fails
Costoclavicular	Compromise of neurovascular bundle as it passes behind clavicle anterior to first rib	Exaggerated shoulder depression that brings clavicle closer to first rib; venography or angiography	Same as for cervical rib but no surgery
Pectoralis minor	Compression of neurovascular bundle between upper anterolateral rib cage and overlying pectoralis minor muscle; occurs when hyperabduction of humerus stretches pectoralis muscle	Venography or angiography; confirmation by electromyography	Exercise to stretch pectoral muscles, improve slumped or round-shouldered posture; avoid activities that require excessive abduction of shoulders

common cause of disabling shoulder pain. If left untreated, tendonitis may calcify and lead eventually to bursitis, a process shown in Fig. 9–13.

Also determine exactly what movements intensify pain. A simple way to distinguish biceps tendonitis from supraspinatus tendonitis is to ask the patient to reach into the back pocket for a wallet; extension of the shoulder will be the most painful position if tendonitis is in the biceps. Then palpate anteriorly over the proximal humerus for the biceps tendon. Tenderness should be localized in this area. The pronounced distal bulging of the biceps muscle clearly distinguishes rupture of the biceps tendon from biceps tendonitis.

A rotator cuff tear is readily detected if it is complete because the patient will be unable to initiate shoulder abduction. A partial tear, however, may be indistinguishable from uncomplicated tendonitis. In this case, confirmation is by shoulder arthrogram.

Scapulocostal syndrome is often confused with cervical root irritation or cervical strain. The patient with scapulocostal syndrome, unlike cervical nerve root compression, will have no sensory, reflex, or motor abnormalities.

Treatment

The chief goals of treating shoulder disorders are to:

1. Reduce inflammation.

TABLE 9–5. *Evaluation and treatment of shoulder pain*

Type of injury	Description and causes	Findings, history, and physical examination	Findings, X-ray, and laboratory tests	Treatment
Supraspinatus tendonitis	Most common cause of disabling shoulder pain; chronic mechanical irritation, with impingement of supraspinatus tendon on overlying coracoacromial ligament, aggravated by round-shouldered posture; sequence of inflammation and engorgement of supraspinatus tendon followed by calcium deposition	Pain poorly localized in lateral upper arm, deep to deltoid muscle, extending halfway down arm to point of deltoid insertion; pain worst at 80–90° abduction; sleeping on involved side increases symptoms, but minimal pain at rest; focal tenderness over greater tuberosity of humerus; may be decreased ROM, usually external rotation lost first; strength of abduction and flexion reduced secondary to pain; normal neurological examination	X-ray of shoulder negative unless progressed to calcification of supraspinatus tendon, then oval island of calcification 2 cm proximal to greater tuberosity; blood chemistry only to rule out systemic rheumatoid disorders	Nonsteroidal anti-inflammatory drugs; ultrasound; superficial heat; active assistive ROM; avoid resistive exercise; pendular exercises; use of pulley mechanism; exercises to improve faulty posture; injection of local anesthetic and 20–30 mg prednisone (or equivalent) along cuff insertion on humerus; avoid injection directly into tendon; control patient's activities
Biceps tendonitis	Inflammation of tendon of long head of biceps	Pain deep to anterior and mid-deltoid muscles, may radiate halfway down upper arm; painful extension of shoulder, abduction, and flexion; tenderness well-localized over biceps tendon when palpated anteriorly over proximal humerus; negative neurological examination	X-ray findings usually negative, but shoulder in internal and external rotation may show soft tissue island of calcification in constant relationship to humerus	Same as for supraspinatus tendonitis; accelerate resolution with local infiltration of local anesthetic and steroid overlying biceps tendon in bicipital groove
Bursitis	Inflammation of subdeltoid bursa; usually secondary to rupture of supraspinatus tendon, when inflammatory debris from tendon enter subdeltoid bursa	Pain aggravated by shoulder movement; tenderness with pressure over deltoid bursa	X-ray may show supraspinatus tendonitis accompanied by enhanced soft tissue shadow at site of bursa; reserve shoulder arthrogram for cases that do	Avoid deep heat, which exacerbates symptoms; use superficial heat; active assistive ROM; inject local anesthetic and steroid into bursa; nonsteroidal anti-

		not respond to conservative measures, dye may be transmitted into subdeltoid bursa	inflammatory drugs
Adhesive capsulitis (frozen shoulder)	Syndrome resulting from any disorder that refers pain to shoulder; caused also by visceral referred pain, reflex sympathetic dystrophy, cervical radiculopathy, brachial plexopathy; muscle spasm leads to immobilization, vasospasm, tissue hypoxia, and edema, which promote fibrosis of soft tissue	Chief complaint pain; loss of motion insidious; intact scapular abduction to compensate for reduced glenohumeral motion; atrophy of spinalis muscles; winging of scapula	X-ray to discover underlying cause; arthrogram in resistant cases	Treat cause; hot packs and ultrasound before active assistive ROM with terminal stretching; home program of wand and pulley exercises; inject steroid into synovial cavity if synovium is not adherent; oral anti-inflammatory drugs; manipulation under anesthesia for resistant cases
Rotator cuff tear	Relatively normal tendon cuff torn by sudden, abrupt forces that may also dislocate shoulder; when inflamed, weak cuff tendons are easily sprained or ruptured by normal forces	Severe shoulder pain; very limited or absent voluntary abduction; sudden onset	Shoulder arthrogram showing escape of dye from glenohumeral synovial cavity into subdeltoid bursa	Depends on severity of injury and age of patient; splint shoulder in abduction and external rotation, immobilize with sling and repair surgically, and limit activities; give anti-inflammatants
Rupture of biceps tendon	Rupture of tendon of long head more common than short head; caused by weak and inflamed tendon or sudden overpowering demand on tendon	Sudden onset of pain in upper arm; weak elbow flexion; accentuated distal bulging of muscle belly compared with opposite extremity; old injury may be found incidentally on examination	None needed	Surgical tenodesis if major disability or cosmetically unacceptable
Scapulocostal syndrome	Painful condition of posterior shoulder region near vertebral border of scapula; caused by chronic strain of levator scapulae muscle; may be secondary to chronic physical or emotional stress and poor posture	Lack of sensory, reflex, or motor findings in upper extremity examination; predictable location of pain and tenderness near insertion of levator scapulae muscle on superior angle of scapula		Ultrasound, short-wave, or microwave diathermy heating of muscle belly and attachment; superficial counterirritant heating; massage and application of fluoromethane spray to help overcome muscle spasm and promote relaxation

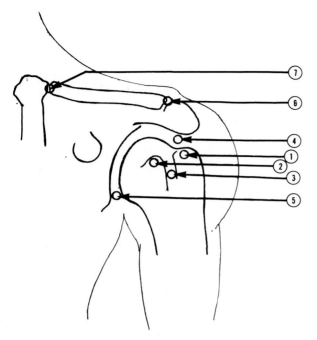

FIG. 9–12. Trigger points. 1, Greater tuberosity and site of supraspinatus tendon insertion. 2, Lesser tuberosity, site of subscapularis muscle insertion. 3, Bicipital groove in which glides bicipital tendon. 4, Site of subdeltoid bursa. 5, Glenohumeral joint space. 6, Acromioclavicular joint. 7, Sternoclavicular joint. [From Cailliet, R. (1981): *Shoulder Pain*, 2nd edit. F. A. Davis, Philadelphia.]

2. Improve faulty posture.
3. Preserve normal range of motion or regain normal motion.
4. Protect against undue stress of the weakened, inflamed connective tissue.

Nonsteroidal anti-inflammatory drugs, beginning with aspirin and other salicylates for mild injuries and a limited course for up to 4 weeks of indomethacin, oxyphenbutazone, or phenylbutazone for more severe injuries, will help relieve pain as well as inflammation. Injection of a local anesthetic and steroid preparation will accelerate resolution of inflammation.

Range of motion (ROM) exercises to counteract disuse should begin in the supine position, which is the least stressful for the upper extremities and shoulder. The patient then progresses through sitting, modified plantigrade, and finally, to the quadruped position, the most stressful of the weight-bearing postures for the shoulder (Fig. 9–14). A home exercise program should consist of gravity-assisted stretching, as in Codman's pendulum exercises (Fig. 9–15), walking the fingers up the wall while the shoulder is held in abduction, and wand-assisted exercises (Fig. 9–16), performed five times each, three times daily.

Recently recommended for the quicker recovery of patients with adhesive capsulitis is prolonged pulley traction accompanied by transcutaneous electric nerve stimulation (TENS) (Fig. 9–17). Application of the TENS unit for 10 min before and after traction reduces the patient's discomfort from the traction. During the first treatment session, 2 to 5 lb of traction is applied, then 7 lb, and increasing up to 15 lb, depending on the patient's tolerance. Treatment sessions are four times weekly during the first 4 weeks, then three times weekly for an additional 4 weeks.

FIBROSITIS: MYOFASCIAL PAIN SYNDROME

Fibrositis, or the myofascial pain syndrome, is characterized by pain and stiffness perceived in a widespread soft tissue distribution and is aggravated by immobility, tension, pressure, and fatigue. Also termed nonarticular rheumatism, fibrositis is further characterized by exquisite tenderness, a ropy feel to the muscles, and dermatographia.

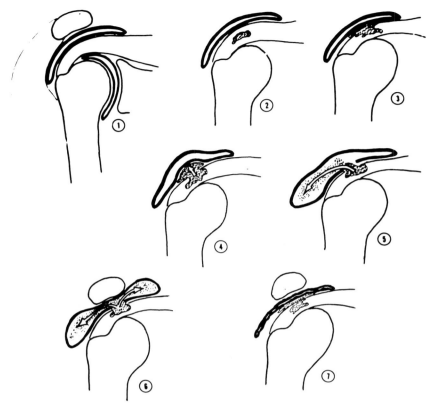

FIG. 9–13. Evolution of calcified tendonitis and formation of bursitis. 1, Normal relationship of supraspinatus tendon (cuff) to coracoacromial arch and head of humerus; intimate relationship of subdeltoid bursa and gleno-humeral joint. 2, Site of calcium deposit in cuff tendon. 3, Bulging calcium has been evacuated from tendon into subbursal space. 4, Partial evacuation into subbursal space with much debris remaining within tendon. 5, Tendon evacuates, with rupture into subdeltoid bursa. 6, "Dumbbell" intrabursal invasion. 7, Adhesive bursitis with thickening of walls of bursa and adhesion between superior and inferior surfaces. [From Cailliet, R. (1981): *Shoulder Pain*, 2nd edit. F. A. Davis, Philadelphia.]

Pathogenesis

Fibrositis is believed to originate in the spine and associated structures. There may be no obvious underlying factors causing this syndrome, or it may occur in association with rheumatoid arthritis, degenerative disk disease, cervical flexion-extension injury, infection, or trauma. More often than by chance alone, fibrositis appears in tense and perfectionistic persons.

Pathological findings are inconsistent. Some reports of muscle biopsy indicate occurrence of inflammatory changes consisting of increased intercellular fluid, fibrosis, and round-cell infiltration. Other biopsy studies show no abnormalities. The clinical and pathological changes may be set up by a deep reflex hyperalgesia mediated by the sympathetic nervous system, which causes local vasoconstriction. It is theorized that muscle ischemia or accumulation of metabolites may cause pain and nodularity.

Evaluation

The clinical picture is one of muscular pain, usually in the posterior neck, upper trapezius, and scapular muscles. In the lower body, similar findings may occur in the lumbosacral para-vertebrals and upper gluteal region (Fig. 9–18). Pain tends to be in a referral pattern of deep structures, not crossing many anatomical bound-

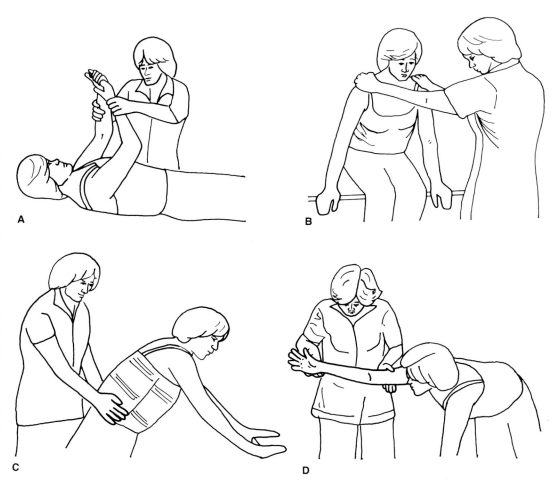

FIG. 9–14. Active assistive shoulder ROM. **A:** Reverse chop in supine position promotes muscular mobility of the involved shoulder. **B:** Sitting position enables less restricted movement of scapulae, promotes controlled mobility, and activates rotator cuff musculature. **C:** Modified plantigrade position, 45°-60° flexion at shoulder. This position increases weight bearing through upper extremity, compared to sitting or standing. Rocking in various directions is easy enough to perform and control for use in home exercise program. **D:** Quadruped position improves control in proximal scapula and shoulder muscles to about 90°. Greatest amount of activity of scapula, rotator cuff, and other shoulder muscles is required in this range to enable functional activities such as dressing and combing hair. (Illustrations by Charlotte Holden.)

aries. It tends to be worse on arising or after prolonged immobility. Exacerbation is caused by exposure to cold. There tend to be predictable, reproducible areas of intense tenderness called "trigger points," which are usually palpable nodules located where the soft tissue is dense, such as muscle insertions. Tendon insertions and soft tissues overlying bony prominences are also very tender. Delineation of nodularity is enhanced by applying a lubricant to the skin, which reduces friction during palpation. Muscles may have a rather ropy consistency instead of a smooth and homogeneous feel. Stroking the skin lightly with the fingernail may result in an exaggerated tissue hyperemia, called dermatographia. Typically, the mid portions of the trapezius muscles, rhom-

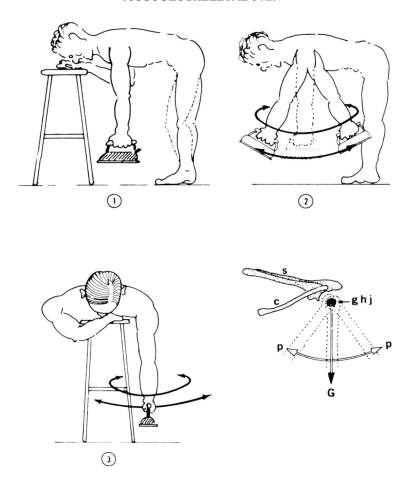

FIG. 9–15. Active pendular glenohumeral exercise. **1,** Posture permits arm to dangle freely, with or without weight. **2,** Arm moves in forward and back sagittal plane, in forward and backward flexion. Circular motion in clockwise and counterclockwise direction is also done in increasingly larger circles. **3,** Front view of exercise showing lateral pendular movement actually in coronal plane. *Lower right* diagram shows effect of gravity (G) on glenohumeral joint (ghj) with an immobile scapula (s). The p to p arc is the pendular movement. [From Cailliet, R. (1981): *Shoulder Pain*, 2nd edit. F. A. Davis, Philadelphia.]

boids, and spinalis have such areas. Neurological examination is negative and muscle strength is not diminished.

Treatment

Although fibrositis tends to be a subacute to chronic condition that is not progressive or crippling, it can be associated with a high level of pain. Acute exacerbations can be treated on an outpatient basis with hot packs, ultrasound to focal tender areas, spray-stretch techniques, and deep fibrositic massage. Narcotics should be avoided whenever possible since symptoms may be prolonged. Salicylates are probably the best first-line drugs, although no specific drug therapy is indicated.

The successful management of fibrositis emphasizes patient education and reassurance. A paradoxical statement may be used to motivate the patient to deal with the tension and stress that aggravate symptoms: Counsel the patient that the level of pain actually may be an index

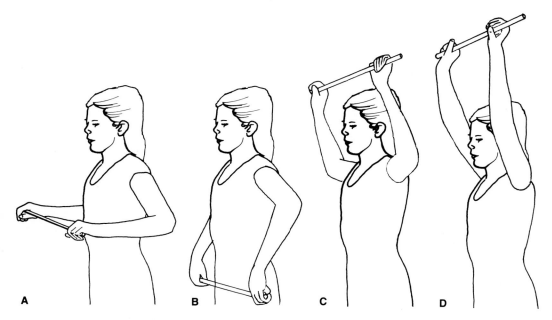

FIG. 9–16. Wand exercises to achieve full range of motion in shoulders. **A,** Internal rotation. **B,** Neutral. **C,** External rotation. **D,** Full forward flexion, made from position B. These exercises permit normal arm to actively or passively assist painful or restricted shoulder. By maintaining flexion and rotation, more painful movement of abduction is gently facilitated. (Illustrations by Charlotte Holden.)

of effort and is perhaps a small price to pay for being a productive and/or perfectionistic individual. Other ways of controlling tension are pacing activities and training in relaxation techniques.

REFLEX SYMPATHETIC DYSTROPHY

Reflex sympathetic dystropy (RSD) is a painful condition arising secondarily to any of several lesions. Prolonged regional sensory input to the central nervous system results in reflex changes seemingly disproportionate to the amount of morbidity. The key features of RSD are altered small vessel circulation (pallor, cyanosis, edema, rubor), trophic changes of the skin (loss of creases, shiny appearance), dysesthesia, and hyperalgesia which result in loss of motion and disuse of the affected portion of the extremity.

Pathogenesis

The most common manifestation of RSD, the shoulder-hand syndrome, has numerous possible origins. Among the most common are cervical spondylosis, coronary insufficiency, and stroke with hemiplegia (see also Chapter 15). As the term implies, many of the changes are reflexive in nature, chiefly vasomotor followed by musculoskeletal and sensory complications. With the altering of circulation, metabolites may build up. These, in turn, cause further vasomotor instability and an increase in tissue fluid (edema), followed by restriction of movement. Trophic changes of the skin also reflect autonomic dysfunction, since it is known that somatosensory endings do elaborate the substances that preserve normal texture and integrity of skin. The pain produces further reflex vasomotor instability accompanied by additional edema, restriction of motion, and pain. Once this cycle is in motion, it may persist for many months unless it is interrupted by aggressive therapy.

Evaluation

Clinical Presentation

In the shoulder-hand syndrome, pain is first perceived in the shoulder region, either by direct

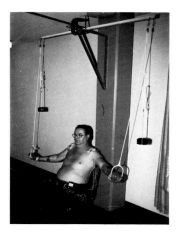

FIG. 9–17. Bilateral pulley traction with placement of TENS electrodes. Place affected upper extremity in as much abduction as tolerated and suspend by pulley rope with weights providing traction during treatment session. Apply traction for 15 min, release patient from pulley handle, and lower extremity slowly to rest in patient's lap for 5 min. Continue procedure until patient ceives total of 2 hr traction. [From Rizk, T., Christopher, R. P., Pinals, R. S., Higgins, A. C., and Frix, R. (1983): Adhesive capsulitis (frozen shoulder): A new approach to its management. *Arch. Phys. Med. Rehabil.*, 64:30.]

injury or by somatic or visceral referral pattern. With prolongation of the sensory input, the condition evolves from diffuse, poorly localized aching in the shoulder to burning or aching beginning distally in the extremity and restricted movement.

Although the cycle may begin in the shoulder, the hand soon becomes painful and sensitive also. Trophic changes in the skin, excessive warmth or coolness, and other stigmata of vasomotor instability also are present. What ensues is a painful, useless extremity that often cannot tolerate even the slightest tactile stimuli. In some cases, the patient may enter the office wearing a glove to provide insulation from unpleasant but common stimuli.

Physical Findings

Comparison proximally shows the typical stigmata of the frozen shoulder syndrome with painful, limited motion. The appearance of the skin distally on the hand shows either arterial constriction with edema and pallor, or arterial venous shunting. Venous constriction manifests as edema with cyanosis or rubor. The skin may correspondingly feel cool or very warm and may be very dry or moist. Skin creases are lost to varying degrees at the metacarpophalangeal and interphalangeal joints, reflecting edema and restriction of usual joint mobility. Tightness or contractures are mostly in extension. These findings distally help to distinguish RSD from the more localized and less complicated frozen shoulder syndrome.

Treatment

Relief of pain, alleviation of sympathetic hyperactivity and circulatory impairment, and improvement of restricted motion are the chief goals of therapy. Since these are closely related, treatment of one favorably affects the others. The best approach is a combined attack, pharmacologically on the sympathetic hyperactivity and physically on the peripheral sequelae of this de-

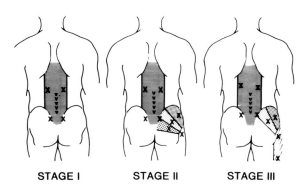

STAGE I   STAGE II   STAGE III

FIG. 9–18. Common areas of pain and muscle spasm in myofascial pain syndromes. *Stage I,* Bilateral paravertebral muscle spasm and tenderness. *Stage II,* Paravertebral muscles and gluteal muscles involved. Sciatica often occurs if pyriformis muscle is involved. *Stage III,* Paravertebral and gluteal muscles and iliotibial tract involved. X, Trigger point. [From Prithvi Raj, P., McLenna, J. E., and Phero, J. C. (1982): In *Chronic Low Back Pain*, edited by M. Stanton-Hicks, and R. A. Boas. Raven Press, New York.]

rangement. When possible, treat the underlying triggering mechanism.

Medication

Oral steroids beginning with moderate to large doses and tapering off over 10 to 14 days will reduce inflammation and provide additional analgesia. This is a good forerunner to aggressive active and passive exercises to regain lost motion. Other analgesics are good adjunctive therapy. Orally administered sympathetic blocking agents can be tried, but these predispose to postural hypotension. Adrenergic blockers such as guanethidine and phenoxybenzamine hydrochloride require between 2 and 7 days to achieve an effect. However, they may eliminate the need for percutaneous stellate ganglion block. This surgical technique is the surest and most direct way to abolish sympathetic hyperactivity temporarily.

Hydrotherapy

Since the hyperesthetic extremity will not tolerate extremes of temperature, a tepid or cool whirlpool will bring about temporary improvement. Immersion of the distal extremity in contrast baths, however, will help stabilize vasomotor function. Immersion is performed alternately in baths of 10 to 16°C and 38 to 40°C.

Massage

Massage of the extremity will increase venous and lymphatic return, thus mobilizing some of the edema and also providing its own counterirritant effect. Tight joints will then tolerate manipulation better. Use of pneumatic massage is a possible alternative to manual massage. The advantage is that it may be used for an hour or longer.

Splinting

Once mobilization is underway and pain is tolerable, dynamic splinting can be used to increase finger flexion. It is an excellent way to preserve motion gained through active assistive

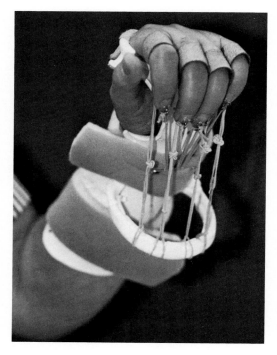

FIG. 9–19. Dynamic finger flexion splint with outrigger finger slings and nail hooks promoting metacarpophalangeal and interphalangeal joint flexion.

stretching. The splint can be applied for increasing periods of time (e.g., 30–90 min) with adjustable tension (Fig. 9–19).

MANAGEMENT IN A MULTIDISCIPLINARY PAIN CLINIC

Any musculoskeletal pain, even from acute injury, can potentially become chronic and recalcitrant. The multidisciplinary pain clinic combines medical and psychosocial approaches to the evaluation and treatment of chronic pain. The primary care physician is one member of the therapeutic team.

Patients with chronic pain should be screened carefully before referring them to a pain clinic to determine whether they are appropriate for a particular pain program. Patients who are receiving workman's compensation or participating in a lawsuit, for example, are less likely to benefit from treatment if they have a vested interest in remaining in pain.

The clinical evaluation emphasizes functional ability and behavioral responses to pain. Each patient completes a pain questionnaire, preferably as a part of the history and physical examination. This questionnaire provides detailed coverage of medication use, psychosocial adjustment, and vocational history.

The treatment objective is to select the appropriate combination of therapeutic modalities for each patient that will reduce pain and increase activity level to improve function yet decrease or eliminate the use of tranquilizing and narcotic medications. Gradual reduction of dependence on medication is facilitated by use of a pain cocktail, in which routinely scheduled doses of analgesics are masked in a liquid form and gradually reduced, or by the self-management approach, in which the patient voluntarily reduces drug dosage under peer pressure. Initially, use traditional physical modalities such as heat, cold, and traction to reduce pain. Then supplement these by TENS and biofeedback. Acupuncture, nerve blocks, and limited surgical intervention are useful in selected cases.

A behavioral modification approach is helpful to increase the activity level of patients who have become physically disabled due to inactivity and "sick-role" behavior. Activities the patient can presently perform constitute a baseline level. Then the activity level is gradually increased by reinforcing successfully completed tasks and withholding response when goals are not reached.

Also modify other pain-preserving behaviors. The patient's behavioral response to pain, as well as the reaction of the patient's family and employer to complaints of pain, must be changed so that improvement will continue when the patient is no longer participating in the pain program. If chronic depression is compounding awareness of pain, the patient should be treated with tricyclic antidepressants, psychotherapy, and involvement in an exercise and activity program. The tricyclics have an analgesic effect of their own. Respond positively to well behavior while limiting response to pain behavior. When the patient is discharged from the program, you can help the family and employers develop insight into the patient's behavior so that the program will be carried out at home and at work.

SUGGESTED READINGS

Cailliet, R. (1977): *Soft Tissue Pain and Disability.* F. A. Davis, Philadelphia.

Cailliet, R. (1981): *Low Back Pain Syndrome*, 3rd edit. F. A. Davis, Philadelphia.

Cailliet, R. (1981): *Neck and Arm Pain*, 2nd edit. F. A. Davis, Philadelphia.

Cailliet, R. (1981): *Shoulder Pain*, 2nd edit. F. A. Davis, Philadelphia.

Jackson, R. (1978): *The Cervical Syndrome*, 4th edit. Williams and Wilkins, Baltimore.

Kessler, R. M., and Hertling, D., editors (1983): *Management of Common Muskuloskeletal Disorders: Physical Therapy Principles and Methods.* J. B. Lipincott, Hagerstown, MD.

Kottke, F. (1961): Evaluation and treatment of low back pain due to mechanical causes. *Arch. Phys. Med. Rehabil.*, 42:426–440.

Ng, L. K. Y., editor (1981): *New Approaches to Treatment of Chronic Pain: A Review of Multidisciplinary Pain Clinics and Pain Centers*, Research Monograph 36. National Institute on Drug Abuse, Rockville, MD.

Rizk, T. E., Christopher, R. P., Pinals, R. S., Higgins, A. C., and Frix, R. (1983): Adhesive capsulitis (frozen shoulder): A new approach to its management. *Arch. Phys. Med. Rehabil.*, 64:29–32.

Stanton-Hicks, M., and Boas, R. A. (1982): *Chronic Low Back Pain.* Raven Press, New York.

Medical Rehabilitation,
edited by L. S. Halstead and M. S. Grabois.
Raven Press, New York © 1985.

CHAPTER 10

Arthritis

Vincent J. Kitowski

Departments of Physical Medicine and Rehabilitation, Baylor College of Medicine, Houston, Texas 77030

Second only to the common cold in contributing to nonfatal ill health and periodic loss of work, the musculoskeletal aches and pains broadly referred to as arthritis compose a large part of the primary care physician's daily work load. Frequently, arthritis becomes a chronic disease that causes significant disability. Over 31 million people in the United States are estimated to have some form of the disease. Although the term arthritis literally refers to the inflammation of a joint, the approximately 100 different conditions involving disorders of the musculoskeletal system include several noninflammatory processes, such as degenerative joint disease.

This chapter focuses on the rehabilitation of arthritis patients. For specific diagnostic methods, refer to one of the rheumatology texts listed under Suggested Readings. The following discussion emphasizes the rehabilitation management of the three major rheumatic disease categories: rheumatoid arthritis (adult and juvenile), degenerative joint disease, and ankylosing spondylitis. Although pathogenesis and manifestations vary, the consequent disabilities of these conditions share much in common. Whether prescribed and implemented by the primary care physician or in concert with the rehabilitation team, many of the same basic rehabilitation treatment principles apply to a wide range of rheumatic disorders:

1. Relieve pain.
2. Prevent joint damage and deformities.
3. Maintain strength and function.
4. Educate the patient and family.

5. Help the patient adapt emotionally to lifestyle limitations imposed by the disease process.

RHEUMATOID ARTHRITIS

Rheumatoid arthritis is a systemic inflammatory disorder of synovial joints and connective tissues. It affects females and males in a ratio of 3 to 1 with a peak incidence of onset during the third and fourth decades. The typical pattern of distribution includes symmetrical involvement of small peripheral synovial joints. Rarely, a single joint can be affected. Signs and symptoms range from mild early morning stiffness to severe, disabling physical deformities.

Relieving Pain

Whether pain is of sudden or gradual onset, relief must often be obtained before other components of the rehabilitation program can be implemented. Initial treatment for pain includes drug therapy and resting the involved joints. Medications of choice are nonsteroidal anti-inflammatory agents such as salicylate preparations, indomethacin, tolmetin, ibuprofen, naproxen, fenoprofen, sulindac, and piroxicam.

Acetylsalicylic acid (aspirin) in doses high enough to reach a therapeutic blood salicylate concentration of 20 to 30 mg/100 ml remains the initial drug of choice for patients with most rheumatic diseases. If the course of treatment is individualized and carefully followed, a majority of patients tolerate and benefit from one of the salicylate preparations (Table 10–1).

What if salicylate therapy cannot be tolerated or supplemental anti-inflammatory action is needed in addition to the optimal salicylate dosage? Try drugs such as indomethacin or one of the propionic acid derivatives (Table 10–2). An increasing variety of these anti-inflammatory drugs are available, and although they all apparently work by the same mechanism, patient response and tolerance vary considerably.

Patients with severe rheumatoid arthritis who are experiencing progressive joint destruction as evidenced by articular erosion on radiographs may benefit from a slow-acting agent such as gold, penicillamine, or hydroxychloroquine sulfate. You should consult with a rheumatologist, however, before initiating this type of therapy due to the prolonged duration of treatment and potentially serious toxicity and side effects of the drugs. With careful monitoring, however, gold has been shown to halt and partially reverse the articular destructive process in about 60% of the patients who receive and tolerate therapy. The patient's basic regimen of nonsteroidal anti-inflammatory drug(s) should be continued in addition to the slow-acting drug.

Because corticosteroids often display extensive and serious side effects with long-term administration, they should seldom be used in patients with rheumatoid arthritis. But seeking a second opinion might help you weigh the risks and benefits of treating a particular patient with oral steroids. Once therapy has started, an immediate attempt at dose reduction and eventual complete withdrawal should be made during the subsequent months.

The pharmacological management of rheumatoid arthritis is outlined in Table 10–3.

Preventing Joint Damage and Deformity

Resting splints, specially designed to protect involved joints, aid in pain relief, the reduction of swelling, the prevention of deformities, and the prevention of trauma to an unstable joint. Used primarily on the hand, wrist, and knee, resting splints are usually indicated during the acute stage of disease and after surgery. They

TABLE 10–1. *Salicylate preparations*

Generic	Trade	Dose	Considerations
Acetylsalicylic acid (ASA), aspirin		2,600–5,200 mg daily, in divided doses; therapeutic salicylate concentration: 20–30 mg/100 ml; children: 80–100 mg/kg/day	Optimal dose is slightly less than dose causing tinnitus
Buffered ASA	Bufferin® Ascriptin®	Same as above	
Enteric-coated ASA	Ecotrin®	Same as above	Less predictable absorption; minimizes gastric distress
Sodium salicylate		2,400 mg/day	
Enteric-coated sodium salicylate	Pabalate®	Same as above	Less predictable absorption; minimizes gastric distress, but does not decrease blood loss
Salsalate	Disalcid®	3,000 mg/day	Does not cause gastrointestinal blood loss, as does aspirin; safe for aspirin-allergic patients; safety and effectiveness for children have not been established
Choline salicylate	Arthropan® Liquid	5–10 cc/day q.i.d.	Use if tablet form cannot be tolerated, as in elderly patient
Choline magnesium trisalicylate	Trilisate® Liquid or Tablets	2,000–5,000 mg/day	Gastrointestinal blood loss is insignificant; not recommended for children under age 12

Therapy with salicylate preparations should be stopped at least 1 week prior to surgery.

TABLE 10–2. *Nonsteroidal anti-inflammatory drugs*

Generic	Trade	Dose	Maximum daily dose	Considerations
Indole derivatives				
Indomethacin	Indocin® Indocid®	25–50 mg q.i.d.	150–200 mg	Adverse side effects, occurring in 36% to 70% of patients, depending on dosage, include neurological reactions, blood loss anemia, gastrointestinal distress; contraindicated in the elderly, as it may precipitate congestive cardiac failure; not good primary agents; prescribe alone whenever possible; some patients are unresponsive
Tolmetin	Tolectin®	200 mg q.i.d. or 400 mg b.i.d.; add 200 mg weekly	1,200–1,600 mg	Useful for patients who benefited from indomethacin but experienced side effects; upper and lower gastrointestinal upset is common
Sulindac	Clinoril®	200 mg b.i.d.	400 mg	Chemical structure similar to indomethacin; neurological reactions and dry mouth are common; no significant blood loss
Propionic acid derivatives[a]				
Ibuprofen	Motrin® Brufen® Advil® Rufen®	400 mg q.i.d. 400 mg q.i.d.	2,400–3,200 mg; children: 100 mg/kg	
Naproxen	Naprosyn®	250 mg t.i.d.	1,000 mg	Effective for children
Fenoprofen	Nalfon® Fenopron®	300–600 mg q.i.d.	1,800–2,400 mg	Less blood loss than aspirin
Phenylacetic acid				
Aclofenac	Mervan® Prinalgin®	500–1,000 mg t.i.d.	3,000 mg	No significant gastrointestinal bleeding; no serious liver, kidney, or bone marrow damage with long-term use; itchy skin rash is common, accompanied by fever and other systemic involvement

[a]Very safe; all compounds exhibit comparable anti-inflammatory properties; side effects are similar to those of salicylates, but less gastric distress makes them more tolerable for long-term treatment; wide range of patient preference is possible.

should not be worn during a time when they would impair function that the patient needs for work.

Resting splints are constructed from a variety of materials, such as plaster of Paris or thermoplastic. They are carefully customized for the individual patient and are usually fitted by an occupational therapist or orthotist. When requesting the fitting of a splint, specify which joints are to be protected and the therapist or orthotist usually will determine the best type of splint for the job, the degree of extension, if

needed, and the fit. Low temperature thermoplastic splints (Fig. 10–1) that you can modify in your own office are commercially available from manufacturers such as Orthoplast or Polyfoam.

Hand splints are usually designed to hold the patient's wrist at 10° to 15° of dorsiflexion with slight flexion of the fingers. This encourages any postinflammatory stiffness, contractures, or fusion to occur in a position that still permits good grip strength. If arthritis is limited to the wrist joint, the splint need only be extended distally

TABLE 10–3. *Pharmacological management of rheumatoid arthritis*

Stage I	Stage II	Stage III

Anti-inflammatory agents
 Aspirin
 Nonsteroidal anti-inflammatory
  drugs
 Occasional intra-articular steroid
  injections
	Remission-inducing agents
	 Gold salt injection
	 Penicillamine
	 Hydroxychloroquine
		Immunoregulatory agents
		 Azthioprine
		 Cyclophosphamide
		 Levamisole

If nonerosive and synovitis resolves, no further drugs may be needed If erosive or synovitis is still active after 4–6 months, then consider proceeding to stage II	If remission occurs, no further drugs may be needed If these agents are ineffective or debility is severe, then consider proceeding to stage III	

to midpalm, leaving the fingers free. Night resting splints are adequate for hands with swelling and pain but minimal or no deformity. Splints that will maintain position, decrease inflammation, stretch the intrinsics, and support the arches are indicated for hands with early ulnar deviation, swan neck, boutonniere, and thumb deformities. Although you may want to prescribe splints to make a dislocated wrist more comfortable, splinting is generally worthless for hands with noncorrectable, fixed deformities.

A long leg splint helps maintain the knee joint in full extension and holds the foot at a right angle in a slightly varus position. If a flexion contracture has already developed, serial splinting combined with exercises may assist in gradually overcoming the deformity. Serial splinting involves the application of a new bivalved plaster

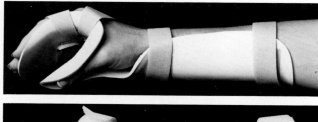

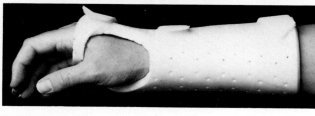

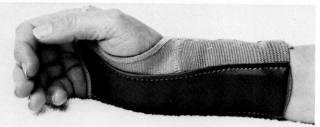

FIG. 10–1. Wrist and finger splints commonly used for patients with rheumatoid arthritis. **Top:** This splint supports the thumb. **Middle:** Working splint supports wrist while enabling free use of hands. **Bottom:** Working splint uses leather and elasticized material incorporating a pliable metal rib. Splint dominant hand in neutral position, nondominant hand in 10% to 15% of extension. [From Bluestone, R. (1980): *Practical Rheumatology: Diagnosis and Management.* Williams and Wilkins, Baltimore, MD.]

of Paris splint every 7 to 10 days as the range of motion improves.

When joints are acutely inflamed, the resting splint should be worn 24 hr a day. Continuous wear is particularly important for the confined patient, although care must be taken to check for skin sores. As the condition improves, many patients need to wear the splints at night only. Supportive wrist splints are often beneficial for patients who have painful instability caused by severe destruction of the wrist. If rheumatoid arthritis affects the cervical spine, a soft felt cervical collar designed to hold the head in a neutral position is used during sleep and for travel in a moving vehicle. When the ankle and foot are involved, custom footwear made by a surgical appliance manufacturer protects the foot and promotes more comfortable ambulation.

Ambulatory aids such as canes, crutches, and walkers alter the distribution of weight-supporting forces and are often useful in assisting ambulation (Fig. 10–2). These devices help protect the traditional weight-bearing joints from damage, but can create extra strain on the equally inflamed or deformed upper extremity joints. Care must therefore be taken to use platform attachments on walkers and crutches to reduce the additional stress to inflamed hands, wrists, elbows, and shoulders. In most cases, the decision to prescribe these devices requires an evaluation of the patient by a physiatrist or physical therapist. Some of the ambulatory aids are available through commercial sources, but others must be custom designed and fitted for the individual patient.

Range of motion exercises are fundamental to the prevention and correction of joint deformity. A physical therapist should tailor exercises of this type to the individual patient and teach the patient and family members a program of daily exercises that can be performed in the home. Initially, when arthritis is acute, gentle passive range of motion exercises are performed on all affected joints by the therapist or family member. The patient should progress quickly to active range of motion.

Maintaining Strength and Function

The most important objective of the entire rehabilitation program is to maintain the patient in a functional state which permits maximum

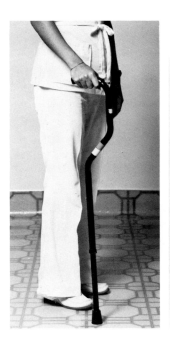
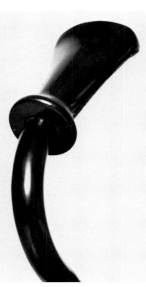

FIG. 10–2. Walking aids designed for arthritic patients. **Left:** Walking stick suited for patients with arthritic hands. **Right:** Handle has large grasping surface which does not require tight grip and can be rotated to suit patient's disability. [From Bluestone, R. (1980): *Practical Rheumatology: Diagnosis and Management.* Williams and Wilkins, Baltimore, MD.]

participation in the activities of daily living. This goal is dependent on the treatment regimen already discussed along with additional muscle-strengthening exercises, altering certain daily activities, and a careful balance between activities and rest.

As soon as the acute stage of the disease is past, the physical therapist instructs the patient in the performance of active extension exercises. When symptoms permit, active resistive exercises are introduced. The goal is to build up muscle groups that oppose the direction of potential deformities and to strengthen extensor, rather than flexor, muscle groups. For a brief overview of therapeutic exercises, see Chapter 4.

A physical or occupational therapist is able to determine how many of the patient's functional needs can be met in the face of progressive or established rheumatoid arthritis and what adaptations can be made to maximize function. Working with you, an experienced therapist is valuable in equipping the patient for a long-term program of self-care. Adaptations such as higher chairs and toilet seats, carts with smooth-running casters for transporting laundry and groceries, and a variety of other self-help devices, can achieve small but significant functional improvements while boosting morale as the patient relinquishes dependency. For example, long-handled, lightweight eating utensils that can be positioned at any desired angle help compensate for limited range of motion (ROM) of the shoulder, and a utensil holder can assist patients with weak hands. A long-handled comb and brush allow independent grooming, a Swedish reacher enables the patient to pick up objects without bending over, and a button hook assists with dressing.

Patients with persistent inflammatory polyarthritis may have to accommodate their lifestyle to periods of rest. The patient and family must be aware, however, that too much rest may result in stiff joints and muscles, while too much activity may damage the joints and increase pain. Several short periods of rest throughout the day are usually recommended. You should encourage the patient to plan activities so that the most important tasks are accomplished first. This type of self-pacing may be difficult for the patient to establish and requires full cooperation from other household members, but the potential for improving physical performance warrants the effort.

Educating the Patient and Family

The functional prognosis of rheumatoid arthritis often depends more on the strength of the patient's personality and the support of a loving family than on the severity of the actual disease process itself. The psychological state of the patient may both affect and be affected by the clinical course of rheumatoid arthritis. While there is no convincing evidence for a premorbid "rheumatoid personality," arthritis is multicausal; psychosocial factors interact with genetic, autoimmune, and infectious factors to produce a "predispositional matrix." Psychological conditions associated with arthritis can be attributed, by and large, to the exacerbations, remissions, pain, crippling, and uncertainty of the disease process.

As the primary care physician and the patient's initial medical contact, you are in the best position to observe the patient's adaptation to the disease and detect signs of emotional disturbance or maladjustment. The following factors are involved in evaluating the mental status of the arthritic patient:

1. Preexisting psychopathology.
2. Character strengths.
3. Precipitating stress.
4. Psychiatric symptoms.
5. Capacity to adapt to the disease and cooperate in treatment.

A period of mourning, which must be distinguished from depression, can be expected as the patient oscillates between intervals of rage, frustration, and desire for revenge and intervals of dependency, regression, and wishes for nurturance. These are predictable reactions to numerous fears about pain and increasing debility. The patient may fear rejection from family, friends, and co-workers due to the changes in physical appearance resulting from swollen joints and drug side effects.

Actual pain may provoke a "chronic pain syndrome" in which the patient limits activity in anticipation of further pain even when it is being successfully alleviated. Weakness, fatigue, and loss of energy, especially since they tend to come and go, may be perceived by the patient and others as character or personality flaws. Maintaining an identity separate from the disease and the accompanying sick role is often difficult. Especially stressful for the patient whose identity is defined primarily by occupation is adapting to the loss of functional ability. Fears may center on job loss and becoming a burden to the family, a dependency on others that produces feelings of humiliation and immaturity. A final source of anxiety is financing the extensive medical treatment of this chronic illness. These concerns will vary according to the patient's personality and age group.

You can help the patient work through and complete the mourning process while maintaining optimal functional ability by:

1. Providing realistic reassurance that crippling and invalidism are not inevitable.
2. Providing symptomatic relief.
3. Setting aside sufficient time to discuss feelings during office visits and to bolster self-esteem.
4. Discussing practical solutions for financing care, as well as for accommodating lifestyle to the demands of the disease.
5. Arranging group conferences with other arthritic patients and their families, as well as with the health care team.
6. Directing the family to information from the Arthritis Foundation, local arthritis clubs, and other community programs available in the area.
7. Educating the patient, family, and employer about the nature and potential consequences of the disease.

Such support not only will facilitate successful completion of the mourning process but also will help alleviate the protracted denial, prolonged intense feelings of guilt and shame, and feelings of hopelessness and helplessness that can escalate into severe depression. Refusal to cooperate with the treatment regimen, seeking constant bed rest, and severe withdrawal from social contact over several months are some indicators that depression or maladjustment is serious enough to warrant referral for psychotherapy.

Throughout this process, you should convey an optimistic attitude. This is not only beneficial to the family but also quite appropriate, because the overall prognosis for the majority of patients with rheumatoid arthritis is good. Approximately one-third experience spontaneous remission; one-third, a low-grade noncrippling course; and only the remaining third, extensive skeletal destruction with progressively impaired function. Even the patients in the latter group, however, can improve significantly; your guidance combined with the cooperation and efforts of the patient and the family can minimize the consequences of the destructive process and help the patient's own tissue resist the long-standing osteoarticular inflammation.

The following steps summarize the supportive management of rheumatoid arthritis:

1. Frequent office visits to assess progress.
2. Education of patient and family.
3. Rest and energy conservation.
4. Physical therapy and exercise.
5. Occupational therapy.
6. Play or recreation therapy.
7. Rehabilitation services.
8. Referral to specialist for consultation when needed.

MODERATELY ADVANCED RHEUMATOID ARTHRITIS

Report of a Case

HISTORY. Two years ago, this 40-year-old white woman developed bilateral pain and early-morning stiffness of finger and wrist joints. A year later, the joints became swollen and increasingly painful. There was bilateral joint involvement in the hands, wrists, and elbows, and especially in the metacarpal phalangeal joints. Joint tightness with limited wrist dorsiflexion followed. The patient lost weight and said at times she had a low-grade fever.

Until recently, aspirin had relieved her symptoms and enabled her to continue working as a secretary for a biochemist. She feared losing her job, which required extensive manuscript typing, because the gradual loss of finger dexterity had severely curtailed her typing speed and accuracy. Another concern was that her husband would be turned off by her deformities. She also believed that her husband and two adolescent sons resented having to perform more of the household chores. Although the patient seemed to be mourning potential social and occupational losses, she was not unduly depressed or pessimistic about the disease outcome. Her attitude was generally cooperative and she seemed eager to play a more active role in minimizing disability and remaining functional.

PHYSICAL EXAMINATION AND LABORATORY RESULTS. The fingers had bilateral fusiform enlargement of the proximal interphalangeal joints with swelling of the metacarpal-phalangeal and wrist joints. Wrist dorsiflexion was limited to 30°. The patient had a weak grip and bilateral atrophic intrinsic muscle. Subcutaneous nodules were present over the elbow extensor surface. Palpation of the involved joints demonstrated tenderness, heat, and swelling. The bilateral metatarsophalangeal joints of the feet were also involved.

Seropositivity for rheumatoid factor, elevated sedimentation rate, and anemia were present. X-rays of the hands, wrist, and feet revealed moderately advanced changes suggestive of rheumatoid arthritis.

REHABILITATION MANAGEMENT. The patient started daily physical therapy on an outpatient basis, and received instructions for home treatment. A paraffin bath (Fig. 10–3) was used for the hands and feet, supplemented by hydrotherapy or moist air cabinet. Following heat application, the patient carried out active joint ROM within pain tolerance. Mild stretching was performed on the contracted wrist joints. A heated therapeutic pool (90–95°F) was used three times weekly for both heat and exercise. Resting splints were used at night to protect and maintain proper positioning of the metacarpophalangeal joints of the hands. Shoes with built-in arch supports, spacious toe cap, wedge heel, and thick crepe sole were custom-made to provide sufficient support and comfort for the metatarsophalangeal areas.

The patient alternated periods of exercise and activity with periods of rest. She took a month's vacation from work, moved her morning arising time from 6:30 a.m. to 9:00 a.m., slept 1 to 2 hr in the afternoon, and retired by 10:00 p.m. With the encouragement of her family physician to find a job involving less strenuous typing, she transferred to a part-time position entering data into a computer for the same

research team. A special reaching device was designed to facilitate key stroke during arthritic flare-ups.

To counteract weight loss, the patient was encouraged to eat four or five meals a day, and aspirin was replaced by sulindac. To minimize gastric distress, she was advised to take pain medications during meal times. Improved relief of pain and inflammation was expected to optimize compliance with the exercise program.

A meeting with the patient's family was scheduled to enlist their cooperation and support and to detect any potential resistance to the patient's treatment regimen. They had to be discouraged from taking over all of the patient's responsibilities; her husband believed that only constant bed rest would prevent his wife from becoming an invalid. His hesitancy to initiate sex with his wife also stemmed from fear that the activity would hurt or unnecessarily fatigue his wife rather than from any loss of sexual desire for her. They eventually discovered that sex was the most comfortable after swimming or a hot bath. The patient was encouraged to clarify for her family which home activities she could do easily and which ones required their assistance. The youngest son, aged 13, was reassured that his mother would not become crippled and bedridden, as he had feared.

The history and physical examination of this patient indicated moderately advanced polyarticular rheumatoid arthritis with some systemic involvement. Replacing aspirin with sulindac, which does not cause significant gastrointestinal blood loss, was expected to help control anemia as well as inflammation. A future need for synovectomy and surgery to remove nodules was anticipated. Despite the progressive nature of this patient's condition, prognosis was considered favorable due to her positive, cooperative attitude and the support of her family.

JUVENILE RHEUMATOID ARTHRITIS

Juvenile rheumatoid arthritis (JRA) is a form of atypical rheumatoid arthritis that can impose tremendous diagnostic difficulties. Unlike the adult form, which is relatively easy to differentiate from other types of arthritis, JRA often mimics other childhood diseases and can present or evolve as one of three clinically definable syndromes: polyarticular, monarticular, or acute systemic. Table 10–4 compares the prevalence, signs and symptoms, and treatment of these three syndromes.

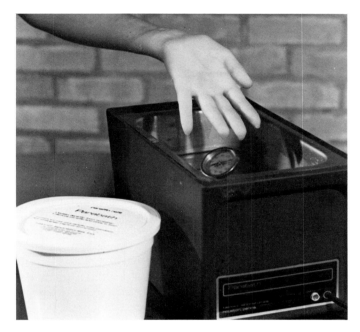

FIG. 10–3. Paraffin bath, applied especially before exercise, helps relieve pain and relax patient while reducing the risk of injury. Paraffin bath. Wax and mineral oil are melted, cooled to 120–125°F, then applied to inflamed hands. (Photo by Gordon Stanley.)

Treatment and rehabilitation management is, for the most part, similar to that described for adult rheumatoid arthritis but more conservative. However, you will need to modify drug selection and dosage for the child's size and age.

Aspirin is generally the drug of choice, while corticosteroids are reserved for only the most intractable cases; steroid-related complications range from growth retardation to mortality in children. Usually, compliance with the rehabili-

TABLE 10–4. *Clinical comparison of juvenile rheumatoid arthritis syndromes*

Syndrome (percent of all cases)	Signs and symptoms	Rehabilitation treatment of all syndromes
Polyarticular (50%, usually girls)	Skeletal distribution similar to adult In early stage, mimics rheumatic fever Cervical apophyseal involvement Temporomandibular joint involvement Low-grade quotidian fever Rash, weight loss, fatigue More common seronegativity	Conservative; aspirin, dose modified to child's age and size; steroids, as last resort due to growth retardation and mortality; paraffin baths; resting splints at night; swimming in heated therapeutic pool; more rest; active joint ROM and stretching of joints; wedge between upper and lower teeth; work closely with family; play therapy
Monarticular (30%, usually girls under age 8) Acute systemic or Still's disease (20%)	Insidious involvement of one to four larger joints Accelerated growth in adjacent bone Chronic iritis, blindness if untreated Widespread inflammation, hectic fever Severe anemia, leukocytosis Lymphadenopathy, hepatosplenomegaly Myocarditis, pericarditis Pneumonitis, pleuritis Rash, weight loss, fatigue	

tation program rests primarily with the parents and/or other family members, although you should include the child in the education effort at a level commensurate with his or her comprehension capabilities.

SEVERE JUVENILE RHEUMATOID ARTHRITIS

Report of a Case

HISTORY. A year ago, this 5-year-old white girl developed symmetrical pain and swelling of wrists, hands, ankles, and feet. She had decreased active joint ROM and quotidian fever ranging from normal to 102°F. She developed a bilateral limp, cervical vertebral involvement, and decreased range of motion in the neck. She lost weight and became listless. At times, there was a migratory pink fading rash over her body.

PHYSICAL EXAMINATION AND LABORATORY RESULTS. Decreased range of motion in the cervical spine, pain, and mild contractures of the knees and wrist were found. The fingers were swollen and had slight radial deviation. On palpation, the joints were tender, warm, and swollen. Involvement of the temporomandibular joint made opening her mouth wide difficult. At times, a migratory, evanescent, discrete, macular, pink-colored rash was seen on various body areas. Laboratory tests revealed a white blood cell count of 13,000/mm³, elevated sedimentation rate, and positive rheumatoid factor. X-rays of the involved joints were suggestive of juvenile rheumatoid arthritis.

REHABILITATION MANAGEMENT. Close medical and rehabilitation supervision was mandatory. Eye examinations were conducted at regular intervals to observe for iridocyclitis and uveitis, conditions that did not develop. Pain and inflammation were controlled by aspirin and other salicylates.

A physical therapist instructed the patient and family members in home treatment. Outpatient physical therapy was employed daily at home until the parents understood the program well enough to supervise it themselves. Paraffin baths for the involved hands and feet were done once or twice daily, followed by active joint ROM with mild stretching of tight joints within pain tolerance. Resting splints were used at night for proper joint positioning of the hands and wrists. A wedge was worn between her upper and lower teeth to reduce pressure on the temporomandibular joint. Outpatient therapy, three times a week, included swimming in a heated therapeutic pool. The parents made sure the child obtained at least 10 hr of sleep nightly and that she took short naps two or three times a day. Two hours a day were spent in play therapy consisting of indoor and outdoor games with other arthritic children.

Treatment of this child employed the simplest, safest, and most conservative measures for managing a refractory case of juvenile polyarthritis with systemic involvement. The presence of a positive rheumatoid factor, which is unusual in children, suggested chronic, moderately severe arthritic involvement. Therefore, long-term therapeutic interventions were avoided that would stunt growth or produce other irreversible side effects. Balancing physical therapy with play and rest, supplemented by aspirin, alleviated pain and inflammation and decelerated progression of the disease, while enabling the development of reasonably normal social, physical, intellectual, and emotional maturation. Compliance with this regimen by the child and her parents was expected to help compensate for the typically unfavorable prognosis associated with this patient's clinical profile.

DEGENERATIVE JOINT DISEASE

Degenerative joint disease (DJD) is a noninflammatory disorder of the synovial diarthroidal joints. Although the term osteoarthritis is often used, it is inaccurate because it implies a prominent inflammatory process. The disease is characterized pathologically by degeneration of articular hyaline cartilage and secondary hypertrophy of the subchondral and marginal bone. The condition is widespread and its frequency increases with age, reflecting the inevitable effects of wear and tear within the joint. Pain, particularly noticeable in the weight-bearing joints, is a major symptom. The chief physical sign is joint enlargement due to bony hypertrophy of the articular margins. Typical skeletal distribution and other signs and symptoms are presented in Table 10–5.

Relieving Pain

As with most forms of arthritis, pain relief is attained through a combination of medications, resting the involved joints, and physical therapy techniques such as the application of heat. Acetaminophen often provides adequate pain relief

TABLE 10–5. *Clinical comparison of degenerative joint disease and ankylosing spondylitis*

	Joint distribution	Signs and symptoms	Rehabilitation treatment
Degenerative joint disease	Distal interphalangeal of hands Around base of thumb Lower cervical spine Lumbosacral spine Hips Knees First metatarsophalangeal joints	Noninflammatory Synovial diarthroidal joint involvement Chondrocalcinosis Pain in weight-bearing joints Joint enlargement and deformity Loss in range of motion, resulting in serious contractures	Long-term Acetaminophen Intermittent courses of anti-inflammatory agents Heat application to involved joints—warm tub baths, heating pads, hot compresses, reflector heat lamps, paraffin baths, hydrocollator packs Short-wave diathermy, ultrasound Daily ROM exercise Ambulatory aids for relief from weight bearing Soft cervical collar Cervical traction
Ankylosing spondylitis	Sternomanubrial Sternoclavicular Symphysis pubis Intervertebral joints of spine Hip synovial Shoulder synovial Sacroiliac	Seronegativity Back pain Neck stiffness Inflammation, fusion of sacroiliac articulations Nongranulomatous acute iritis Lumbar lordosis loss Increased thoracic and cervical kyphosis Early flexion contacture of hip Impaired trunk flexion "Poker-back" fusion	Nonnarcotic analgesics Antispasmodics Hot showers Locally applied hot and cold packs High doses of anti-inflammatory agents Phenylbutazone Avoid prolonged periods of bed rest Postural, trunk extension, and ROM exercise Walking and swimming

when used in fairly large doses of up to 12 tablets per day, although many patients require something stronger. The effectiveness of propoxyphene is sometimes disappointing and habituation can occur.

Individuals often benefit from the use of salicylates or nonsteroidal, anti-inflammatory agents. In addition to their analgesic properties, these drugs help control the transient inflammation sometimes contributing to the articular pain of DJD. The large doses required for patients with rheumatoid arthritis are seldom indicated when treating patients with DJD. Intermittent courses of submaximal doses frequently provide the patient with significant pain relief. After finding the drug that is most effective and preferred by the patient, you can prescribe the agent from time to time, or continuously if required for symptomatic relief.

Because DJD requires long-term treatment, an emphasis on nonpharmacological approaches is preferred. The application of heat to the involved joints usually provides symptomatic relief, although it does not alter the progression of the disease. Using heat immediately before ROM exercises is particularly beneficial. Heat can be applied at home for 20 min, from one to three times per day. Outpatient physical therapy offers the additional benefit of short-wave diathermy or ultrasound treatment. Hydrocollator packs (Fig. 10–3) can be used during outpatient physical therapy or at home.

Although resting or protecting the involved joints is important in any pain relief regimen, undue immobility must be avoided. Therefore, the patient is encouraged to continue using the hands and lower extremities actively while limiting the work load to pain tolerance. Partial

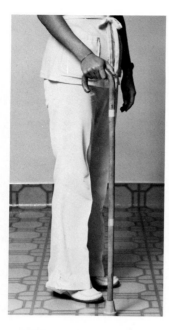

FIG. 10–4. Standard round-handled cane useful for patients with DJD affecting the hip or knee. [From Bluestone, R. (1980): *Practical Rheumatology: Diagnosis and Management.* Williams and Wilkins, Baltimore, MD.]

relief from weight bearing can be obtained by the use of ambulatory aids, either canes or walkers (Fig. 10–4), and a four-point gait pattern.

When the cervical spine is involved, a soft felt cervical collar provides support. Constant or intermittent cervical traction, applied as the patient is sitting in a chair inclined slightly backward so that the head is flexed about 20° to 25°, can relieve muscle spasm and pain.

Constant traction assists in elongating muscles and ligaments while reducing cervical or lumbar spasm and unnatural straightening. You should apply constant traction twice a day for 10 to 15 min when the patient is in severe pain or confined to bed. Weight is usually limited to 8 to 12 lb to avoid displacement of the temporomandibular joint. Constant traction has the advantage of adaptability to home treatment (Fig. 10–5). Applying hydrocollator packs during traction can help extend tolerance by relieving pain, as well as by increasing blood supply, metabolism, and the elasticity of soft tissue.

Intermittent traction consists of alternating 6- to 8-sec periods of weight application with 6- to 8-sec periods of rest. This alternation enhances patient tolerance, enabling longer traction sessions and weight application up to 20 lb.

Preventing Joint Damage and Deformity

Loss of ROM in DJD usually results in impaired strength and function, but rarely produces the contracture deformities seen in rheumatoid arthritis. The joint deformities that do develop from this disease are secondary to joint destruction and, as such, cannot be prevented.

Maintaining Strength and Function

The key to maintaining strength and function for the patient with DJD is to remain physically active within reasonable limits of pain tolerance. Daily ROM exercises are crucial to this goal. The recommended exercise regimen includes strengthening the musculature surrounding the involved joints. An exercise program of this type is particularly important if you are considering referring the patient for surgical treatment. Postoperative rehabilitation is greatly enhanced by the presence of strengthened muscle groups around the operation site. Good posture helps maintain range of motion and decreases the strain on joints and soft tissues. Adaptive devices, such as those used by rheumatoid arthritis patients, enhance function and encourage independence.

ANKYLOSING SPONDYLITIS

Another distinct group of rheumatic diseases are the chronic, nonspecific, inflammatory spondyloarthropathies, which include ankylosing spondylitis, Reiter's syndrome, and psoriatic arthritis. Ankylosing spondylitis is the most common example of these seronegative spondyloarthropathies. The majority of patients with this disease are young men who complain of back pain and stiffness in the neck associated with clinical and radiographic features of inflammation within the large cartilaginous and small synovial joints of the axial skeleton. The typical

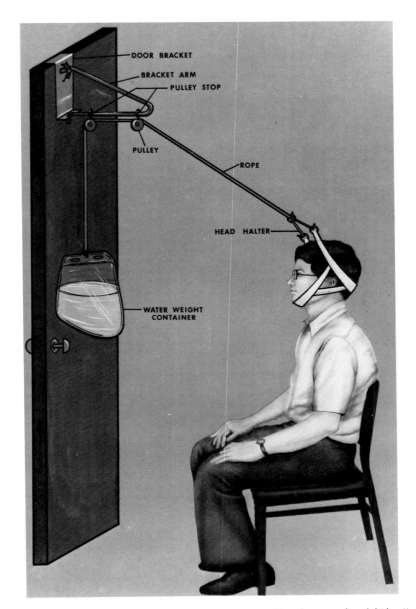

FIG. 10–5. A method of home traction for treating DJD with cervical involvement. A weight is attached through a pulley to a halter and the neck pulled into slight flexion. The weight may be constant or intermittent, slowly lifted and lowered by the patient or an attendant. [From Waylonis, G. W. et al. (1982): Home cervical traction: Evaluation of alternate equipment. *Arch. Phys. Med. Rehab.*, 63:388.]

osteoarticular distribution of ankylosing spondylitis is described in Table 10–5. Widespread involvement of the small synovial joints is uncommon. Approximately 25% of patients with this arthropathy at some time develop a nongranulomatous acute iritis.

Relieving Pain

Pain during the early stages of ankylosing spondylitis results from the inflamed joints and associated paraspinal muscle spasm, often preventing maximum range of motion and compliance with the prescribed exercise program. Treatments used to lessen the painful muscle spasm and thus permit a progressively intense exercise program are listed in Table 10–5. The drugs most frequently used for ankylosing spondylitis differ substantially from those normally used for rheumatoid arthritis. Phenylbutazone is the preferred drug, although one of the nonsteroidal, anti-inflammatory drugs such as indomethacin is often quite effective in patients who cannot tolerate phenylbutazone. Salicylates, slow-acting agents, and corticosteroids are rarely effective in controlling the symptoms of this disease.

Phenylbutazone, given orally in doses of 100 mg three to four times per day, is remarkably predictable in relieving the inflamed spine. You can monitor the safety of the drug by alerting patients to a possible idiosyncratic reaction during the first few weeks of therapy and suspending therapy at the first sign of a sore throat, fever, or skin rash. If the drug is well-tolerated, a complete blood cell count performed every 6 to 8 weeks throughout therapy provides an early clue to development of any bone marrow aplasia. Once the initial benefits of therapy are felt and the exercise program is underway, many patients will respond favorably to lower doses of the drug.

Preventing Joint Damage and Deformity

Fusion of the cartilaginous and small synovial axial skeleton joints often follows the inflammatory process, leaving some loss of mobility. Prolonged periods of bed rest are avoided to prevent intensification of the symptoms and skeletal fusion that would substantially impair function. Deformities can range from minor changes such as loss of normal lumbar lordosis to a severe end-state deformity in which the patient is fixed in a stooped position and walks with a slow shuffling gait. If physical therapy is initiated to guide the patient in establishing good posture and complying with a specially designed lifelong exercise program, the risk of severe deformity can be decreased. Although a classical "poker-back" fusion may occur even in an individual who follows an exercise program and maintains

good posture throughout the day and night, he can still remain functionally independent.

Maintaining Strength and Function

The functional prognosis for most patients with ankylosing spondylitis is excellent if an appropriate rehabilitation program is initiated in the early stages of the disease. The exercise program, preferably designed and implemented by an experienced physical therapist, includes movements that encourage trunk extension and maintenance of maximum mobility within the axial skeleton, the adjacent rib cage, and the pelvic and shoulder girdles. Instruction also is required to ensure good upright posture while sitting or standing and a continuation of the flat, fully extended position when sleeping. Range of motion exercises are necessary for the cervical spine, shoulder and hips. In addition to the standard range of motion exercises, walking and swimming are excellent ways to preserve range of motion.

Educating the Patient and Family

You must make the patient fully aware that the ultimate prognosis of ankylosing spondylitis depends heavily on compliance with the exercise program structured to counteract the contractures and deformities of the disease. This understanding is particularly important in patients who are relatively asymptomatic, because they are still at risk of developing severe functional disabilities. Occasionally, you may need to recommend an occupational change if the work prevents frequent changes of position or demands prolonged periods in a stooped posture. The family's cooperation in encouraging the patient to comply with the prescribed exercise regimen is invaluable. Due to the nature of this disease, many of the major lifestyle adjustments required by families of patients with rheumatoid arthritis are not necessary with ankylosing spondylitis. Nevertheless, you will need to reassure both the patient and family members that, in most cases, the patient's posture and level of function can be preserved to a degree sufficient for engaging in a virtually normal lifestyle.

SURGICAL TREATMENT FOR ARTHRITIS

Treatment of arthritic conditions exclusively by surgery is rarely indicated. However, operations properly timed and spaced during the course of the disease can relieve incapacitating pain, restore stability of the joint, improve function, correct or prevent deformity, alleviate joint stiffness, prevent harmful stress on uninvolved joints, arrest progressive synovitis, and improve appearance when other therapeutic interventions are no longer effective. There is controversy as to whether surgery for arthritis should emphasize prevention or merely correction and reconstruction. Common prophylactic procedures include synovectomy, release of a trapped nerve, local excision of a nodule, and fusion of the cervical spine. Restorative or reconstructive procedures are arthrodesis, arthroplasty, and joint replacement.

When synovectomy is indicated, usually when erosions appear on the roentgenogram after 24 to 30 months, it should be performed as early as possible to arrest the otherwise inevitable progression of the disease. The danger of postoperative complications contraindicates major surgery unless the potential benefits are very clear to the patient and family.

It is up to you, as the primary care physician, to choose an orthopedic surgeon whom you can trust to weigh carefully the risks and benefits of surgery for your patient and who can determine the best timetable for each operative procedure. If you refer the patient for surgery too late in the progression of the disease, the operative intervention becomes more difficult, the complication rate from postoperative stiffness increases, and arthritis may be eliminated without halting the progress of concomitant DJD.

The major goals for all reconstructive joint surgery in arthritic patients are to alleviate pain and to decelerate joint deterioration. Other considerations include tendon rupture, nerve compression, troublesome rheumatoid nodules, and possible impairment of healing in patients receiving steroids, penicillamine, and immunosuppressive agents. All considerations other than pain, however, should be secondary to the maintenance of function, especially when correction of a deformity may impair a function critical to the patient's occupation. Another important factor in patient selection is motivation, which strongly affects rate of recovery.

Therefore, the foremost contraindication for surgery is lack of motivation. Other contraindications include severe generalized disease, an extremely active arthritic condition involving most of the joints, as disease can be expected to recur within a short time, successful adaptation to severe deformities in an elderly patient, and depression. In general, unless consistent drug therapy has been unsuccessful, patients with fewer than six of the American Rheumatism Association's criteria for rheumatoid arthritis—morning stiffness, muscle pain, pain on motion in one joint, swelling of one joint, swelling of an additional joint, and symmetric swelling of joints—should delay surgery until radiological signs of progression become visible.

Arthritically involved joints are treated by numerous surgical procedures. The preeminent type of preventive operation is synovectomy. The arthroplasties, including excision, interposition, and partial or total joint replacement, are reconstructive. Osteotomy and arthrodesis are preventive as well as partially reconstructive. The type of procedure selected depends primarily on the stage of the disease and secondarily on the number of joints involved and the idiosyncracies of the patient's personality. Multiple joint contractures and involvement of both the upper and lower extremities would mandate selecting a procedure to make the patient ambulatory. When ambulation is not a realistic goal, the next priority is restoration of the upper extremities to enable self-feeding and self-care of other personal needs.

Patients who are poorly motivated would benefit the most from operations requiring little self-effort to regain function. Impressive results may even restore a more optimistic outlook and cooperative attitude favorable to the successful outcome from future operations requiring greater rehabilitative participation by the patient. Motivation can also be enhanced by inviting the patient to participate in the decision about what surgical procedures would be most beneficial, especially if numerous joints have been destroyed. The surgeon can inquire about what results the patient expects and explain what is realistic.

SUGGESTED READINGS

Baum, J. (1982): A review of the psychological aspects of rheumatic diseases. *Semin. Arthritis Rheum.*, 11:352–361.

Bluestone, R. (1980): *Practical Rheumatology: Diagnosis and Management*. Williams and Wilkins, Baltimore, MD.

Capell, H. A., Daymond, I. J., and Dick, W. C. (1984): *Rheumatic Disease*. Springer Verlag, New York.

Donovan, W. H. (1977): Physical measures in the treatment of juvenile rheumatoid arthritis. *Arthritis Rheum.*, 20(Suppl):553–557.

Ehrlich, G. E. (1980): *Rehabilitation Management of Rheumatic Conditions*. Williams and Wilkins, Baltimore.

Gschwend, N. (1980): *Surgical Treatment of Rheumatoid Arthritis*. W. B. Saunders, Philadelphia.

Melvin, J. L. (1982): *Rheumatic Disease: Occupational Therapy and Rehabilitation*. F. A. Davis, Philadelphia.

Moskowitz, R. W. (1982): *Clinical Rheumatology: A Problem-Oriented Approach to Diagnosis and Management*. Lea and Febiger, Philadelphia.

Riggs, G. K., and Gall, E. P., editors (1984): *Rheumatic Disease: Rehabilitation and Management*. Butterworth, Boston.

Medical Rehabilitation,
edited by L. S. Halstead et al.
Raven Press, New York © 1985.

CHAPTER 11

Rehabilitation of the Patient with Amputation

Robert H. Meier

Departments of Rehabilitation, Physical Medicine, and Orthopedic Surgery, Baylor College of Medicine, and Houston Center for Amputee Services, The Institute for Rehabilitation and Research, Houston, Texas 77030

Rehabilitation of the amputee involves the prescription and fitting of a prosthesis to replace the missing limb, as well as training to diminish the physical loss and restore function. The physician must also help the amputee deal with the change of body image imposed by the absence of a limb, whether congenital or acquired. Therefore, the management of amputation should include evaluating the meaning of the amputation to the individual in relation to his or her environment. Also, an essential goal of an amputee rehabilitation program is the education of the patient and family regarding realistic ideas and attitudes about the disability.

PREVALENCE AND ETIOLOGY

Approximately 400,000 amputees are presently living in the United States. The greatest cause (60%) of limb loss today is occlusive arterial disease. Amputation in patients with vascular disease, often associated with diabetes mellitus, has its highest incidence in the 60 to 70 year age bracket. Trauma accounts for 30% of amputations and occurs most commonly in the 17 to 55 year age group. Of this group, 71% are males. The trauma usually affects the lower extremity, with a ratio of ten lower extremities to every upper extremity amputated. Another 5% of amputations are related to tumor and are seen primarily in the 10 to 20 year age group. The final 5%, related to congenital birth defects, account for the majority of amputated limbs seen in the age range from birth to 16 years.

GOALS OF AMPUTATION SURGERY

Amputation surgery is a plastic and reconstructive technique that will fashion a limb suitable for fitting a comfortable and functional prosthesis. The goal of the surgeon is to produce a firm, cylindrical limb that is free of sensitive scar tissue, with bone that is well padded by muscle and subcutaneous tissue along its length. The end of the stump should be covered by healthy, nonadherent muscle, fascia, subcutaneous tissue, and skin. The suture line should be located as far as possible from the prosthetic pressure areas.

Levels of acquired amputation are classified in Fig. 11–1.

PATIENT ASSESSMENT FOR PROSTHETIC USE

In order to determine if the patient is a candidate for a prosthesis, the cardiovascular, central nervous, and musculoskeletal systems must be evaluated thoroughly. These considerations are especially relevant to lower extremity amputation.

Cardiovascular Function

Use of a lower extremity prosthesis increases the amount of energy expended during ambulation when compared with the same speed of ambulation with normal lower extremities. Use of a unilateral, below-knee prosthesis requires about 25% to 45% more energy than normal,

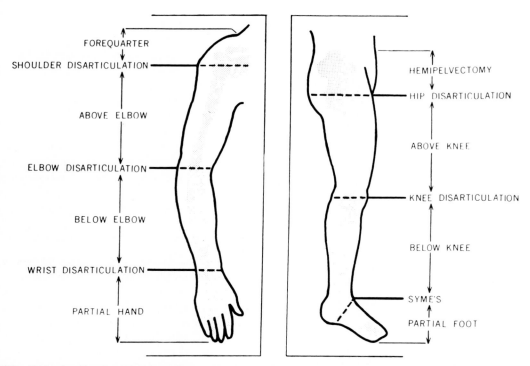

FIG. 11–1. Levels of amputation of upper and lower extremities. [From Garrett, J. F., and Levin, E., editors. (1973): *Rehabilitation Practices for the Physically Disabled.* Columbia University Press, New York.]

while an above-knee prosthesis requires 65% to 100% more energy. In some patients, these increases in energy may place excessive stress on the myocardium, with some ischemia. Hence, the use of a prosthesis may precipitate congestive heart failure or lead to myocardial infarction.

Occlusive vascular disease in the remaining lower extremity may render the patient unable to tolerate the increased work load necessary to walk using a prosthesis. A patient with intermittent claudication in the remaining leg prior to prosthetic training may have increased claudication when using a prosthesis. In fact, prosthetic usage may precipitate vascular insufficiency in the remaining extremity. Therefore, following lower extremity amputation, the opposite leg must be closely examined for signs of vascular compromise. These signs include loss of hair, shiny skin, decreased capillary filling, venous guttering, and hypertrophic nails.

Central Nervous System

Rule out cerebrovascular insufficiency resulting in organic brain syndrome. If short-term memory and the ability to learn new motor skills are impaired, the ability to learn to use the prosthesis may be compromised.

Vision

Adequate visual acuity is important, since visual feedback helps to substitute for sensation lost in the amputated body part. The abilities to read large newspaper print and to see the placement of a foot on the floor are simple visual criteria for successful prosthetic training.

Musculoskeletal Function

Muscle strength and joint range of motion should be evaluated on the amputated and nonamputated sides. Proximal muscle strength, especially for hip extension and abduction, is important in the above-knee amputee. In addition to good strength in these muscles, the below-knee amputee needs strong knee extension for satisfactory prosthetic function. Normal or nearly normal joint range of motion, with maintenance of hip and knee extension, also is essential for good prosthetic function.

PHASES OF MANAGEMENT

Care of the patient with amputation can be handled conveniently in four phases: acute post-surgical, preprosthetic, prosthetic, and follow-up. In ideal circumstances, each phase flows into the subsequent one, and successful prosthetic function is obtained within 1 to 2 months of amputation. Management requires close cooperation and communication between the patient and the health professionals involved.

Acute Postsurgical Phase

While the sutures are still in place, encourage the patient to do active range of motion exercise of the proximal joints. Hip and knee flexion contractures can be prevented by having the patient lie prone at least 4 hr per day. To avoid hip or knee contractures, do not place pillows under or between the legs. Encourage the recent amputee to exercise actively the remaining leg musculature. The following exercises should be done every few hours, gradually increasing the number of repetitions:

1. *Gluteal setting:* Lie prone and pinch buttocks together for a slow count of five.
2. *Hip extension:* Lie prone, raise the stump off the mattress as high as possible, and hold for a slow count of five.
3. *Quadriceps setting:* Lie supine and hold knee as straight as possible for a slow count of five.
4. *Hip abduction:* Lie on the side with the hips extended, lift the stump toward the ceiling and hold for a slow count of five.

Patients with upper extremity amputation will benefit from the following exercises involving the shoulder complex:

1. *Scapular abduction:* Reach as far forward as possible with both arms.
2. *Scapular adduction:* Try to pinch the spine with both scapulae.
3. *Shoulder elevation:* Shrug the shoulders as high as possible.
4. *Humeral flexion:* Lift the arm as far forward and above the head as possible.
5. *Humeral extension:* With the arm at the side, reach as far backward as possible.
6. *Humeral abduction:* Move the arm straight out to the side and above the head.
7. *Humeral rotation:* Rotate the humerus inward and outward.

Hold each exercise for a slow count of five. These exercises should be done every few hours in repetitions of ten, with deliberate motion. Below-elbow amputees should be taught elbow flexion and extension, forearm pronation, and supination exercises.

Preprosthetic Phase

The preprosthetic phase usually follows suture removal, while the patient is awaiting scar maturation, and precedes wearing the prosthesis.

Stump Wrapping

Elastic bandages will not only help control edema but also shrink and shape the residual limb prior to prosthetic casting. To help suspend the bandage, a figure-eight wrap usually incorporates the proximal joint closest to the stump. Wrapping from the distal to proximal site should provide distal compression. The stump should be rewrapped every 4 hr or whenever the bandage loosens, slips, or bunches. An elastic stump shrinker may be used if elastic wrapping is impractical.

Skin Care

Before the incision is completely healed, a whirlpool often is helpful in slowly healing limbs or wounds that are draining. Schedule hydrotherapy for 20 to 30 min once or twice daily. A detergent or antiseptic additive such as Betadine® may be helpful for cleansing. Closely monitor the water temperature to avoid scalding, especially if there is dysvascular disease. In this case, keep the water temperature below 90°F.

After the incision is healed, soften the skin with a water-soluble cream or lanolin preparation three times daily. Gentle massage of the distal soft tissues helps keep them mobile over the end of the bone. Tapping the scar and distal soft tissue four times a day often helps desensitize these areas prior to wearing the prosthesis. Tap with the finger tips, starting lightly and increasing pressure for about 5 min until mild discomfort is produced.

Good skin hygiene should be taught, using mild soap to work up a lather and then rinsing with lukewarm water. The skin should be patted, not rubbed dry. Cleansing is recommended daily in the evening.

Ambulation

The patient with a unilateral leg amputation usually can begin walking before a prosthesis is fitted by balancing on one leg with the support of forearm or underarm crutches. The bilateral amputee is trained in wheelchair transfers.

Prosthetic Phase

The first step in the prosthetic phase is developing a prosthetic prescription. This is best done by a team of experienced rehabilitation professionals who can follow the patient through the pre- and postprosthetic fitting periods. The physician is encouraged to discuss the various prosthetic components with the amputation team so that the options in prosthetic prescription are considered. The prescription should contain specific prosthetic component parts instead of merely stating "one below-knee prosthesis." The following characteristics of the amputee should be considered when prescribing a prosthesis:

1. Size.
2. Level of amputation.
3. Previous occupation and future vocation.
4. Avocational interests.

5. Preference for functional or cosmetic device.
6. Secondary diagnoses.
7. Psychological adjustment to amputation.

Prosthesis Fabrication

The prosthesis is a custom-fitted artificial limb and hand fabricated by a certified prosthetist who is a health professional and a craftsperson. The phases of prosthetic fabrication include:

1. Plaster cast made of the residual limb.
2. Plaster representation of the amputated limb made from the plaster mold.
3. Plastic laminate socket made over the plaster limb.
4. Components added to the socket.
5. Fitting adjustments.

In some centers, immediate postoperative rigid dressings are applied over the fresh amputation to decrease edema, promote wound healing, and decrease pain. In lower limb amputation, a pylon and prosthetic foot can be attached to this rigid dressing to begin early ambulation within 2 to 3 weeks of the operation. In upper limb amputation, the terminal device and control cables can be attached to the rigid dressing within 24 hr of the operation (Fig. 11–2).

If immediate postoperative dressings are not used, a temporary or preparatory prosthetic socket can be applied to hasten shaping and shrinking of the stump (Fig. 11–3). More often, shaping and shrinking are accomplished by wrapping the stump with elastic bandages or using a shrinker made of elasticized fabric.

Prosthesis Check-Out and Training

A comfortable fit is even more essential for successful prosthetic wearing than function. Prosthetic sockets are made to distribute weight on pressure-tolerant areas and to relieve the pressure on intolerant areas.

During the early period of use, give the patient a specific schedule for wearing the prosthesis. For example, the patient may begin by wearing the prosthesis, without weight bearing, for 15-min intervals and increasing this time as the skin tolerates it. Frequent skin checks for

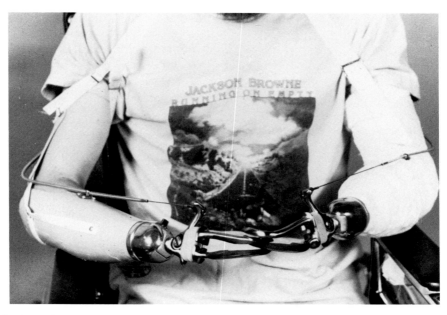

FIG. 11–2. Immediate postoperative rigid dressing with terminal device and control cable for bilateral below-elbow amputee.

areas of redness are also necessary. Reddened areas that do not clear within 20 to 30 min may preclude further wear without modifications of the prosthesis.

Training should be done by an experienced therapist, not left to the motivation of the patient. Prosthetic training should involve patient education regarding the use and care of the prosthesis. This training can increase the confidence the patient gains using the prosthesis. The ultimate aim of prosthetic training is the restoration of lost or difficult function that would be impossible without the prosthesis.

Performing Activities of Daily Living

The unilateral upper extremity amputee undergoes training in occupational therapy 2 hr daily to shift hand dominance, if necessary, for such activities of daily living as eating, dressing, personal hygiene, and communication. Performance of these activities may be facilitated by using the prosthesis with terminal devices such as various hooks and the myoelectric hand shown in Fig. 11–4. The more proximal the upper ex-

tremity amputation, the more difficult it is to restore bilateral skills. Bilateral shoulder disarticulation amputees have the most serious problems with self-care and may never become independent, even with a prosthesis.

Follow-Up Care

Initially, follow-up care should be done at regular intervals—every 1 to 3 months—in order to evaluate the patient for gait deviations, maintenance problems, poor fit, skin problems, and bone problems. Gait deviations should be corrected immediately because they quickly become habitual and are difficult to correct once they appear. Another common early problem is shrinkage of the soft tissue of the stump; this usually can be corrected by adding an additional ply of stump sock. Poor fit, which may lead to skin irritation or ulceration, must be corrected quickly by the prosthetist. Bone overgrowth may also cause pain and skin problems. Prosthetic socket modifications may be necessary to alleviate this problem. Occasionally, additional surgery is required.

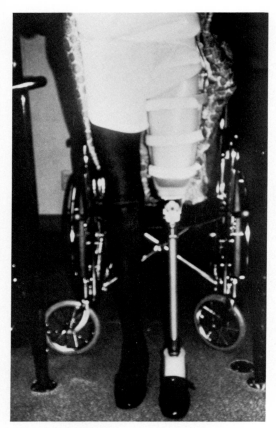

FIG. 11–3. Preparatory adjustable polypropylene socket with aluminum pylon and foot for left above-knee amputee.

COMMON COMPLICATIONS OF AMPUTATION

Skin Disorders

Any minor skin irritation should be viewed as a potentially dangerous sign and dealt with as early as possible. The management of common skin problems of amputees is discussed in Table 11–1.

Weight Changes

Amputees frequently lose substantial weight before and/or after amputation. Since prosthetic socket shape remains constant while the residual limb shape fluctuates, a weight gain or loss of only 5 lb may change the proper fit of the pros-

thesis and lead to skin problems. Therefore, the amputee should be encouraged to stay within 5 lb of the fitting weight if it is medically sound to do so.

Joint Contractures

In the lower extremity, contractures of the hips are very limiting because they make it difficult to extend the hip and to keep the center of gravity in the normal location. If the center of gravity is displaced, more energy is required for ambulation. A knee flexion contracture may limit the successful fitting of a prosthesis. Treatment consists of early range of motion exercise at the proximal joints and proper bed positioning.

In the upper extremity, scapular limitation of motion can affect the appropriate activation of prosthetic arm components. Intact scapular motion is especially important in the patient with bilateral upper extremity amputation. Glenohumeral contracture may limit the use of the arm prosthesis as a functional assistive device. Early range of motion exercises of the entire shoulder girdle, described earlier in this chapter, will help prevent such contractures.

Energy Expenditure

The most important determinant of functional wear of a lower extremity prosthesis is whether or not the amputee can safely expend the energy required for ambulation. Too many geriatric amputees have been fitted with prostheses only to be confined to a wheelchair because they had insufficient cardiovascular reserve to tolerate the increased energy expenditure required to walk while wearing the prosthesis. Wheelchair ambulation may be the most practical and safest level of function for such patients.

Intermittent Claudication

The major cause of lower extremity amputation is generalized occlusive arterial disease. If one lower extremity is amputated because of vascular disease, chances are the remaining extremity is also at risk for amputation. If substantial claudication, ulceration, or pregangrenous

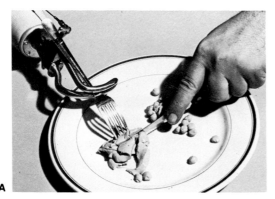

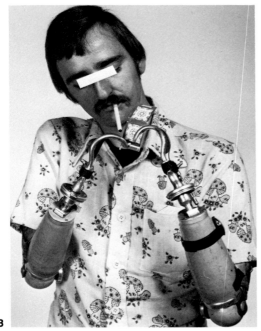

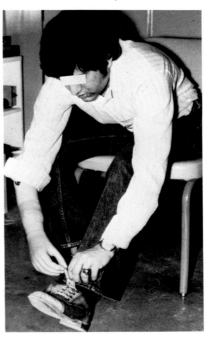

changes exist in the remaining extremity, ambulation with the prosthesis may place too much demand on impaired circulation and produce severe pain in the remaining extremity. Thus, use of the prosthesis may hasten the need for amputation of the "normal" extremity—amputation that would not have been required as quickly had the patient continued to function using a wheelchair.

Neuroma

Any nerve that is cut forms a distal neuroma as it heals. In some cases, these nodular bundles of axons in connective tissue cause pain as the prosthesis applies pressure. Initially, relief may be obtained by modifying the socket. The neuroma may be injected locally with 50 mg lidocaine hydrochloride (Xylocaine®) and 40 mg triamcinolone acetonide (Kenalog®). These injections can be combined with ultrasound therapy. Phenolization of the neuroma may relieve pain for a longer period. Desensitization of the neuroma can be aided sometimes by tapping and vibration. Surgical excision with phenolization and silicone capping has been advocated for some cases.

TABLE 11–1. *Common skin problems of amputees*

Skin problem	Characteristics, probable causes	Treatment
Edema	Proximal choking of stump by socket	Modification of prosthesis
Contact dermatitis	Sensitivity to skin cream, soap, stump sock wool, plastic resins in prosthetic socket	Cool compresses; antipruritic lotions; steroid cream
Posttraumatic epidermoid cysts	Long-term prosthetic wear in above-knee amputee, occurring near proximal medial portion of prosthesis; usually staphylococcal infection	Warm compresses; systemic antibiotics; surgical excision of chronic uninfected nodules
Folliculitis	Staphylococcal infection of hair follicle producing inflammatory papule or pustule; aggravated by prosthetic wear; maceration of skin with bacterial invasion due to warmth and perspiration in summer months	Thin nylon sheath worn between skin and stump sock; more frequent changes of stump socks; discontinue wearing prosthesis until problem subsides
Furuncles	Staphylococcal infection of pilosebaceous apparatus, producing larger and more painful papules than in folliculitis	Warm compresses; incision; drainage; discontinue wearing prosthesis; may need systemic antibiotics
Nonspecific eczema	Weeping, itching, nonhealing plaque of dermatitis over distal aspect of stump; may be dry and scaly, then moist; may wax and wane over many years; may be secondary to edema and congestion of distal residual limb; poorly fitting prosthesis	Modification of prosthesis; local steroid application
Intertriginous dermatitis	Irritation of skin surfaces that are in constant apposition, compounded by excessive sweating and constant moisture, in inguinal region or infolding of redundant skin at end of limb	Instruction in proper hygiene—cleaning apposing folds of skin, applying drying powders
Adherent scars	Constant rubbing of scar tissue on prosthesis leads to skin breakdown and ulceration	Prevention by massage; cream preparations to soften scar tissue; modification of prosthetic socket to relieve pressure or friction on scar
Callus formation	Elevated area of hyperkeratosis at point of friction or pressure	Socket modification if calloused area is sensitive or ulcerating
Ulceration	Excessive socket pressure or motion of limb in socket	Socket modification; adding or reducing thickness of stump socks; keeping base of ulcer clean; discontinue wearing prosthesis until ulcer is healed

Phantom Pain

Phantom pain may have a delayed onset compared with phantom sensation. Most phantom pain decreases in intensity and then disappears within a few weeks to months. However, varying degrees of incapacity accompany pain in the few amputees for whom it is a persistent problem.

Chronic, troublesome phantom pain appears more often in amputees with the following characteristics:

1. Pain persisting more than 3 weeks following amputation.
2. Compulsive, self-reliant personality.
3. Amputation following a disease process present for more than 1 year.
4. Unemployment for more than 1 year after limb loss.

Phantom pain occurs much less frequently in patients under 35 years of age than in older patients. It also may be triggered by autonomic functions such as micturition, defecation, and ejaculation.

Successful management of phantom pain has been irregular and unpredictable, despite the numerous remedies that have been attempted. These include wearing of a prosthesis, local injections at phantom pain trigger points, chemical or surgical sympathectomy, transcutaneous nerve stimulation, behavior modification, and psychosocial counseling.

PSYCHOSOCIAL ADJUSTMENT

Needs and Perceptions of the Amputee

Amputation rehabilitation, as in other areas of disability, must consider both the expressed and the covert needs of the patient. The physician must consider the amputation experience within the patient's own terms and relate the experience to the patient's environment. If the usual goal of rehabilitation is to assist the patient to become incorporated as a worthwhile person into an able-bodied world, then medical care necessarily includes restoration of useful function, restoration of normal appearance, and reduction of pain. But helping the patient achieve maximum vocational, avocational, and economic potential also helps to restore self-worth and self-esteem.

Phases of Adjustment to Amputation

The phases of adjustment to amputation frequently include shock, defensive retreat, acknowledgment, and adaptation. The initial reaction to a physical catastrophe such as amputation is often shock, which leaves the individual with a feeling of overall helplessness. Shock is more marked in the traumatic amputee, who had no psychological preparation for the limb loss. As the patient begins to mobilize his resources, the phase of defensive retreat is prompted by a need for anxiety reduction and accomplished by using avoidance mechanisms such as fantasy, denial, and magical or rigid thinking. During the period of acknowledgment, the patient begins to deal realistically with the change in his or her body. This frequently results in a period of stress characterized by depression and mourning. The process of adaptation involves a reorganization whereby the patient develops a renewed sense of self-respect, productivity, achievement, and social acceptance.

Not all patients will progress sequentially through these phases. Early fitting of a prosthesis with restoration of function may help to reduce the initial shock and hasten the process of acknowledgment and adaptation. The amputee's reaction to amputation usually reflects other patterns of reaction to prior life crises. There is seldom a direct relationship between the extent of physical loss and the patient's psychological difficulties. These difficulties depend more on individual personality than on the type of amputation sustained. Many patients perceive the amputation as a punishment, which produces feelings of guilt and shame. Introversion, self-pity, feelings of inferiority, and social isolation may result.

Adaptation is facilitated by a combination of individual and group therapy to educate as well as provide support. Individual therapy typically consists of emotional support by a psychologist, social worker, or other health care professional to work through feelings of loss, anger, and grief. Relaxation and assertiveness training may also be helpful. The therapeutic group should be limited to 5 to 10 inpatients and outpatients. It focuses on dealing with feelings of helplessness, isolation, and depression. The group is also an effective means of educating patients about issues shared by all of them, including:

1. Stump care.
2. Home exercise and fitness.
3. Prosthetic selection and operation.
4. Prevention of further amputations.
5. Assistive devices for activities of daily living.
6. Government assistance programs.

In addition, a family conference may be useful during the preprosthetic phase and prior to discharge. The family should be reassured that the considerable anxiety the patient may demonstrate on discharge is normal. In fact, it is common for the amputee to have regressed to a less functional level by the time of the first follow-up appointment after discharge. Setting up community support before discharge will help minimize anxiety and regressive behavior.

Vocational Implications

Most amputees who had professional, managerial, or executive careers before amputation are able to return to their former employment with the aid of prostheses. Amputees with a lower educational level, especially if their work involved heavy lifting and other manual labor, generally need training and education to prepare for a different job.

The person with unilateral arm amputation may desire to change the terminal device attached to the prosthesis for different vocational, recreational, and social activities. Office work is best performed with an aluminum hook or functional hand, factory or manual labor with a voluntary opening steel hook, and jobs involving frequent public contact with a cosmetic hand. Regardless of the job task performed, the prosthesis is used to assist as the normal hand is used for manipulation.

The occupation of the leg amputee may need to be adapted to any impairment in walking, climbing, standing, pushing, pulling, and balancing. The extent of impairment depends on the level of amputation and whether it is unilateral or bilateral. At the above-knee level, jobs should be avoided that require frequent stair climbing or walking up and down ramps, uphill, and over sand or mud. A unilateral below-knee amputee can drive an automatic or standard transmission vehicle, while a unilateral above-knee amputee should only drive an automatic vehicle.

Another consideration when the amputee returns to work is the climate of the work environment. A hot, humid environment promotes skin maceration, friction between the stump and socket, and prosthetic deterioration.

Recreation

Participation in recreational activities not only promotes emotional well-being but also helps prevent the adverse consequences of a sedentary lifestyle. Excessive weight increases the load at the stump-socket interface of the lower extremity. Physical fitness is vital for preventing amputation of a second limb in patients with dysvascular disease.

Special prostheses and equipment are available to enable amputees to participate in the sports they enjoyed before amputation or in undertaking new endeavors. These include:

1. Above-knee and below-knee water-resistant prostheses for swimmers (Fig. 11–5A).
2. An adjustable, foot-ankle unit for the proficient swimmer and scuba diver.
3. Prostheses and equipment for skiers (Fig. 11–5B).
4. Devices for golfers with upper and lower extremity amputation.
5. Terminal devices to enable bowling, holding a rod and reel (Fig. 11–5C), playing baseball, holding tools, firing a pistol, or swimming.

Wheelchair sports—basketball, tennis, racing, field events, and weight-lifting—are also open to amputees.

CONGENITAL LIMB DEFICIENCY

The management of congenital limb deficiency is quite different from dealing with an adult who has an acquired amputation. The effect of the limb deficiency on the infant is nil, but frequently the parents experience guilt, pity, or rejection. Guilt feelings should be discussed openly with the parents. Point out that the causes of congenital limb defects, as well as preventive measures, are rarely known. However, as these children grow, they will become aware of the difference between themselves and their peers. Preparing the child, the family, and other caretakers to deal with a different body image is an important rehabilitation goal.

The child with a congenital limb deficiency should be evaluated by a prosthetic team as soon after birth as possible. Most congenital upper extremity amputees should be fitted with a prosthesis in the first 4 to 6 months of life to facilitate gross two-handed activities. A child with a congenital lower extremity deficiency should be fit-

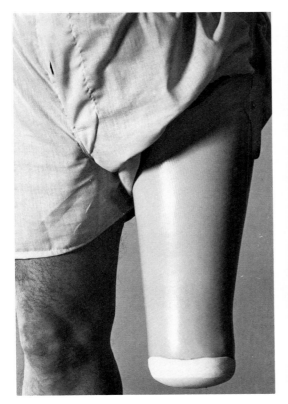

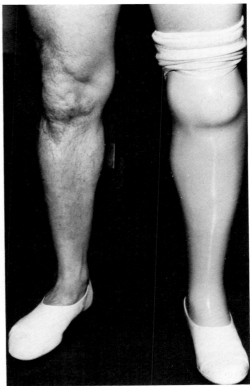

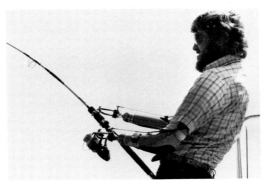

FIG. 11–5. Devices that enable amputees to participate in sports. **Upper right:** Water-resistant prosthesis aligned for walking with thin rubber slipper, which allows walking to beach or pool, showering while standing, or swimming. **Upper left:** Special pad attached for snow skiing and protective socket on stump lessens tendency to injure stump if amputee falls. [From Rubin, G., and Fleiss, D. (1983): Devices to enable persons with amputation to participate in sports. *Arch. Phys. Med. Rehabil.*, 64:37,39.] **Bottom:** Conventional body-powered prosthesis enables bilateral upper-limb amputee to manipulate fishing rod.

ted as soon as he shows signs of wanting to pull up to stand—usually at about 9 months of age. The development of muscle coordination and other milestones should be the same as for nondisabled children. Thus, children fitted at an early age are given the chance to incorporate the prosthesis into their natural body image.

Most children can be treated on an outpatient basis; parents usually make the best therapists because they spend much more time with the child than a health professional does. Usually, the lower extremity amputee has fewer problems wearing a prosthesis than the child with an upper extremity amputation. Since trying to walk is natural for children, and the prosthesis enables walking, adaptation is usually quick. In some upper extremity amputees, however, a great deal of encouragement is necessary to get the child to wear the prosthetic arm. At first, the upper extremity prosthesis may be more of a deterrent than an aid, but with time and family encouragement, this trend reverses.

Whenever possible, the juvenile amputee should take an active part in school, sports, community, and family activities. Most children who are amputees go on to achieve an optimum level of function, and the transition through life is easier if they are not set apart at an early age or given unnecessary special attention as they mature.

CARE OF STUMP SOCKS AND PROSTHESES

Stump Socks

Except in the case of a suction socket, a sock is usually worn over the skin of the amputated extremity, inside the socket of the prosthesis. Socks are worn to give additional padding, to allow for slight changes in stump size and shape, and to absorb perspiration. Although usually made of wool, they also may be acrylic fiber or cotton. Socks come in various thicknesses, designated by the number of ply. The most commonly used are 3-ply and 5-ply. A new prosthesis should fit comfortably when the patient is wearing a 3-ply sock. Usually, the socket needs modification if more than 10 to 15 plies of socks are needed for the patient to wear the prosthesis comfortably.

The amputee should wear a fresh sock daily and have a sufficient supply of socks to be able to store them for several days after washing to ensure thorough drying. Wool stump socks should be washed in lukewarm water using a mild soap, or in cold water using Woolite. Suds should be squeezed into the socks—never rubbed. Lifting the socks out of the water will cause them to stretch, and excessive wringing or twisting should be avoided. Drying can be hastened by rolling the sock in a towel to remove excess water. The socks should be dried at a moderate temperature and never against direct heat or in sunlight.

Prostheses

The prosthetic socket should be cleansed daily, preferably at night. The socket should be washed with warm water and a mild soap, wiped out with a cloth dampened in clean water, and allowed to dry thoroughly before the prosthesis is worn. Longevity of the prosthesis depends on many factors, including wear and tear on component parts, quality of prosthetic workmanship, and change of stump size, shape, and length. In general, the first prosthesis will usually need to be replaced within 18 months, but thereafter, prostheses should require less frequent replacement. Lower extremity prostheses require more frequent replacement than upper extremity prostheses because the lower extremity bears the body weight. Once the amputee has had the first prosthesis replaced, a lower extremity prosthesis should last an average of 2 to 4 years. An upper extremity prosthesis should be satisfactory for 3 to 5 years.

UNILATERAL BELOW-KNEE AMPUTATION IN A GERIATRIC PATIENT WITH PERIPHERAL ARTERIAL DISEASE

Report of a Case

HISTORY. This 66-year-old, overweight man was admitted to a general hospital for a gangrenous right leg with sepsis, ulcers, and intractable pain at rest. He had a 15-year history of maturity-onset diabetes mellitus that was being controlled with tolazamide, 250 mg/day. Two years ago, he had lymphedema, and 8 months ago, cellulitis of the right leg treated with systemic antibiotics. Diminished femoral and popliteal pulses were compatible with a 5-year history of intermittent claudication.

The gangrenous right leg was amputated at a mid-length below-knee level, and after suture removal, the stump was wrapped twice daily with 4-inch, elastic, compression bandages. He spent 3 weeks in the hospital, including regular visits to the physical therapy department for a preprosthetic program.

REHABILITATION MANAGEMENT. The primary therapeutic goal was to provide this patient with the most effective means of ambulation that would enable him to pursue retirement activities, without endangering the remaining leg.

Techniques of good skin hygiene were applied to the remaining leg, as well as to the stump. He was instructed to inspect his left leg and foot daily for signs of skin irritation or injury. Elastic support stockings were worn on the left leg to minimize edema and improve leg comfort.

The patient was put on a weight-reduction program with the goal of losing 50 lb. This included a diet with restricted caloric intake, which would still provide the 50% carbohydrate, 30% fat, and 20% protein required to prevent hypoglycemia while adequately controlling his diabetes. To aid not only in weight loss but also in preventing contractures, he began a program of water exercise that minimized weight-bearing on the stump and on the remaining leg.

During the second week of hospitalization, he experienced phantom pain, a common phenomenon in elderly patients with a preexisting disease process. It was managed successfully with TENS applied to the stump.

PROSTHETIC FITTING AND AMBULATION. Prosthetic fitting was postponed until the patient lost weight because the prosthetic socket would no longer fit properly after substantial weight loss. In addition, his excess weight would overtax his compromised vascular system during gait training. The patient was trained to ambulate with a walker and then crutches prior to discharge from the hospital. He was sent home on an active exercise program for both legs but emphasizing right knee and hip extension. He returned 6 months after amputation and a below-knee prosthesis was fitted. The prosthetic prescription was a patellar tendon bearing prosthesis with a supracondylar cuff to hold the prosthesis in place. The foot was a solid-ankle-cushion-heel (SACH) design bolted to the leg. This prosthetic prescription should allow him to return to most if not all previous home, work, and recreational activities.

The patient received 12 training sessions altogether, three times a week, on an outpatient basis. Gait training began with short periods of prosthetic wearing and static standing. As the skin tolerated the intimate fit of the prosthesis and no significant pain occurred, active walking was begun. He was advised to limit prosthesis wearing time whenever he experienced unusually severe pain in his left leg. He was fitted with special protective shoes with Plastiazote insoles to prevent injury to the left foot.

After discharge, the patient visited the physical therapist and prosthetist for follow-up of functional prosthetic goals and his family physician for evaluation of his vascular condition. During the first year following amputation, the condition of his remaining leg remained stable despite occasional episodes of intermittent claudication.

SUGGESTED READINGS

Banerjee, S. N., editor. (1982): *Rehabilitation Management of Amputees.* Williams and Wilkins, Baltimore.

Bender, L. F. (1974): *Prostheses and Rehabilitation after Arm Amputation.* Charles C Thomas, Springfield, Ill.

Friedmann, L. W. (1978): *Psychological Rehabilitation of the Amputee.* Charles C Thomas, Springfield, Ill.

Goldberg, R. T. (1984): New trends in the rehabilitation of lower extremity amputees. *Rehabil. Lit.,* 45:2–11.

Kegal, B., Webster, J. C., and Burgess, E. M. (1980): Recreational activities of lower extremity amputees: Survey. *Arch. Phys. Med. Rehabil.,* 61:258–264.

Kostiuk, J. P. (1981): *Amputation Surgery and Rehabilitation: The Toronto Experience.* Churchill Livingstone, New York.

Levine, A. M. (1984): The elderly amputee. *Am. Fam. Physician,* 29:177–182.

Miroslaw, V. (1978): *Amputations and Prostheses.* Bailliere Tindall, London.

Redhead, R. G. (1984): The place of amputation in the management of the ischaemic lower limb in the dysvascular geriatric patient. *Int. Rehabil. Med.,* 6:68–71.

Thompson, D. M., and Haran, D. (1983): Living with an amputation: The patient. *Int. Rehabil. Med.,* 5:165–169.

Wolfgang, G. L. (1984): Complex congenital anomalies of the lower extremities: Femoral bifurcation, tibial hemimelia, and diastasis of the ankle. Case report and review of the literature. *J. Bone Joint Surg.,* 66:453–458.

Medical Rehabilitation,
edited by L. S. Halstead et al.
Raven Press, New York © 1985.

CHAPTER 12

Disabilities Caused by Cancer

Raul Villaneuva

University of Texas Medical School, Houston, and Private Practice, McAllen, Texas 78501

Rehabilitation of the cancer patient with the goal of restoring function and improving the quality of life is becoming more critical as more patients survive beyond 5 years. Like other chronic illnesses or severe injury, either primary tumor or metastasis may produce significant disability. The type and stage of the tumor has a profound effect on what therapeutic modality is selected at any given stage of the cancer's progression or remission. Therefore, disability such as hemiplegia resulting from cancer is treated differently than if it had resulted from vascular insufficiency or thrombosis, and often with dramatic improvement. Constant contact with the oncologist, whether a surgeon, radiotherapist, or chemotherapist, must be coordinated with the efforts of the primary care physician and other members of the therapeutic team.

CARCINOMA OF THE BREAST

The treatment plan for rehabilitating the patient with carcinoma of the breast depends on how far advanced the disease is on diagnosis. Will she require radiotherapy and chemotherapy before surgery, or mastectomy alone? The patient who postponed seeking treatment until her disease was far advanced will require palliative radiotherapy followed by chemotherapy. Depending on the tumor's response to treatment, her rehabilitation program will need frequent readjustment as she experiences markedly limited shoulder range of motion, varying degrees of neurological involvement of the brachial plexus, edema and lymphedema, disabling pain, and ulceration of the skin.

Presurgical Evaluation

As you take the history, note any underlying conditions that could interfere with rehabilitation after mastectomy. Is there a history of trauma, injury, or disease of the bony or soft structures of the shoulder that may have limited its range of motion? Investigate the possibility of fractures, subluxation, dislocation, muscle tears, tendonitis, bursitis, capsulitis, myofascitis, or arthritic conditions. During the physical examination, record any signs of limited range of motion, muscle atrophy, or nerve impairment. Goniometric measurements are taken at the initial visit and periodically during the course of radiotherapy.

Managing Complications of Radiotherapy

Special precautions must be taken in planning a rehabilitation program for patients who underwent radiotherapy prior to mastectomy, or lumpectomy. Because resulting decreased tissue vascularization delays healing, the patient should be constantly supervised and exercise should be less forceful than in other medical conditions. Avoid heat treatments to the irradiated area, which may produce severe burns.

Throughout the period of radiotherapy, the patient performs range of motion (ROM) exercises with the help of her family. Because irradiated structures may fibrose in a shortened position at any time within this period, the exercises should be performed two or three times a day for 6 months and then at least once a day for a period of 1 to 2 years. The patient who had limited range of motion before diagnosis of cancer or who is markedly depressed or anxious may benefit from daily supervision in a program that also includes massage and active-assistive range of motion exercises to avoid development of contractures or pain. When radiotherapy is completed, the patient is sent home for approximately 3 months and then returns for surgery. Continuing to perform the prescribed exercises during this interval is critical for successful post-surgical outcome.

Exercise After Mastectomy

A patient can begin exercising while bedfast as early as the third day after mastectomy. Passive flexion, abduction, and abduction-external rotation are done to evaluate the mobility of the shoulder, without mobilizing the skin flaps or applying undue tension on the surgical wound. Mobilization of the flaps while the suction catheters are in place may cause the separation of a portion of the flaps, the formation of seromas prone to infection, and the early formation of lymphedema.

At this time, the patient is instructed in:

1. Positioning to avoid stress on the shoulder or undue pressure on the ulnar nerve at the elbow.
2. Relaxation exercises to avoid tightness of the shoulder girdle.
3. Active ROM for the elbow, wrist, and fingers of the involved extremity.
4. One-handed activities of daily living.

By the fifth postoperative day, if the suction catheters have been removed, new goniometric measurements are taken with passive range of motion. Take baseline circumferential and volumetric measurements of both arms and provide guidelines for proper skin and hand care. In addition, check for any possible tightness of the shoulder girdle musculature, i.e., the trapezius, the levator scapulae, and the rotator cuff. These muscles are more or less tender at palpation in the early postoperative phase. The frequency and severity of tenderness tend to increase when the patient is anxious or depressed, indicating myofascitis. Because myofascitis interferes with

rehabilitation, it should be treated specifically with massage, muscle relaxants, ultrasound, and moist heat if the patient did not undergo radiotherapy before mastectomy.

If the serratus anterior muscle is weak, instruct the patient to avoid lifting, pushing, or pulling. In addition, she should do all exercises for shoulder ROM in the supine position to minimize strain against the weak muscle, which could result in a tight and painful rotator cuff and limited range of motion in the shoulder.

Activities of Daily Living

Because complete healing may take several weeks, the patient and family are instructed in one-handed activities or the use of adaptive equipment. In addition, the patient is told to avoid activities against resistance. For the homemaker, we suggest the use of a serving cart to carry meals or other objects, walking with the vacuum cleaner rather than pulling and pushing it, and the use of a long-handled sponge. Participation in such activities as drawing and painting, weaving on an upright loom, macrame, lacing leather articles, and weaving with a Turkish knot frame will help increase the ROM of the affected shoulder. When the stitches have been removed and the patient is ready to be discharged, the rehabilitation program may be continued under the supervision of the primary care physician and a visiting nurse, physical therapist, or occupational therapist, as needed.

Preventing Lymphedema

Patients who have undergone a radical mastectomy or dissection of the axillary or inguinal lymph nodes are especially susceptible to developing lymphedema. Although therapeutic exercise promotes normal range of motion necessary for good fluid exchange in the limb, exercises against resistance and work activities may increase the edema. This results from increased circulation and muscle activity byproducts combined with decreased lymphatic flow. In most instances, kneading massage is contraindicated because it may damage the already overloaded and insufficient lymphatic vessels and valves, and because it is difficult to obtain equal amounts of pressure as the massage progresses from the distal to the proximal end of the extremity.

Early treatment of lymphedema is crucial. The following are some specific steps that can be used to prevent and treat lymphedema:

1. Avoid infection of involved extremity, burns, cuts, and insect bites, exposure of arm to intense oven heat, ingrown nails or cuticles, and excessive exercise.
2. Prescribe antibiotics for early postoperative period.
3. Mobilize arm to prevent seromas and accelerate healing of surgical wound.
4. Show patient how to squeeze skin of arm and compare its fullness with that of unaffected side.
5. Prescribe diuretics during postoperative period, especially if patient has cardiovascular problems or lives in hot, humid area.
6. If lymphangitis or cellulitis appears, completely rest limb, prescribe antibiotics, apply mild heat, discontinue pneumomassage, and apply elastic support.
7. When infection has subsided, apply pneumomassage for 3 hr twice a day for about 5 days or until lymphedema is reduced.
8. Fit Jobst elastic support after reduction has been accomplished.
9. Correct cardiac or renal insufficiency and hypertension to maximize benefits of pneumomassage.
10. At each visit, weigh patient and measure circumference and volume of affected limb.
11. Teach the patient and a family member how to measure the affected limb at least once a week; an office visit in 30 days is indicated if edema is increased by 25%-30%.
12. Continue pneumomassage at home, or use elastic wrapping. If edema remains greater than 30%, browning has occurred, and adequate reduction was not obtained during the final days of circulator treatment.

CANCER OF THE HEAD AND NECK

Of all cancer patients, those with cancer of the head and neck pose the greatest challenge.

Chronic smoking, alcoholism, loneliness, and aging interact to make the rehabilitation of these patients more difficult. Involved in their care are several specialists in addition to the primary care physicians and usual rehabilitation specialists (see Chapter 2). These specialists include head and neck surgeons, plastic surgeons, maxillofacial prosthodontists, intravenous hyperalimentation specialists, cosmetologists, and stomal therapists. Patients who require radiotherapy or neck surgery in addition to the primary surgery to remove the tumor from the face or mouth will require more extensive rehabilitation.

Impaired Speaking and Swallowing

Early rehabilitation of patients who will have structures necessary for speech or swallowing removed minimizes dysfunction. If properly trained, even a patient who has 50% of the tongue removed can speak with only a slight defect. In addition to speech problems, swallowing difficulty is experienced by patients who are left with 80% or all of the tongue removed, part of the mouth floor removed, or a flaccid cheek.

Prior to laryngectomy, audiological screening is performed. The patient's voice is taped, and a former patient who has become proficient at esophageal and artificial-larynx speech visits. Good diagnostic indicators of the patient's future ability to speak include motivation level, ability to understand and follow instructions, and hearing acuity. The operation and speech training are discussed with the patient and family to dispel fears and answer any questions.

Patients who undergo neck surgery that affects swallowing should be evaluated by serial electrodiagnostic studies. Strength duration and nerve irritability tests should be performed early and repeated daily or weekly, depending on the patient's status. Electromyographic studies should be done as early as 8 days postoperatively for the facial nerve and 12 days for the accessory nerve.

After a total glossectomy, the patient can facilitate swallowing by moving the head backward and contracting the musculature of the floor of the mouth. This technique moves the bolus to the oropharynx, where the soft palate descends over it and pushes it down into the esophagus. A small bolus with a good degree of moisture and consistency is preferred over a liquid for swallowing retraining.

Managing Muscle Weakness

When the posterior triangle of the neck is entered during a node biopsy or a modified or radical neck dissection, damage to the accessory nerve or its complete severance is possible. Paralysis usually results regardless of the degree of nerve damage. Another complication is bilateral sectioning of the jugular veins during surgical treatment of cancer. To prevent rupture of the carotid artery and the development of facial edema, these patients should avoid the Valsalva maneuver and should not be positioned face down for postural drainage.

Evaluation

Patients with a temporarily or permanently damaged accessory nerve are evaluated by measuring the space between the scapular border and the spine. Asking the patient to shrug the shoulders is not sufficient for evaluating the function of the trapezius muscle, although this

method has been recommended. The following procedure is more accurate:

1. View patient from behind, arms at the side and all clothing removed.
2. Observe location of scapula; if trapezius is weak, vertebral border of scapula will be displaced laterally and upward with a downward rotation.
3. Note space between vertebral border of scapula and vertebral spine; space will be wider on involved side if trapezius is weak.
4. If test is positive (2 and 3), ask patient to abduct the arm; abduction is usually limited to 90° and affected shoulder drops.
5. Patients with abnormal innervation of upper trapezius by upper cervical plexus are able to abduct to 160° by rotating and horizontally elevating the clavicle.
6. Weak midtrapezius muscle prohibits horizontal abduction against resistance.

Therapeutic Exercise

Early in the postoperative course, treatment indications and contraindications are similar regardless of the degree of nerve damage because, from a kinesiologic point of view, the pectoralis group is the main antagonist of the trapezius muscle (Table 12–1). Since each muscle that is

TABLE 12–1. *Kinesiology of the trapezius muscle*

Functions	Synergistic muscles	Antagonistic muscles
Elevation of shoulder and scapula by upper fibers	Levator scapulae Rhomboideus major Rhomboideus minor	Pectoralis major, lower fibers Pectoralis minor Subclavius Serratus anterior
Upward rotation of scapula by its upper and lower fibers	Serratus anterior	Anteriorly: Pectoralis major, lower fibers Pectoralis minor Posteriorly: Levator scapulae Rhomboideus minor Latissimus dorsi Rhomboideus major
Scapula and shoulder retraction by its middle fibers	Rhomboideus major Rhomboideus minor	Pectoralis major Pectoralis minor Serratus anterior

Adapted from Hollinshead, W. H. (1960): *Functional Anatomy of the Limbs and Back*, 2nd edit., W. B. Saunders, Philadelphia.

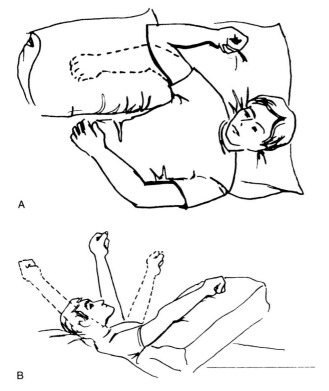

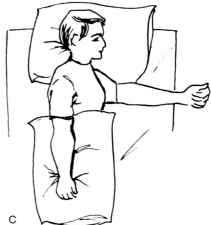

FIG. 12–1. Passive or active exercises done in the supine position. **A:** Patient changes from 45° of internal rotation to 45° of external rotation. **B:** Patient performs arm flexion; some manual resistance may be added 15-21 days after surgery. **C:** Patient lies on side opposite to the surgical site with hand positioned on a pillow for elevation and to avoid shortening of internal rotators.

synergistic with the trapezius in one motion is antagonistic in another, muscle substitution or replacement is impossible.

Table 12–1 illustrates how the different muscles contribute to shoulder dysfunction when the trapezius muscle is temporarily or permanently paralyzed. The pull against the remaining shoulder girdle muscles is further compounded if contractures of the pectoralis muscles are also present. Consequently, the following types of exercises are contraindicated in trapezius weakness or paralysis because they will worsen disability:

1. Any exercise while the patient is sitting or standing.
2. Codman's exercises (pendulum, finger ladder, or circumduction).
3. Any carrying, pulling, or pushing with the affected extremity.

All therapeutic exercises, therefore, are done in the supine position to avoid unnecessary pull against the involved musculature (Figs. 12–1, 12–2, and 12–3). Passive exercises are accomplished from the second through the fifth postoperative day, either while the patient is in bed or in the physical therapy department. During this time, emphasis is placed on proper positioning while in bed (see Fig. 12–1C), maintenance of full stretch of the pectoralis muscle, and attention to the surgical flaps.

For patients receiving radiotherapy to the head and neck, special precautions must be taken because irradiated tissue takes 7 to 14 days longer to heal than normal tissue, and the carotid artery has been denuded of its cover. Unusual pull at this time may result in seroma formation or wound dehiscence. Nevertheless, early mobilization of all joints involved is imperative. When the temporomandibular joint lies within the radiation field, complete contracture (trismus) may set in, making it impossible for the patient to open the mouth. The fibrosis resulting from irradiation

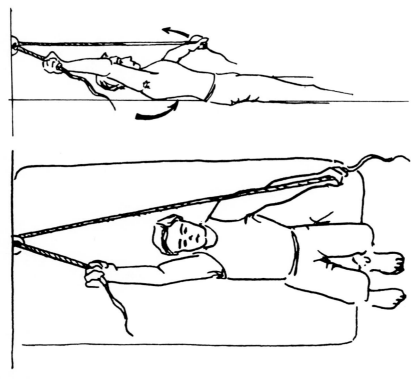

FIG. 12–2. Home pulley exercises for shoulder range of motion, always performed lying down, after mastectomy or mechanical dissection, or with weakness of the serratus anterior muscles. **Top:** Pulley at center of patient's midline to produce arm flexion. **Bottom:** Pulley away from the midline, to produce arm abduction.

of the neck can limit the ROM of the cervical spine, resulting in secondary pain. All of these patients should be evaluated early and placed in a preventive program of ROM and massage with gradual skin mobilization. Due to the increased risk of burn, they should not undergo any heat treatments.

Active-assistive, ROM exercises performed in the prone position may be added to the passive program 6 days after surgery. After the 15th day, the patient begins active range of motion exercises for the shoulder (see Figs. 12–1A, B, and 12–2), isometric exercises for the rhomboid muscles (see Fig. 12–3), and shoulder shrugging. Active flexion, extension and lateral flexion, and rotation of the neck with gradual passive stretch to gain neck mobility are performed, but constantly observe the skin flaps during these exercises. Add passive stretch of the pectoralis groups 3 weeks postoperatively, and add grad-

ual, manual resistive exercises to strengthen the rhomboids, levator scapulae, and serratus anterior the second month after surgery.

Gradually increase resistance with weights, as tolerated by the patient, to increase strength and endurance (Fig. 12–4). Although muscle substitution is not expected when the trapezius muscle is paralyzed, a balance between a stretched-out pectoralis muscle and the attainment of the best strength possible by the levator scapulae, rhomboids, and serratus anterior will undoubtedly result in a more functional and cosmetically acceptable shoulder.

Activities of Daily Living

Beginning on the second day after neck surgery, activities of daily living are allowed with the unaffected arm. The affected extremity, however, should be used only to assist. Patients should wear a sling while they are up and about except

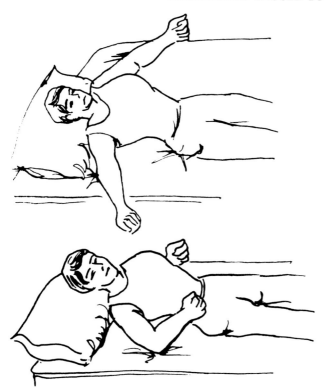

FIG. 12–3. Isometric exercises. **Top:** Patient pushes arms against mattress to gain shoulder retraction and reinforce midtrapezius and rhomboideus muscles. **Bottom:** Patient pushes elbows against mattress to gain strength in midtrapezius and rhomboideus muscles.

when they are performing activities of daily living. Because the sling eliminates the gravitational pull on the shoulder musculature caused by the weight of the arm, it not only minimizes shoulder drop and pain but also eliminates the unnecessary stretching of the levator scapulae and the rhomboid muscles. At this time, the patient and the family are given a list of precautions:[1]

1. Maintain good posture to prevent chest muscles from tightening and pulling against weaker muscles on back of shoulder and to minimize discomfort when wearing brace.
2. Avoid sitting for long periods, and use chair with straight back.
3. Wear arm support at all times when sitting, standing, or walking.

4. Lie on your back as much as possible when sleeping and place back pillow under your spine between your shoulder blades and neck pillow under your neck.
5. Do not use your (involved) arm until advised to do so.
6. Do not lift or carry objects weighing more than 3 lb with your (involved) arm.
7. Do not lie on your (involved) side.
8. Place your (involved) hand on your hip to relieve pressure under the arm, whenever necessary, when wearing the brace.

On the sixth postoperative day, the patient may begin such activities as weaving on a floor or upright loom, painting, sanding, working with ceramics, or typing. To eliminate gravitational pull, an overhead, counterbalanced sling is worn as the patient performs these activities (Fig. 12–5).

Orthoses

If the patient's vocation requires prolonged, unsupported use of the affected arm in front of

[1]From Villaneuva, R., Drane, J. B., Gunn, A. E., Brandon, B., Knight, N., and Bell K. (1976): Rehabilitation of the cancer patient. In: *Cancer Patient Care at M. D. Anderson Hospital and Tumor Institute*, edited by R. L. Clark and C. D. Howe. Year Book, Chicago.

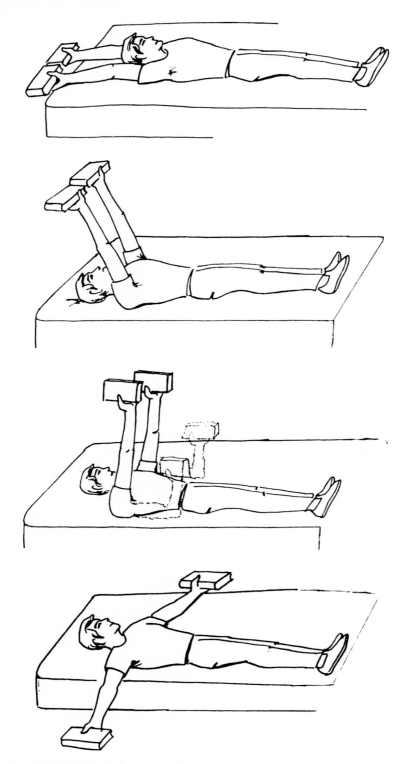

FIG. 12–4. Supine patient performs resistive exercises using weights to strengthen the rhomboideus, levator scapulae, and serratus anterior muscles.

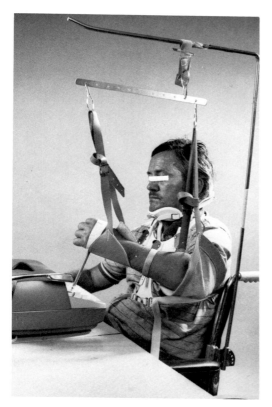

FIG. 12–5. Overhead sling supports patient's upper extremity as he touches typewriter keys with pencil.

the body, wearing an orthosis will result in a more functional shoulder that is less painful at the end of the day (Fig. 12–6). Patients who would especially benefit from an orthosis are teachers, beauticians, welders, carpenters, painters, butchers, cooks, and anyone whose job requires a considerable amount of carrying, lifting, pushing, or pulling.

Maxillofacial Rehabilitation

As more patients survive head and neck cancer for longer periods of time, the use of functional and cosmetic prostheses in the rehabilitation of surgically treated cancer patients with gross defects and deformities is becoming more common. The maxillofacial prosthodontist can repair oral and facial defects resulting from orbital exenteration, removal of the external ear, and loss of the entire nose that cannot be repaired

satisfactorily by the plastic surgeon alone. Prosthetic appliances are also constructed to cover a surgical defect that the surgeon does not want covered with skin grafts, enabling adequate inspection of the treated areas during follow-up examinations. The objectives of using maxillofacial prosthetics in rehabilitating head and neck cancer patients include: improving appearance; restoring function; protecting tissues; and, facilitating psychological adjustment. These prosthetic aids, especially obturators, may obviate the need for subsequent surgical procedures, hasten healing, facilitate eating, improve the patient's emotional well-being, and shorten hospitalization. There are numerous advantages of using a maxillofacial prosthesis immediately after surgery (Table 12–2):

1. Serves as matrix for surgical dressing.
2. Protects wound from food debris.
3. Supports oral and facial structures in normal positions by minimizing scar contracture.
4. Protects wound from trauma.
5. Reduces possibility of postoperative hemorrhage by maintaining pressure directly or indirectly on split-thickness skin graft used to line cheek flap.
6. Improves patient's speech and prevents formation of compensatory speech habits requiring correction later.
7. Enables patient to take food by mouth postoperatively, obviating need for nasogastric feeding tube.

Before any patient with head and neck cancer is treated by surgery, radiotherapy, and/or chemotherapy, the required prostheses are designed, fitted, and fabricated, according to measurements taken from cephalometric lateral head roentgenograms, occlusal intraoral roentgenograms, and impressions of the face, cranium, and jaws. These include surgical splints, stents, surgical obturators, and implant prostheses for use during the primary surgical procedure. During preoperative planning for using prostheses, consider the availability of adequate soft tissue for primary closure without tension, the ease of adjusting the size and configuration of the pros-

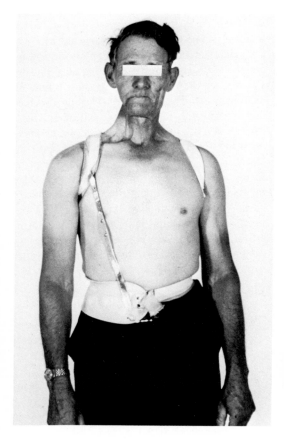 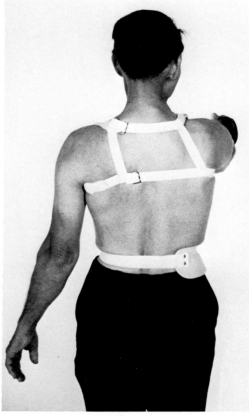

FIG. 12–6. Patient wears orthosis to compensate for trapezius weakness. **Left:** Front view. **Right:** Back view.

thesis during the operation, and the ability to secure the prosthesis to the remaining portions of the mandible. The successful use of prostheses depends on these and other critical factors. Avoid using metal implant prostheses in patients who will undergo radiotherapy.

ADJUSTMENT TO MAXILLOFACIAL DEFORMITY

Report of a Case

HISTORY. This 62-year-old man was admitted to a hospital in the sun belt that specialized in treating cancer. The diagnosis was advanced basal cell carcinoma. He reported a long history of prolonged sun exposure from outdoor work, including 26 years of highway construction as a project engineer. There was also a strong family history of the disease; both of his parents, of northern European descent and light complected, had been treated for basal cell carcinoma.

The patient's basal cell carcinoma first occurred at age 30 and was treated by cauterization; 18 months later, the condition recurred and he underwent several operations over the next 15 years as the disease invaded his upper jawbone and blinded his right eye.

SURGICAL AND PROSTHETIC MANAGEMENT. The first operation was done to remove a tumor from his right eye socket. Subsequent surgery was more radical; his hard palate, 80% of his upper jawbone, septum, sinuses, and the left side of his face were excised, resulting in the loss of most of his eyesight in the left eye. Two weeks after surgery, he received his first obturator, which enabled him to eat, drink, and talk. Application of a temporary prosthetic device to cover the surgical area enabled him to appear in public and return home to visit his family.

REHABILITATION MANAGEMENT. Because the patient's deformities and disease preempted returning

TABLE 12–2. *Maxillofacial prostheses used in management of cancer patients*

Type of prosthesis	Time of application	Purpose
Surgical implant	Immediate—during operation	Replaces portions of mandible removed surgically
Cone locator, docking device, intraoral cone	During radiation treatments	Enables decreased daily set-up time on machine; improves accuracy of daily duplication of field of radiation; eliminates passage of rays through major salivary glands and muscles of mastication, which prevents development of xerostomia and trismus
Radiation stent	During radiation treatments	Displaces normal tissue from fields of radiation; shields underlying tissues; holds jaws open; maintains movable tissue (tongue, cheeks, lips, soft palate, floor of mouth) in static position
Fluoride carrier	During radiation involving major salivary glands	Applies 1% sodium fluoride gel topically to prevent radiation-induced dental caries and, ultimately, necrosis and loss of mandible
Interim obturator	After initial healing of wound, usually 6–8 weeks after operation	Extends into palatal defect to improve voice quality and enhance retention and stability of immediate prosthesis; includes artificial teeth to aid in masticating food and improve articulation and appearance
Removable mandibular resection appliance	Same as obturator	Corrects centric relationship between mandible and maxilla following resection of one side of mandible, thereby preventing malocclusion and inability to chew food well; removed after remaining muscles of mastication have been retrained
Dynamic bite opener	Same as obturator	Prevents trismus after operation around temporomandibular joints and muscles of mastication by applying light, continuous pressure on jaws
Temporary facial prosthesis	Same as obturator	Compensates for facial defects when surgeon elects to delay surgical correction of facial defect

to his former lifestyle, rehabilitation focused on creating a new lifestyle that would accommodate continued treatments. After the surgical wounds had healed, the patient was referred to a cancer rehabilitation center for recuperation and readjustment. He reported that the handicrafts, gymnastic facilities, relaxing in the gardens, and discussions with other demoralized patients helped alleviate his depression and anxiety and prepare him to enter social interactions despite his severe facial deformity. He felt, however, that adjustment to his previous cancer treatments would have been facilitated if the surgeons and other physicians had been able to take the time to explain the reasons for the tests and the various types of chemotherapy. Patient education was a vital component of the rehabilitation program, but, unfortunately, not of his acute care in the hospital.

Because of his restricted eyesight and limited ability to travel, the patient was unable to resume gainful employment. The constant changes in eyesight compounded by frequent updating of his prostheses would have required absence from work for a week at least

every 3 months. Recreation was somewhat restricted for financial reasons, causing the family to forfeit vacation trips. After returning home, however, he often visited the family lake house to fish and enjoy nature with his cat as a companion. He was able to complete light construction tasks such as building a carport for his boat.

PSYCHOSOCIAL ADJUSTMENT. Sessions with a psychiatrist who specialized in therapy for cancer patients helped him cope with the various phases of disease progression and deformity. The psychiatrist suggested that as an outdoor, physical type of person, he could channel his rejection-related anger away from his loved ones and caretakers by boxing, hitting a punching bag, and hitting a chain-link fence with a baseball bat to relieve tension.

Because his wife was an art teacher and strongly affected by aesthetics and physical appearance, she had a difficult time adjusting to his facial deformity even while he wore his lifelike prosthesis. Although she no longer desired sexual relations or other physical contact with him, they were able to preserve their relationship as a close friendship. He was gradually able to accept the rejection of his family and friends as a "knee-jerk" rather than intentional response. However, he remained hesitant about public appearances and exposure to new acquaintances.

OSTEOGENIC SARCOMA WITH AMPUTATION

Rehabilitation of patients who require amputation due to cancer differs from that of patients who require amputation for other reasons. Because the entire host bone must be removed in osteogenic sarcoma, the level of amputation is generally higher. Consequently, hemipelvectomy or interscapulothoracic amputations are more common than below-knee or below-elbow amputations. In addition, amputees with cancer are usually younger than other amputees.

Managing Lower-Extremity Amputation

While most amputees are able to be fitted for a prosthesis immediately after surgery, followed by application of a permanent prosthesis, fitting may have to be delayed for patients with amputations above the knee. Chemotherapy may cause weight loss with corresponding rapid changes in stump size, as well as decreased strength and endurance. If these patients do not wait until their weight stabilizes, the socket will require several adjustments and become obsolete in a short time. Fitting conventional prosthetic components and gait training can be implemented once weight is stable (see Chapter 11).

Greater mechanical loss and muscle imbalance result from hip disarticulation, modified hemipelvectomy, or hemipelvectomy than from above-knee or below-knee amputation. These mechanical problems, which often impede sitting and walking, can be corrected with the help of a molded laminated socket with a flat base as well as ambulatory aids and gait training (Table 12–3).

The home program should include adaptive equipment for proper grooming and toiletry (see Chapters 5 and 6) and exercises to maintain spinal mobility, prevent scoliosis, and relieve low back pain. Persistent pain mandates evaluation to rule out metastasis.

Managing Upper-Extremity Amputation

Interscapulothoracic and shoulder disarticulation are the most common levels of amputation in treating cancer. Although few of these patients can be expected to wear an upper-extremity prosthesis for a long time, fabricating a cosmetic shoulder from liquid foam may make the prosthesis more acceptable. The cosmetic shoulder usually is constructed from a cast of the patient's shoulder made preoperatively or from reversing a cast made of the remaining shoulder. A combination breast and shoulder prosthesis is available for the female patient who also has undergone a mastectomy. Fitting the prosthesis as soon as the stitches are removed enables the patient to wear it at discharge from the hospital. Once sufficient healing has occurred, a terminal device (see Chapter 11) can be ordered and the patient can begin lessons in one-handed activities of daily living (see Chapters 5 and 15).

TUMORS OF THE CENTRAL NERVOUS SYSTEM

Two to five percent of all tumors are primary tumors of the central nervous system; 80% of these affect the brain, while 4,000 new cases of primary spinal cord tumor are detected every year. Half of all primary brain tumors are gliomas, mostly glioblastomas, with meningiomata the most prevalent nongliomatous tumors. Pituitary adenomas account for 12% to 18% of intracranial neoplasms. Children, however, are most likely to have medulloblastomas (30%) and astrocytomas (30%) located in the posterior cranial fossa.

In comparison, most primary spinal cord tumors are meningiomas and neurofibromas (50%), usually at the thoracic levels, while gliomas represent another 23%, half of which arise at the filum terminale or conus medullaris.

Systemic neoplasia more frequently metastasizes to the brain than to the spinal cord, with cerebral metastasis the most frequent neurological complication of systemic cancer regardless of origin. From 20% to 40% of all tumors eventually metastasize to the brain, most commonly originating from the lung or breast,

TABLE 12–3. *Management of mechanical imbalance in high-level amputation*

Level of amputation	Effect on balance and gait	Correction
Hip disarticulation	Abdominal and hip-elevating muscle retention enables correct gait, free of vaulting	Cane needed only when walking on uneven ground, grass, or thick carpet
	Added thickness of prosthetic bucket elevates hip on amputated side more than on normal side, upsetting balance when sitting	Place small foam cushion under normal side
Modified hemipelvectomy	Loss of ischial tuberosity and iliac crest to symphysis pubis results in loss of abdominal musculature needed for pelvic tilt and impairment of hip-elevating muscle; patient cannot clear floor during swing phase of gait	Functional gait requires vaulting with assistance of cane or crutch.
	Soft tissue remaining on amputated side compresses within prosthetic bucket more than on normal side	Place cushion under prosthesis
Hemipelvectomy	Lost function of abdominal and hip-elevator muscles makes walking and sitting very fatiguing	Fit patient with endoskeletal type of prosthesis; crutches or canes always needed for vaulting and walking

and secondarily from the large bowel, pancreas, or kidney. More than half of all patients with malignant melanoma also develop brain metastases.

The most common primary sources of epidural metastases with spinal cord compression are breast, lung, Hodgkin's disease, and prostatic carcinoma. Ninety percent of these patients initially present with pain localized to the site of spinous metastasis.

Managing Spinal Cord Tumor

Since there is little difference between the symptoms caused by primary tumors and metastatic involvement of the vertebral body or canal, rehabilitation for both types is similar.

A thorough survey of the patient admitted with neurological symptoms related to the spinal cord or cauda equina includes one or more of the following: bone survey, CT scan, myelography, and electromyography. If the symptoms are of short duration, and evaluation confirms the presence of an incomplete lesion or an incomplete block, a decompressive laminectomy usually is performed. After complete postsurgical healing, irradiation may begin. If complete

paraplegia with loss of bladder and bowel control lasts for more than 24 hr, however, radiation and chemotherapy may be the treatment of choice.

Progressive Mobilization

After decompressive laminectomy, motor strength in the lower extremities of patients with incomplete lesions gradually returns within a short time. The rehabilitation program for these patients begins at bedside after the laminectomy. It usually consists of active-assistive to active exercises for the lower extremities, strengthening of the upper extremities, and training in activities of daily living. Depending on the level of functional return, some patients may require adaptive equipment to gain independence. These patients are measured for the appropriate brace within 72 hr after laminectomy, and the patient and family are instructed in how to align and use it.

The program progresses gradually to include transfer activities, the use of parallel bars, and ambulation with assistive devices (see Chapter 15). The patient who does not regain sufficient strength for ambulation is taught to perform all activities of daily living using the wheelchair

(Fig. 12–7). The majority of these patients become ambulatory in 2 to 3 weeks after surgery, while the others may require 2 or 3 months.

Some of the patients whose neurological deficit was complete and/or lasted for more than 24 hr regain some motor activity many months after treatment. This partial return of function can be used in transfer activities and in taking a few steps without bracing. The bladder and bowel program prescribed for these patients is the same as that outlined for patients with lesions to the spinal cord resulting from trauma (see Chapters 17 and 25).

Selecting Orthoses

Cancer patients usually require fewer orthoses than do patients with spinal impairment from other causes. For instance, the SOMI brace alone is often sufficient for patients with lesions from the basilar apophysis of the occiput down to T2 (Fig. 12–8). This brace facilitates not only mobilization of the patient but also the administration of radiotherapy. For patients with lesions at the thoracolumbar level, the braces most frequently prescribed are Jewett hyperextension, long Taylor-Knight, and chairback. (Indications for the use of these and similar orthoses are described in more detail in Chapter 6.) A butterfly band is preferred at the top of the latter two orthoses. This arrangement enables two or three higher levels of support to be attained. The lower end of the band should reach just below the costal margin at the intersection with the top of the lateral bar. This modification is particularly needed in cases of metastasis from rib 8 to rib 12 to provide protection for the ribs and thereby prevent the abdominal pad from exerting pressure against the lower costal cartilage.

When prescribing orthoses, also consider the progression of metastasis, which may occur in more than one area of the body. In a patient with a 60% collapse of T10, for example, review not only the X-ray films of the entire spine, but also those of the ribs, pelvis, sternum, clavicle, and scapula. These structures are used for support or counterpressure by the different braces.

A brace that can be modified as the disease progresses is the most practical choice. If the tumor produces new lesions at the spine of the scapula or clavicle, the uprights of a long Taylor-Knight brace can be removed, and the "cow horns" can be added to apply pressure over the tendon of the pectoralis major under the clavicle.

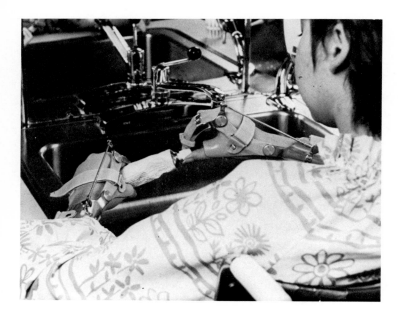

FIG. 12–7. Wheelchair-dependent patient with spinal tumor learns to brush teeth with splints compensating for upper extremity weakness.

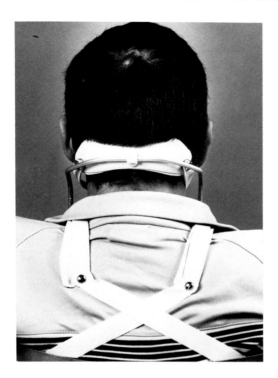

FIG. 12–8. SOMI brace supports neck and upper back without interfering with mobilization or radiotherapy.

Managing Tumors of the Brain

Tumors of the brain can cause such symptoms as monoplegia, paraplegia, quadriplegia, and speech and language disabilities that may subside when the tumors are surgically removed or reduced by irradiation. In many of these cases, the neurological deficit resolves and arm function, speech, or the ability to ambulate with minimal assistance returns from 2 weeks to several months after treatment is initiated.

Since functional status may change every few days, the patient should be reevaluated frequently. Despite possible recurrence of the tumor, functional restoration lasting for months or years may gain the patient enough time to become fully independent in activities of daily living or even return to previous employment. By contrast, most patients with damage to the central nervous system due to accident, trauma, or vascular disease seldom experience this degree of recovery and usually require more pro-

longed rehabilitation and hospitalization. Unlike the stroke patient, for example, the cancer patient does not necessarily require bracing of the lower extremity, although a hand orthosis usually is needed.

LEUKEMIA AND LYMPHOMA

Several degrees of paraplegia or quadriplegia may be produced when leukemia or lymphoma cells invade the cerebrospinal fluid. Since both leukemia and lymphoma respond well to chemotherapy and radiotherapy, these symptoms are usually of short duration, and the patient has a good recovery. The guidelines mentioned for patients with brain tumors apply to these patients as well. In addition, when leukemic cells invade the marrow of long bones, they produce a moderately severe pain that discourages ambulation. These patients should begin a bedside program of passive or active-assistance, ROM exercises, and the nursing staff should be instructed in proper positioning techniques to avoid skin problems, contractures, or pressure on the peripheral nerves.

SOFT TISSUE SARCOMA

Sarcomas arise from connective and supportive tissues: bone, cartilage, nerve, or fat. The disabilities produced by soft-tissue sarcomas are closely related to their location and include peripheral neurological involvement of an isolated nerve, nerve trunk, or plexus, or loss of joint mobility in the case of synovial sarcomas. As the sarcoma progresses, serial electromyographic studies are essential for localizing neuropathy and related weakness. When the sarcoma involves the lower extremities, a bivalve orthosis may be needed in addition to bracing to protect a weak area in a long bone. Active-assistive, ROM exercises, passive stretch, and a three-point extension orthosis are also required when the tumor is close to a joint, such as the elbow, wrist, knee, or ankle, where a contracture could develop.

PSYCHOSOCIAL ADJUSTMENT

Some of the issues the patient with cancer must face differ markedly from issues faced with any other chronic illness. A common social stigma is that the patient is responsible for getting cancer and thus equally responsible for curing himself or herself. Unlike those who undergo amputation or other disfiguring treatments for other reasons, the patient with cancer often feels permanently contaminated by disease, a stigma too often confirmed by some degree of social ostracism that lasts beyond remission. Great strength of will is needed to move again into daily social interactions with a face disfigured or a body marred by the removal of limbs or organs. Although many of these patients are capable of meeting some occupational demands after rehabilitation, former or potential employers may perceive them as terminally ill and too debilitated to be productive.

The cancer patient must cope with a great deal of uncertainty and ambiguity. From now on, the possibility of death remains a formidable issue even during remission; the patient cannot predict if, when, or where the disease might recur. A major decision must be made whether to live with therapy, associated with disfigurement and additional discomfort that often severely compromises the quality of life, or to die without treatment. Treatment not only produces distressing side effects, but also a financial burden to the family that may seem futile if the patient's disease is terminal. The patient and family will benefit from knowing what community resources are available for financial as well as emotional support.

The primary care physician plays five major roles in helping the cancer patient adjust to the illness and its treatment:

1. Often the first to confront the patient with the diagnosis of cancer.
2. Makes the appropriate referrals and arrangements for care.
3. Consults with the family throughout treatment.
4. Interprets the oncologist's therapeutic decisions to the patient and family.

TABLE 12–4. *Behavioral response to cancer*

Normal, adaptive	Abnormal, maladaptive
Prediagnostic Phase	
Denial of disease presence and delay in seeking treatment	Development of cancer symptoms without having the disease
Diagnostic Phase	
Shock	Complete denial with treatment refusal
Disbelief	Fatalistic treatment refusal with belief death is inevitable
Initial, partial denial	
Anxiety	
Anger, hostility, persecutory feelings	Search for other opinions and/or unproven cures
Depression	
Initial Treatment Phase	
Surgery	
Grief reaction to changes in body image	Postoperative reactive depression
Postpone surgery	Severe, prolonged grief reaction to changes in body image
Seek nonsurgical alternatives	
Radiotherapy	
Fear of X-ray machine and side effects	Psychotic-like delusions or hallucinations
Fear of being abandoned	
Chemotherapy	
Fear of side effects	Residual drug-induced psychoses
Change in body image	Severe isolation-induced psychotic disturbances
Anxiety, isolation	
Altruistic feelings and desire to donate body or organs to science	Severe paranoia
Follow-up Phase	
Return to normal coping patterns	Mild depression and anxiety
Fear of recurrence	
Recurrence and Retreatment Phase	
Shock	Reactive depression with insomnia, anorexia, restlessness, anxiety, and irritability
Disbelief	
Partial denial	
Anxiety	
Anger	
Depression	

From Dixon, E. A. (1982). *Diagnosis and Treatment of Cancer.* Addison-Wesley, Menlo Park, CA.

5. Manages the terminal phase of illness and arrangements surrounding the patient's death.

While undertaking these roles, the physician must answer the patient's questions without conveying undue pessimism about the prognosis of the disease, even in the face of potential fatality.

In addition, the primary care physician should try to identify the patient at high psychosocial risk of maladaptation to cancer. The patient who has experienced life as a series of alienating, depriving, depressing, and destructive episodes is likely to fare worse than the person with a more optimistic outlook. An unhealthy response to cancer is any behavior that shortens the patient's chances for survival so that experiences of self-defeat, isolation, and despair increase. A patient who espouses life by paying lip service to the rehabilitation program while emotionally seeking death will derive limited benefits from therapy. Throughout the phases of cancer diagnosis, treatment, and follow-up, certain behaviors are considered normal psychosocial responses to the illness while other maladaptive responses should alert the physician to the need for psychiatric evaluation. These behaviors are contrasted in Table 12–4.

Self-help groups led by patients who have had cancer for some time may help the new patient adapt to the potential functional limitations associated with the various types of cancer. New patients have an opportunity to express their fears and to find out how the old patients have been coping with cancer. Before surgery, a new patient can also be paired with an individual cancer patient who has already undergone surgery for the same condition. New patients about to undergo mastectomy, colostomy, or laryngectomy may derive hope from the old patient's physical survival and restoration to full function. Cancer patients can also depend on each other for emotional support through shared experiences and learn new coping skills in supportive group therapy meetings led by psychologists and psychiatrists.

SUGGESTED READINGS

Cohen, J., Cullen, J. W., and Martin, L.R., editors. (1982): *Psychosocial Aspects of Cancer*. Raven Press, New York.

deFries, H. O. (1979): Rehabilitation of patients following surgery for oral malignant disease. *Otolaryngol. Clin. North Am.*, 12:227–234.

Dietz, J. H. (1981): *Rehabilitation Oncology*. John Wiley, New York.

Dolinka, M. K., Eideken, J., and Finkelstein, J. B. (1974): Complications of radiation therapy: Adult bone. *Semin. Roentgenol.*, 9:29–40.

Friedenbergs, I., Gordon, W., Hibbard, M., Levine, L., Wolf, C., and Diller, L. (1982): Psychosocial aspects of living with cancer: A review of the literature. *Int. J. Psychiatry Med.*, 11:303–329.

Grabois, M. (1976): Rehabilitation of the postmastectomy patient with lymphedema. *Cancer Ann.*, 26:75–79.

Gunn, A.E. (1984): *Cancer Rehabilitation*. Raven Press, New York.

Lehmann, J., Justus, F., DeLisa, J.A., and Warren, C. G. (1978): Cancer rehabilitation: Assessment of need, development, and evaluation of a model of care. *Arch. Phys. Med. Rehabil.*, 59:410–419.

Marchant, J. (1978): *Rehabilitation of Mastectomy Patients: A Handbook*. Heinemann, London.

Nealon, T. F., Jr., editor. (1976): *Management of the Patients with Cancer*, 2nd edit. W. B. Saunders, Philadelphia.

Nixon, D. W. (1982): *Diagnosis and Management of Cancer*. Addison-Wesley, Menlo Park, CA.

Peterson, L. G., Popkin, M. K., and Hall, R. C. W. (1981): Psychiatric aspects of cancer. *Psychosomatics*, 22:774–793.

University of Texas M. D. Anderson Hospital and Tumor Institute. (1984): *Rehabilitation of the Center Patient* 2nd edit. Year Book Medical Publishers, Chicago.

Vanderpool, H. Y. (1978): The ethics of terminal care. *JAMA*, 239:850–852.

Villaneuva, R., ed. (1977): Rehabilitation of the patient with head and neck cancer. *Cancer Bull.*, 29(2):22.

Villaneuva, R., and Ajmani, C. (1977): The role of rehabilitation medicine in physical restoration of patients with head and neck cancer. *Cancer Bull.*, 29:46–54.

West, D. W. (1977): Social adaptation patterns among cancer patients with facial disfigurement resulting from surgery. *Arch. Phys. Med. Rehabil.*, 58:473–479.

Medical Rehabilitation,
edited by L. S. Halstead et al.
Raven Press, New York © 1985.

CHAPTER 13

Pulmonary Rehabilitation

*Dan K. Seilheimer and **Rogelio M. Borrell

*Private Practice and Department of Pediatrics, Baylor College of Medicine, Houston; and
**St. Anthony Center, Houston, Texas 77030

CHRONIC OBSTRUCTIVE PULMONARY DISEASE

Chronic obstructive pulmonary disease (COPD) is the second leading cause of permanent disability in the over 40 age group. While treatment of COPD is not known to decrease morbidity or mortality, an aggressive program of pulmonary rehabilitation can improve the quality of life for these patients. Chronic obstructive pulmonary disease is a general term applied to a group of diseases that include chronic bronchitis, emphysema, and asthma. Patients with COPD may have elements of any or all of these diseases.

Evaluating Pulmonary Function and Disability

Table 13–1 compares the clinical features and diagnostic criteria for chronic bronchitis, pulmonary emphysema, and asthma. Since these diseases are not mutually exclusive, the main objective of evaluation is assessment of the extent of pulmonary dysfunction rather than differential diagnosis among the three diseases. Table 13–2 describes the tests of pulmonary function that are used to detect, identify, and differentiate respiratory disabilities that may result from COPD as well as estimate their severity. Note that vital capacity (VC) is the difference between total lung capacity (TLC) and residual volume (RV). In obstructive disease, VC will decrease either if the RV increases

and TLC remains unchanged or if RV increases more than TLC (Fig. 13–1).

These tests also enable the physician to evaluate response to treatment and to follow the course of the disease. Pulmonary function tests are not sensitive enough, however, to detect early localized changes, and interpretation must take into consideration inconsistencies in patient cooperation and effort.

The degree of functional disability experienced by a patient is generally predictable from the severity of dyspnea. As the following classification shows, disability can range from mild to very severe:

1. **Class I:** Not significantly restricted in normal activities; dyspnea occurs only during unusually strenuous activities; employable.
2. **Class II:** Independent in essential activities of daily living but restricted in some other activities; dyspneic when climbing stairs or incline but not when walking on level surface; employable if job is sedentary.
3. **Class III:** Dyspnea occurs during usual activities such as showering or dressing; not dyspneic at rest, can walk several blocks at own pace, but cannot keep up with others of own age; does not require physical assistance; probably not employable in any occupation.
4. **Class IV:** Dependent on some help in performing essential activities of daily living; dyspneic with minimal exertion and must pause after climbing one flight of stairs,

TABLE 13-1. *Differential diagnosis of chronic obstructive pulmonary disease*

Disease	Clinical features	Causes	Diagnostic criteria
Chronic bronchitis	Overproduction of mucus; chronic cough productive of sputum; may progress to severe exercise limitation and shortness of breath due to hypoxia, hypercapnia, and increased work of breathing from marked airway obstruction; "blue bloater"	Smoking; asthma; frequent respiratory tract infections in childhood; air pollution; occupational exposure to dust, fumes; impaired tracheobronchial host defenses	Productive cough for at least 3 months of year during 2 successive years; obstruction indicated by pulmonary function tests; improvement with bronchodilators indicates concomitant asthma; marked hypoxemia with carbon dioxide retention; diffuse rhonchi, musical squeaks, coarse rales, and wheezes in chest; possibly cardiomegaly and cyanosis
Pulmonary emphysema	Distal airways narrow on expiration; gradually increasing shortness of breath and exercise intolerance; tissue destruction decreasing elastic recoil of lung; "pink puffer"	Alveolar destruction leads to enlarged air sacs and poor structural support of distal airways	Decreased expiratory flow but normal airway resistance measurements of large airway function; increased total lung capacity; decreased single breath diffusing capacity for carbon monoxide; hyperlucent lung fields, flattened diaphragm, increase in A-P diameter of thorax, or normal chest roentgenograms; mild decrease in arterial P_{O_2}; normal P_{CO_2}; hypertrophied sternocleidomastoid and scalene muscles; barrel-shaped chest; low diaphragms; markedly diminished breath sounds; distant heart sounds
Asthma	Intermittent episodes of coughing, wheezing, and shortness of breath; widespread narrowing of airways reversed spontaneously or by bronchodilators	Increased responsiveness of trachea and bronchi to allergens, exercise, strong odors, viral and other infections, changes in environmental temperature, and emotional stress	Tests of expiratory flow and airway resistance demonstrate airway obstruction; test results improve when repeated after administration of bronchodilator; normal P_{O_2} and P_{CO_2} between episodes; hypoxemia and gradually rising P_{CO_2} with progression of attack

TABLE 13–2. *Common measures of pulmonary function*

Standardized term	Symbol	Definition
Lung volumes		
Inspiratory reserve volume	IRV	Maximal volume of gas that can be inspired from end tidal inspiration
Tidal volume	TV	Volume of gas inspired or expired during each respiratory cycle
Expiratory reserve volume	ERV	Maximal volume of gas that can be expired from resting expiratory level
Residual volume	RV	Volume of gas remaining in lungs at end of maximal expiration
Lung capacities		
Total lung capacity	TLC	Amount of gas contained in lungs at end of maximal inspiration
Vital capacity	VC	Maximal amount of gas that can be expelled from lungs following maximal inspiration
Inspiratory capacity	IC	Maximal amount of gas that can be inspired from resting expiratory level
Functional residual capacity	FRC	Vital capacity performed with expiration as forceful as possible
Ventilatory measurement		
Forced vital capacity	FVC	Vital capacity performed with expiration as forceful as possible
Forced expiratory volume	FEV_T	Volume of gas exhaled over given time interval during performance of forced vital capacity (e.g., $FEV_{1.0}$ is forced expiratory volume of 1 sec)
Forced expiratory flow	FEF_{v1-v2}	Average rate of flow for specified volume segment of forced expiratory spirogram (e.g., $FEF_{200-1200}$ and $FEF_{0-25\%}$)
Forced mid-expiratory flow	FMF	Average rate of flow during middle two quarters of volume segment of forced expiratory spirogram (i.e., from 25% to 75% of volume, or $FEF_{25-75\%}$)
Maximal voluntary ventilation	MVV	Amount of air that subject can breathe with voluntary maximal ventilatory effort per unit of time

walking more than 100 yards, or dressing; often restricted to home if living alone.

5. **Class V:** Entirely restricted to home and activity often limited to bed or chair; dyspneic at rest; dependent on help for most of needs.

Therapeutic modalities in a rehabilitation program should be custom selected according to the patient's ability to reduce dyspnea and economize the exertion needed to perform activities of daily living.

Preventing Exacerbations

A pulmonary rehabilitation program for patients with COPD is designed to halt or delay progression of the disease, reduce airway obstruction, relieve hypoxemia, treat complications, educate the patient and family, and provide psychosocial support.

Patients with impaired respiration reap the most benefits from rehabilitation if they stop smoking. As a result, coughing and sputum production decrease. Furthermore, expiratory flow rates decrease at a slower rate in COPD patients who stop smoking than in those who continue. Air pollution and occupational inhalants should also be avoided even if changes in residence or employment are necessary.

Since intercurrent infections may worsen the disability or even cause death from respiratory failure, COPD patients should avoid individuals with viral respiratory infections (cold and flu). Immunization with influenza and polyvalent pneumococcal vaccines according to the current recommendation of the Communicable Disease Center also is indicated.

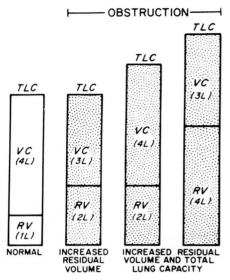

FIG. 13–1. Factors in COPD that decrease vital capacity. [From Tashkin, D. P., and Cassan, S. M. (1978): *Guide to Pulmonary Medicine.* Grune & Stratton, New York.]

Relieving Bronchospasm

While the benefit of bronchodilators in asthma is obvious, the need for bronchodilators in patients with chronic bronchitis or emphysema may not be as apparent. When bronchospasm is clearly contributing to disability, and expiratory flow rates improve following bronchodilator use, the COPD patient should receive a trial of treatment with these agents. Even patients who do not show immediate spirometric improvement may have objective and subjective evidence of improvement following a few weeks of receiving theophylline or theophylline salts orally. Newer, sustained release preparations allow convenient twice daily dosage. Regardless of the theophylline preparation prescribed, plasma levels of the drug should be maintained in the therapeutic range of 10 to 20 mg/ml.

Aerosolized bronchodilators often have been administered by intermittent positive pressure breathing (IPPB) in the past. Hand-held nebulizers and metered dose inhalers may be used to deliver these agents without the expense and the risk of alveoli overdistention associated with IPPB.

Alone or in combination with theophylline, sympathomimetic agents may be given orally or by aerosol. The newer beta–2 agonists, metaproterenol and terbutaline, are recommended; they have less cardiac toxicity and a longer duration of action than the older agents.

The role of corticosteroids in relieving bronchospasm in asthma is well known. Their role in other forms of COPD is controversial. A 2- to 3-week trial of oral steroids is warranted in disabled patients if symptoms are not controlled by conventional bronchodilators. Beclomethasone, an inhaled corticosteroid hormone, is recommended because its lack of systemic side effects enables steroid benefits without complications. Steroid use should be stopped if no improvement occurs. Otherwise, maintain the patient on the lowest dose that adequately relieves bronchospasm.

Reducing Secretions

Patients with COPD have occasional episodes of increased cough and sputum production, apparently due to respiratory infection. Such episodes should be treated with a 7- to 10-day course of oral tetracycline or ampicillin. Several agents aid in thinning and removing bronchial secretions. Although expectorants, mucolytic agents, detergents, and proteolytic enzymes may help some patients, side effects prohibit the routine use of any of these agents. Discourage the development of viscid and crusted secretions by ensuring a fluid intake of 2 to 3 liters per day and maintaining humidity in the home above 50%.

Avoid dehydration, which may thicken secretions. On the other hand, there is no reason to believe that overhydration is beneficial. Attempts at deposition of water in the tracheobronchial tree by jet or ultrasonic nebulizer, mist tent, and steam inhalation result mostly in swallowed water. However, some patients do seem to benefit from such topical hydration.

Although postural drainage and chest physical therapy have not been objectively evaluated in COPD, patients who have difficulty expectorating large amounts of sputum or those with bronchiectasis may benefit from these modalities. Positioning the patient for 5 to 10 min with the affected lobe or lung uppermost, percuss the chest using rapid, repetitive strokes, at least three or four times daily (Fig. 13–2). When coughing is too shallow to expel sputum, manually compress the patient's lower thorax and upper abdomen after maximal inspiration to vigorously expulse air and expectorate sputum.

Breathing Retraining

There is little objective evidence that breathing exercises are helpful in improving functional ability and relieving dyspnea in COPD patients, yet many physicians and patients have claimed substantial subjective improvement. Breathing exercises do have the following benefits:

1. Prevent atelectasis.
2. Increase efficiency of accessory muscles so that oxygen cost of breathing is reduced.
3. Replace forced breathing, which actively compresses airways, with relaxed breathing, which maximizes airway opening.
4. Reduce gross hyperinflation of lung by increasing expiration.
5. Reduce sensation of breathlessness by increasing diaphragmatic excursion and reducing thoracic movements.
6. Mobilize and maintain mobility of chest wall.
7. Enhance clearing and defense of airways by increasing cough efficiency.

A trial of abdominal breathing with pursed lips expiration is not only warranted in dyspneic patients but may also improve exercise tolerance. A physical therapist can instruct the patient to inhale slowly and deeply by moving the

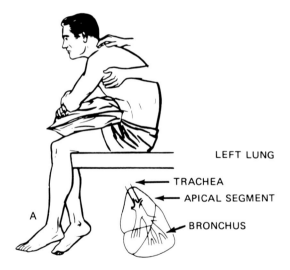

LEFT LUNG

← TRACHEA

← APICAL SEGMENT

← BRONCHUS

A

FIG. 13–2. Two positions and percussion sites for draining lung congestion. **A:** Drainage of apical (uppermost) segment of left upper lobe. **B:** Drainage of medial segment of right middle lobe. [From Barnes, T. A., and Israel, J. S. (1980): *Brady's Programmed Introduction to Respiratory Therapy*, 2nd edit. Robert J. Brady, Bowie, MD.]

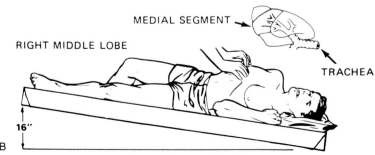

MEDIAL SEGMENT →

RIGHT MIDDLE LOBE

TRACHEA

16"

B

abdomen outward (diaphragmatic breathing) and to exhale slowly against pursed lips (Fig. 13–3). The patient learns to breathe in a more efficient manner by following a program of progressive training sessions based on the following steps:

1. Teach physical relaxation.
2. Relax short, tight muscles of shoulder girdle and upper chest.
3. Correct faulty posture of high, hunched shoulders, thoracic kyphosis, compensatory lumbar lordosis.
4. Increase mobility of rib articulations between cervical and thoracic vertebrae and loosen scapulae.
5. Show patient how to press on lower ribs to assist deeper expiration and resist inspiration.
6. Teach voluntary control of abdominal respiration.

Exercise Conditioning

Improvement in the patient's exercise ability not only increases functional ability and reduces the occurrence of acute chest illnesses but also promotes a feeling of well-being. A graded exercise program lasting at least 2 to 6 weeks may enable previously chairbound patients to engage in normal activities of daily living or even to resume gainful employment. This greater independence, in turn, counteracts depression and promotes self-confidence. The endurance of COPD patients can be increased by a program of gradually escalating exercise such as walking, stair climbing (Fig. 13–4), and pedaling a stationary bicycle. Encourage the patient to breathe slowly and deeply through pursed lips to gradually increase the duration and speed of walking. Severely affected patients may require supplemental oxygen, at least at the beginning of the exercise program (Fig. 13–5).

Teach specific exercises to strengthen abdominal muscles and improve chest mobilization (Fig. 13–6), especially if the patient has a tight barrel chest. Holding a cane or wand while exercising provides clearer guidelines for movement (Fig. 13–7). Modified or conventional sit-ups will help strengthen abdominal muscles. The patient flexes the knees, takes a deep breath, and pulls the knees toward the chest while exhaling. The patient then inspires while extending back to a supine position.

Oxygen Therapy

Recent advances in oxygen delivery systems have made the outpatient use of low-flow oxygen more practical and economical. In addition to the bulky compressed gas cylinders, liquid oxygen containers that can be carried by the patient and stationary concentrators that extract oxygen from room air are commercially available (see Appendix). Patients likely to benefit from low-flow oxygen usually have a resting arterial PO_2 less than 50 mm Hg. Low-flow oxygen therapy is particularly indicated when chronic bronchitis or emphysema is complicated by pulmonary hypertension and right heart failure. Low-flow oxygen use has several potential benefits:

1. Decreases pulmonary vascular resistance in patients with cor pulmonale.
2. Reduces exercise intolerance that is due to hypoxemia.
3. Relieves neuropsychiatric symptoms caused by hyoxemia, e.g., headaches, impaired mentation, depression, irritability.
4. Decreases polycythemia due to hypoxia-induced erythrocytosis.

To avoid depressing the respiratory drive of patients with chronic hypercarbia, always limit oxygen flow to 3 liters/min or less by nasal cannula. Arterial blood gases should be determined along with the patient's clinical response when assessing the efficiency of this therapeutic modality.

Common Complications

Cor Pulmonale

Chronic hypoxemia in COPD may lead to cor pulmonale. Indications that this complication has developed include worsening dyspnea and ex-

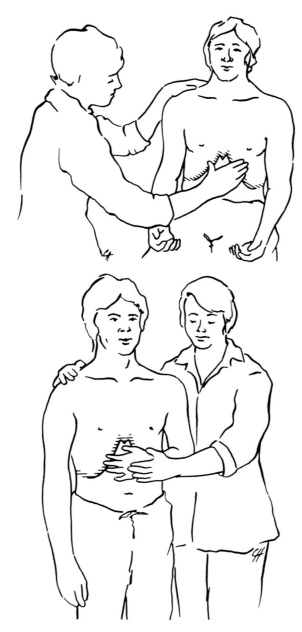

FIG. 13–3. Training in diaphragmatic breathing. **Top:** With shoulders and hands relaxed, patient practices breathing in sitting position as therapist places hand over diaphragm. **Bottom:** Patient observes movement of chest and abdomen in full-length mirror as therapist places his hand over diaphragmatic movements. [From Frownfelter, D. L. (1978): *Chest Physical Therapy and Pulmonary Rehabilitation: An Interdisciplinary Approach.* Year Book Medical Publishers, Chicago.]

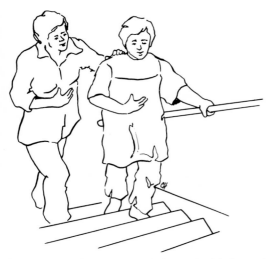

FIG. 13–4. Patient pauses slightly as he inhales and exhales as he climbs one or two stairs. [From Frownfelter, D. L. (1978): *Chest Physical Therapy and Pulmonary Rehabilitation: An Interdisciplinary Approach.* Year Book Medical Publishers, Chicago.]

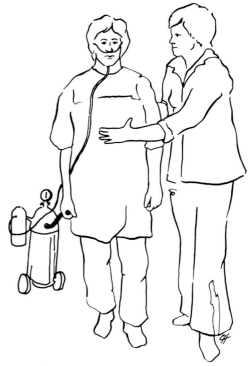

FIG. 13–5. Diaphragmatic breathing assisted by low-flow oxygen as COPD patient practices walking, taking long, slow steps. [From Frownfelter, D. L. (1978): *Chest Physical Therapy and Pulmonary Rehabilitation: An Interdisciplinary Approach.* Year Book Medical Publishers, Chicago.]

ercise intolerance. When heart failure occurs in COPD, fluid accumulation in the lungs inhibits gas exchange. The cautious use of diuretics and salt restriction aid in removing excess fluid and usually lessen disability. They may, however, cause a significant hypokalemic, hypochloremic metabolic alkalosis. Spirolactone or oral potassium supplements help to correct and prevent this side effect of diuretic use.

The use of digitalis in cor pulmonale is controversial. Since patients with cor pulmonale have an increased tendency to develop digitalis toxicity, this drug should be used cautiously and only when heart failure is not responsive to other therapy. Cor pulmonale in COPD is an indication for long-term administration of low-flow oxygen therapy, both in the hospital and at home.

Respiratory Failure

Acute respiratory failure may be caused by infections in patients with advanced COPD. Patients experiencing exacerbations should be monitored for this life-threatening complication. Mechanical ventilation in an intensive care setting may be needed to support patients during these acute episodes. Long-term mechanical

ventilation should be continued, however, only according to the patient's and family's wishes, the prospects for disease progression, and the patient's chances for recovery.

Educating the Patient and Family

Relatively few people are aware of the disabling aspects of COPD. Patients and their families need to be familiar with the nature of the disease, the rationale for the individual rehabilitation program, and possible complications for which medical attention should be sought. Provide written instructions and illustrations of postural drainage positions and discuss with the patient how to adapt or provide home equipment, such as tilting the bed and using appropriate pillows. An inexpensive exercise slant board can be purchased for doing postural drainage at

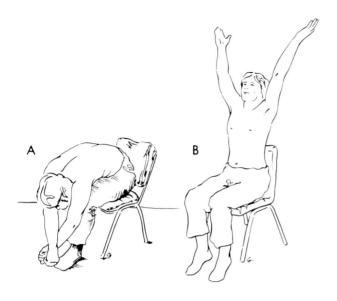

FIG. 13–6. Chest mobilization exercise. **A:** Patient exhales as he bends forward to touch floor. **B:** Patient inhales as he stretches his arms up and out to a "V" over his head. [From Frownfelter, D. L. (1978): *Chest Physical Therapy and Pulmonary Rehabilitation: An Interdisciplinary Approach.* Year Book Medical Publishers, Chicago.]

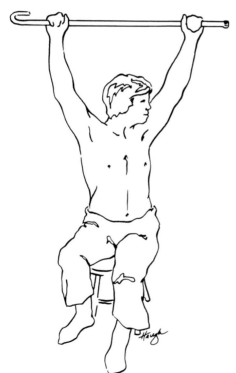

FIG. 13–7. Chest mobilization exercise with assistance of cane. Patient exhales as he rotates his trunk. [From Frownfelter, D. L. (1978): *Chest Physical Therapy and Pulmonary Rehabilitation: An Interdisciplinary Approach.* Year Book Medical Publishers, Chicago.]

home. Whenever possible, teach a member of the family how to perform the therapeutic techniques involved.

Discussions about prognosis and expected improvement in vocational, recreational, and self-care functioning should be realistic. Frequent follow-up allows the physician not only to assess and modify the patient's program but also to encourage continued efforts toward the goals that have been mutually agreed upon.

Psychosocial and Vocational Management

The personality characteristics typical in patients with COPD are depression with associated feelings of hopelessness and worthlessness, hysteria, and hypochondriasis. Dyspnea can be a frightening, distressing experience and awareness of the downhill course of the disease promotes depression. Anxiety, depression, and somatic concern are significantly reduced, however, in patients who participate in a respiratory rehabilitation program.

The asthma sufferer may have incurred additional psychosocial disability if the attacks began in childhood. Although functional disability would have occurred only during acute episodes, the resulting delay in social maturation, inadequate basic education, and limited life experience often impoverish interpersonal skills and lead to passivity, dependency, a lack of self-confidence, and chronic depression. Such patients may benefit from long-term or short-term psychotherapy.

Depending on the severity and types of symptoms exhibited by the patient with COPD, he or she may have to train for a more sedentary occupation or change the responsibilities required of a current job. Often, employers are willing to restructure a job for a senior, trusted employee. In the work environment, COPD patients should avoid sudden changes in temperature, as well as exposure to adverse weather conditions, extreme dryness or humidity, atmospheric dust, and irritating gases. Recurrent infection may mandate moving to a warmer, drier climate.

In addition to dyspnea, a chronic cough and absenteeism often interfere with job performance. Expectoration may be a cosmetic impairment to jobs requiring close interpersonal interaction such as sales and public relations. Absenteeism is a greater problem in the "blue bloater" with bronchitis, who suffers periodic exacerbations from infection, bronchospasm, and fatigue.

Reassure the patient's employer that moderately severe shortness of breath may be uncomfortable but does not damage the patient. Also emphasize that since the rate of deterioration is extremely slow in moderate COPD, 5 years or more of continued employment can be expected. Patients with severe COPD, however, can expect 1 to 2 years of sedentary employment. Continued smoking reduces this outlook.

In general, the patient who has a normal spirogram, normal resting and exercise blood gases, and the capacity to climb four flights of stairs without distress can even perform heavy physical labor. Patients able to climb three flights can perform medium work, while those limited to two flights are still capable of homemaking. The person with a Po_2 of 60 mm Hg and a Pco_2 of 80–90 mm Hg may be able to walk several blocks slowly, drive a car, and remain at work in a sedentary job. Although stair climbing limited to one flight designates severe respiratory impairment, such patients may be able to drive a cab or operate an industrial sewing machine; homemaking, however, is too strenuous.

CHRONIC OBSTRUCTIVE PULMONARY DISEASE WITH BRONCHITIS AND CLASS III DISABILITY

Report of a Case

HISTORY AND EVALUATION. This 54-year-old man was admitted to the intensive care unit with acute respiratory failure and cor pulmonale secondary to bronchitis. He had a 40-year history of smoking one to two packs of cigarettes a day. When bronchitis had been diagnosed 3 years ago, he had tried unsuccessfully to switch to a pipe. He also had a 10-year history of hypertension for which he takes prazosin, 1 mg t.i.d.

Over the past 2 years, he has been able to walk three or four blocks slowly, continue driving, and climb two flights of stairs. Since retiring on disability a year ago from his job in mobile home sales, he has kept occupied with gourmet cooking and gardening. He has experienced some dyspnea while performing activities of daily living. Just prior to hospitalization, respiratory infection had reduced his class III functional status to class V disability.

Physical examination revealed fever of 102°F, productive cough with discolored sputum, increased breathlessness, tachypnea, suprasternal retractions, tachycardia, elevated pulmonary blood pressure of 140/25 mm Hg, cardiomegaly, diaphoresis, central cyanosis, papilledema, and asterixis. Ulcers were noted on the third and fourth digits of the right hand, suggesting thromboangiitis obliterans induced by smoking. Arterial Po_2 was 40 mm Hg and arterial Pco_2 was 70 mm Hg. Sputum culture indicated *Streptococcus pneumoniae* infection.

INPATIENT MANAGEMENT. Respiratory infection was treated with cefazolin, 1 g every 6 hr intravenously. Polythiazide, 1 mg, was combined with prazosin, 2 mg t.i.d., to relieve pulmonary congestion and peripheral edema. To lower pulmonary artery pressure, low-flow oxygen was administered by molecular sieve at 2 liters/min continuously for at least 15 hr daily. Aminophylline, 200 mg every 6 hr, was administered for bronchodilation. Intravenous and oral fluid therapy helped prevent dehydration. Additional measures to reduce airflow obstruction included liquefaction of thick bronchial secretions with mist therapy, mobilization of secretions through controlled coughing, postural drainage with chest percussion and vibration, and breathing retraining. To prevent elevating his blood pressure any further, head-down postures were avoided. A respiratory therapist taught the patient's wife the techniques of chest physiotherapy so that the maneuvers could be performed properly at home.

OUTPATIENT MANAGEMENT. He was discharged on continuous home oxygen therapy using a portable, lightweight liquid oxygen walker unit. His wife helped him with chest physiotherapy daily. As he reclined in the semi-Fowler's position for 10 min, she percussed over the area of the anterior upper lobes. As he exhaled through pursed lips, she then vibrated over the drainage area for six expirations. After he rested briefly, the process was repeated as he leaned forward to drain the apical and posterior segments of the upper lobes. He coughed up secretions whenever he felt the need.

Daily relaxation exercises consisted of head rolls, shoulder shrugs, and shoulder rolls. The patient was encouraged to practice breathing with an incentive spirometer whenever he felt the urge for a cigarette. Having been unable to smoke while in the hospital, he enrolled in a behavioral program at a hospital-affiliated preventive medicine center with a group of smokers to discourage resumption of his habit.

For several weeks, he was able to take walks only with the assistance of low-flow oxygen. However, he was able to increase his distance one block each month and within 6 months could walk several blocks without supplemental oxygen.

DYSFUNCTION OF VENTILATORY MUSCLES

The muscles of respiration are necessary for the movement of air into and out of the alveoli, where gas exchange occurs, for coughing, which clears the airways of secretions that impair gas exchange and increase the work of breathing, and for sighing, which is thought to help prevent atelectasis. Dysfunction of the inspiratory or expiratory muscles is a major cause of morbidity and mortality in a variety of neuromuscular diseases (Table 13–3). The comprehensive management of several of these diseases is discussed in Chapters 15, 17, 18, and 19. Some patients with respiratory muscle disease are able to maintain the normal work of breathing indefinitely unless a metabolic rate accelerated by exercise or fever, lower respiratory infection, or atelectasis makes their muscle function inadequate. Atelectasis and infection also develop in patients with impaired neuromuscular mechanisms of the upper airway that protect against aspiration.

In traumatic quadriplegia, the cause of death is usually pulmonary. Ventilatory muscle paral-

TABLE 13–3. *Classification of neuromuscular diseases affecting the respiratory system according to site affected*

I. Peripheral receptors or afferent nerves
  A. Familial dysautonomia (Riley Day syndrome)
  B. Bilateral globectomy or bilateral carotid endarterectomy
II. Central receptors and central respiratory integrating neurons
  A. Ideopathic hypoventilation in nonobese (Ondine's curse)
  B. Pickwickian syndrome
  C. Bilateral high cervical cordotomy
III. Diffuse central nervous system
  A. Sedative or narcotic overdosage
  B. Cerebral vascular accidents and tumors
IV. Central motor neurons
  A. Poliomyelitis
  B. Progressive muscular atrophy (Wernig-Hoffman disease)
  C. Amyotrophic lateral sclerosis
V. Peripheral efferent nerves
  A. Polyneuritis
    1. Guillain-Barré syndrome
    2. Acute intermittent porphyria
  B. Phrenic nerve paralysis—surgical trauma or tumor
  C. Tetanus
VI. Motor end plate dysfunction
  A. Myasthenia gravis
  B. Curare, succinylcholine, other neuromuscular blockers
  C. Botulism
VII. Muscle disease (polymyopathy)
  A. Polymyositis and dermatomyositis
  B. Muscular dystrophy (Duchenne type)

From Tashkin, D. P., and Cassan, S. M., editors. (1978): *Guide to Pulmonary Medicine.* Grune & Stratton, New York.

ysis may impair rehabilitation, which involves treating and preventing acute pulmonary complications and providing adequate ventilation for the patient to function up to his or her full potential.

Evaluating Muscle Function

Fatigue of the respiratory muscles should be suspected in patients with neuromuscular disease who have symptoms of shortness of breath, exercise intolerance, somnolence, cough, and/or sputum production. The physical findings of hypoventilation may include tachypnea with very shallow respiration, tachycardia, use of accessory muscles of respiration, anxiety, altered mental state, and cyanosis. If atelectasis consolidation is present, there is dullness to percussion, egophony, and a marked decrease in breath sounds over the affected area. Retained secretions and lower respiratory infection usually produce rhonchi, rales, and fever.

Laboratory evaluation of ventilatory muscle dysfunction may include chest fluoroscopy to assess diaphragmatic excursion and chest roentgenograms to detect peripheral complications. Arterial blood gas measurements are necessary for determining the adequacy of ventilation and of oxygenation. An elevated PCO_2 (>45 mm Hg) indicates that alveolus ventilation is inadequate and that assisted ventilation is probably needed. A PO_2 of less than 60 mm Hg is an indication for supplemental oxygen delivery. Elevated hemoglobin and serum bicarbonate levels suggest that hypoxia and hypoventilation, respectively, have been present long enough for compensatory mechanisms to occur.

Although usually done in special laboratories, simple pulmonary function tests may be performed at the bedside. A hand-held spirometer measures the patient's vital capacity. A simple monometer and mouthpiece determine the maximum amount of pressure the patient is able to generate with the respiratory muscles (negative inspiratory force). These measurements should be done at frequent intervals in patients at risk for ventilatory muscle dysfunction to monitor changes and anticipate respiratory failure. A vital capacity less than 10 to 15 cc/kg of body weight or a negative inspiratory force of less than -20 to -30 cm/H_2O indicates that the patient is at risk for respiratory muscle failure.

Reducing Secretions

As in patients with COPD, respiratory infections may lead to respiratory failure in patients with neuromuscular disease. Tetracycline is given to adolescents and adults and ampicillin to children with lower respiratory infections while awaiting the results of the sputum culture and sensitivity tests.

Weakness of the respiratory muscles impairs the patient's ability to take a deep breath, to cough, and to expectorate secretions. IPPB given three or four times daily and followed with postural drainage is recommended for neuromuscular patients who have lower respiratory tract infection or atelectasis associated with copious airway secretions. If secretions are a recurrent problem, daily IPPB and chest physiotherapy consisting of frequent movement and turning, postural drainage, percussion, vibration, cough training, and breathing exercises may be preventative. Percussion and vibration can be performed by machine or manually.

Patients with marked expiratory muscle dysfunction may not be able to generate the necessary expiratory force to cough up secretions. They can be assisted to cough while in the supine position by a nurse, therapist, or family member. Following a maximum inspiration, the patient closes the glottis and performs a Valsalva maneuver. The assistant aids in generating pressure by placing the hands over the abdomen and pressing firmly. The glottis is suddenly opened to produce a cough.

Respiratory Muscle Retraining

Since neuromuscular patients do not suffer from expiratory air flow obstruction, the breathing retraining techniques such as pursed lip breathing used in obstructive lung disease are not applicable to neuromuscular dysfunction. However, improving the endurance and strength of respiratory muscles in neuromuscular patients may be possible through several muscle training techniques. Two of these techniques are particularly easy to learn and perform at home.

Exercising against weights placed on the mid-upper abdomen increases diaphragm muscle strength because diaphragm contraction is responsible for protrusion of the abdomen during inspiration. Twice a day for 15 min, the patient forcefully protrudes the abdomen against the weights during inspiration and contracts the abdomen during expiration. While monitoring the patient for undue fatigue, gradually increase the weight during these sessions from 2 to 20 lb.

Also, for 10 to 15 min twice a day, have the patient breathe through a mouthpiece in which the orifice is constricted. This exercise places a resistive load on the respiratory system, which may increase muscle strength. Make the orifice small enough so that the load is significant but large enough that the patient can maintain adequate ventilation.

Preventing Aspiration

When the patient's neuromuscular impairment involves the pharyngeal or laryngeal muscles, aspiration may occur. The gag reflex should be evaluated during routine examinations and whenever lower airway secretions increase. An artificial airway by endotracheal or tracheostomy tube may be necessary to protect the lungs from aspiration. Other indications for airway placement are copious tracheobronchial secretions that the patient is unable to cough up, the need for positive pressure mechanical ventilation, and upper airway obstruction (e.g., tracheal stenosis).

Most patients with neuromuscular disease do not require inflation of the tube's cuff. The inflated cuff increases the likelihood of tracheal granulation tissue and stenosis. When continued aspiration or poor ventilation due to leakage around the tube makes inflation necessary, the cuff should be inflated to a low pressure, about 20 mm Hg as measured with the bedside monometer, such that a minimal air leak is present around the tube.

When an artificial airway will be needed for no longer than 2 or 3 weeks, however, nasotracheal intubation is preferred over tracheostomy. Some patients who aspirate may be fed via a nagogastric or gastrostomy tube. If this tube successfully controls aspiration, the patient's home and hospital care will be simpler than if a tracheostomy is required.

When a tracheostomy is necessary, provide some means for the patient to speak. For chronic use, a tracheostomy tube with a large air leak around it may allow enough air to pass through the vocal cords on expiration to enable speech (Fig. 13–8A). Some patients may require a fenestrated tracheostomy (Fig. 13–8B) or a "Trach-Talk" attachment (Fig. 13–8D).

Avoiding Respiratory Acidosis

When the ventilatory muscles are unable to maintain adequate alveolar ventilation, the P_{CO_2} rises, causing respiratory acidosis and a fall in P_{O_2}. The decreased P_{O_2} can be treated with supplemental oxygen; however, oxygen does not improve the respiratory acidosis. Assisted ventilation is necessary to decrease the P_{CO_2} and avoid the possibly fatal consequences of respiratory acidosis.

Negative pressure ventilators such as the tank respirator (iron lung, Fig. 13–9) and cuirass (see Chapter 18, Fig. 18–4) are preferred for those patients who are able to breathe spontaneously for part of the day but who need mechanical ventilatory assistance for the rest of the time. While negative pressure ventilators have the disadvantages of bulkiness and noisiness, they have the advantages of not requiring a tracheostomy to connect them to the patient and of being easier to operate and maintain than positive pressure ventilators.

Positive Pressure Ventilators

Most hospitals have positive pressure ventilators, but their disadvantage for home application is their immobility. Compact ventilators powered by an internal, rechargeable battery or by a standard 12-volt automobile battery may be placed on a rear platform of a wheelchair (Fig. 13–10). Such ventilators allow patients mobility in the hospital during rehabilitation and can be used for outpatient ventilatory support of patients with chronic, severe respiratory muscle dysfunction.

IPPB is essential to sustain life in apneic patients or in those with severe respiratory distress. Patients at risk for ventilatory muscle failure should be followed closely for evidence of impending failure so that IPPB can be instituted before the crisis of severe respiratory acidosis develops. A P_{O_2} above 45 mm Hg is usually an indication for IPPB. When the vital capacity falls to less than 10 to 15 cc/kg of body weight and

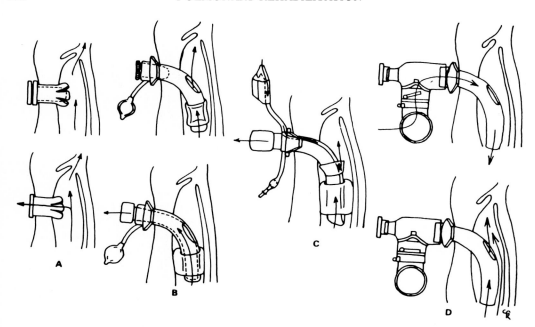

FIG. 13–8. Special tracheostomy appliances to facilitate speech. **A:** Tracheostomy button. Obturator directs air through larynx for speaking *(upper left).* Removing obturator enables suctioning *(lower left).* **B:** Fenestrated tracheostomy tube. When stoma is plugged, air can pass through fenestration between trachea and larynx *(upper).* Insertion of inner cannula occludes fenestration such that air must pass through stoma. **C:** Pitt speaking tracheostomy tube. Air passes through tube while stream of gas passes from small base tube past larynx, permitting speech. **D:** Trach-Talk attached to tracheostomy tube. During inspiration, air is drawn past one-way through stoma *(upper).* During expiration, valve closes, causing expired gas to exit through larynx. Trach-Talk can be used only with uncuffed or fenestrated tube. [From Shapiro, B. J. (1982): Pulmonary rehabilitation of the neuromuscular patient. In: *The Practice of Rehabilitation Medicine*, edited by P. E. Kaplan and R. S. Materson. Charles C Thomas, Springfield, Illinois.]

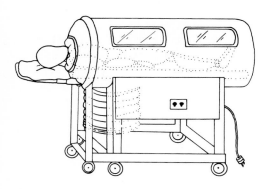

FIG. 13–9. Tank ventilator. Bellows at bottom expands, creating negative pressure inside tank for inspiration. [From Shapiro, B. J. (1982): Pulmonary rehabilitation of the neuromuscular patient. In: *The Practice of Rehabilitation Medicine*, edited by P. E. Kaplan and R. S. Materson. Charles C Thomas, Springfield, Illinois.]

the negative inspiratory force decreases to less than -20 to -30 cm/H_2O, IPPB should be considered. The more rapidly the vital capacity and negative inspiratory force deteriorate, the earlier IPPB should be started.

Patients with acute, reversible pulmonary disease may be weaned from IPPB when the process has abated. Patients who are ventilated for ventilatory muscle dysfunction secondary to an irreversible neuromuscular disease usually require long-term IPPB. Since IPPB can be provided at home, it should not prevent an active rehabilitation program. Cautious efforts should be made to wean patients with some ventilatory muscle dysfunction to find the maximum amount of time that spontaneous ventilation can be maintained. Patients allowed gradually increasing periods of spontaneous breathing by T-tube tire should be reconnected to the ventilator

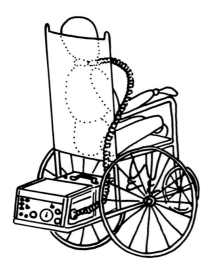

FIG. 13–10. Portable, battery-operated, positive pressure ventilator attached to wheelchair. [From Shapiro, B. J. (1982): Pulmonary rehabilitation of the neuromuscular patient. In: *The Practice of Rehabilitation Medicine*, edited by P. E. Kaplan and R. S. Materson. Charles C Thomas, Springfield, Illinois.]

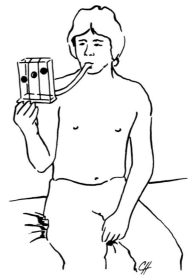

FIG. 13–11. Inspiratory incentive spirometer. Patient is encouraged to hold maximal inspiration long enough to elevate spheres for a few seconds, thus improving distribution of ventilation. [From Frownfelter, D. L. (1978): *Chest Physical Therapy and Pulmonary Rehabilitation: An Interdisciplinary Approach.* Year Book Medical Publishers, Chicago.]

before respiratory distress and respiratory muscle exhaustion occur. Weaning patients with neuromuscular disease by gradually decreasing the number of breaths per minute given the patient (IMV mode) is not usually successful. Prolonged periods of rest will facilitate weaning and help avoid chronic fatigue in patients with limited respiratory muscle endurance.

Inspiratory Incentive Spirometry

More effective than IPPB in conscious and alert patients, inspiratory incentive spirometry over increasing time periods may also help wean patients from IPPB. This method is indicated for any patient who cannot prevent alveolar collapse by taking deep breaths or yawning. Unlike other expiratory methods, such as blow bottles, it does not aggravate atelectasis. A typical schedule is five or six maximal inspirations once per hour, with resting between attempts. The patient is encouraged and motivated by being able to observe directly daily improvement. Another advantage of the inspiratory incentive spirometry is its adaptability to home use. Hand-held spirometers are available that can measure the vol-

ume of air inspired up to 4,000 ml (Fig. 13–11).

Obstacles to Independent Ventilation

Patients with neuromuscular disease may be very difficult to wean from mechanical ventilation. Before deciding that the patient cannot be weaned, every reversible factor contributing to decreased respiratory muscle function or to increased work of breathing must be corrected. Patients often become malnourished when an acute illness becomes protracted. Poor nutrition limits respiratory muscle endurance. Patients with nasotracheal or tracheostomy tubes can eat, but their spontaneous intake may be inadequate. Maintenance nutrition and any deficits should be met by nasogastric tube or total parenteral feedings. Respiratory muscle activity may also be affected by electrolyte disorders or drugs that act on the respiratory system, especially narcotics and sedatives.

The work of breathing may be increased by complicating lung disease (e.g., atelectasis, pneumonia, bronchitis, asthma), left ventricular failure with pulmonary edema, failure to control tracheobronchial secretions, an airway tube that is too small, or increased oxygen needs due to fever. Correct these factors before concluding that the patient cannot be weaned from IPPB.

Common Complications

Respiratory Failure

The most common complication of ventilatory muscle dysfunction is acute respiratory failure. If respiratory infections cannot be prevented, they should be treated daily and aggressively while monitoring the patient for signs of respiratory failure.

Although good nursing care and alarm systems will help prevent life-threatening technical problems in ventilator-dependent patients, unavoidable accidents may still occur. Problems to be anticipated include mechanical breakdown, ventilator disconnection from the patient, mucous plugging of the tracheostomy tube, and power failure.

Scoliosis

Scoliosis often develops in patients with chronic neuromuscular disease. This spinal deformity decreases lung volumes and increases the work of breathing by putting the ventilatory muscles at a mechanical disadvantage. Scoliosis can be detected on the physical examination, but should be verified by 36-inch gravity-loaded spine films. Bracing or surgery may be necessary to arrest the progression of scoliosis before it worsens ventilatory ability.

Cor Pulmonale

Cardiac muscle involvement of the primary disease (e.g., muscular dystrophy) must be ruled out if cor pulmonale is suspected. Unless severe kyphoscoliosis is present, cor pulmonale usually can be reversed by long-term maintenance of adequate ventilation and oxygen.

SUGGESTED READINGS

Agle, D. P., and Baum, G. L. (1977): Psychological aspects of chronic obstructive pulmonary disease. *Med. Clin. North Am.*, 61:749–758.

Barnes, T. A., and Israel, J. S. (1980): *Brady's Programmed Introduction to Respiratory Therapy*, 2nd edit. Robert J. Brady, Bowie, MD.

Epstein, J., and Gaines, J. (1983): *Clinical Respiratory Care of the Adult Patient*. Robert J. Brady, Bowie, MD.

Frownfelter, D. L. (1978): *Chest Physical Therapy and Pulmonary Rehabilitation: An Interdisciplinary Approach*. Year Book Medical Publishers, Chicago.

Haas, A., Pineda, H., Haas, F., and Axen, K. (1979): *Pulmonary Therapy and Rehabilitation: Principles and Practice*. Williams & Wilkins, Baltimore.

Lertzman, M. M., and Cherniack, R. M. (1976): Rehabilitation of patients with chronic obstructive pulmonary disease. *Am. Rev. Resp. Dis.*, 114:1145–1165.

Shapiro, B. J. (1982): Pulmonary rehabilitation of the neuromuscular patient. In: *The Practice of Rehabilitation Medicine*, edited by P. E. Kaplan and R. S. Materson. Charles C Thomas, Springfield, IL.

Tashkin, D. P., and Cassan, S. M., editors (1978): *Guide to Pulmonary Medicine*. Grune & Stratton, New York.

Medical Rehabilitation,
edited by L. S. Halstead et al.
Raven Press, New York © 1985.

CHAPTER 14

Cardiac Rehabilitation

William P. Blocker, Jr.

Rehabilitation Medicine and Cardiac Rehabilitation Program, Veterans Administration Medical Center, and Departments of Physical Medicine and Rehabilitation, Baylor College of Medicine, Houston, Texas 77030

An estimated 454.3 million of the world's population have or will develop coronary heart disease. The Scandinavian countries and the United States still lead the world in the prevalence of heart disease, but the rate is increasing in the developing countries. In the United States alone, approximately 5 million persons have coronary heart disease, and more than one-fifth of them will die from the disease each year. Autopsies on young Americans killed in the Korean War showed an alarming prevalence of heart disease, dispelling the illusion that coronary heart disease occurs only in old age. During the last two decades, women also have experienced a sharp rise in myocardial infarctions, producing a 20-fold increase in deaths compared to previous decades.

CAUSES OF FUNCTIONAL DISABILITY

Patients with cardiac disease have little, if any, impairment in ambulation, and none in eating, dressing, personal hygiene, or communication skills. However, they do suffer the consequences of heart failure, angina, and cardiac arrhythmia. In heart failure, the reduction in the amount of blood pumped produces symptoms of fatigue, lethargy, weakness, apathy, poor memory, and depression. If secondary lung congestion is also a problem, shortness of breath will make lying flat difficult, limit exertion, and lead to frequent awakening during the night due to paroxysmal nocturnal dyspnea and coughing.

Relief is obtained through administration of diuretics to decrease the circulating blood volume, potassium to replace loss through urine, digitalis to increase the force of contraction of the failing heart, and long-acting blood vessel dilator medications to decrease the resistance against which the heart must pump. In addition, salt and fluid intake should be restricted.

Angina pectoris is usually experienced as a sensation of pressure, tightness, or heaviness behind the breastbone radiating down the inner arm and through to the back or upward toward the jaw. Shortness of breath, nausea, vomiting, and a cold, clammy sweat may accompany the pain. Physical exertion, abnormalities of heart rhythm, cigarette smoking, exposure to cold air, and emotional upset often precipitate angina attacks. After the pain has gone, patients usually can resume their usual activities because there is no damage to the heart muscle. The physician should not only prescribe nitroglycerine and propranolol for angina but also identify those environmental factors that trigger attacks and encourage the limitation of these activities.

Because abnormalities of heart rhythm may decrease the blood supply to any of the body's organs, arrhythmias may result in a wide variety of symptoms, including palpitations, angina pectoris, heart failure, and such neurological symptoms as faintness, focal or diffuse transient muscular weakness, and visual and speech difficulties.

OBJECTIVES

The main objectives of cardiac rehabilitation, which includes assessment and management, are:

1. Primary prevention of coronary heart disease in the high-risk, cardiac prone person.
2. Treatment of patients who have had a myocardial infarct to reduce the length of hospitalization, accelerate the return to work safely, reduce the number of recurrent myocardial infarctions, and improve the chance of surviving subsequent infarctions.
3. Secondary prevention of graft occlusion in patients who have had coronary bypass surgery.

ASSESSMENT

Indications and Contraindications

Any patient with one or more major cardiac risk factors (Table 14–1) should be enrolled in a cardiac rehabilitation program, as should anyone with ischemic heart disease and stable angina pectoris. Also, consider the coexistence of other possible risk factors, including the following:

1. Heredity.
2. Hypothyroidism.
3. Oral contraceptives.
4. Oral hypoglycemic agents.
5. Ethnic cultural factors.
6. Abnormal platelet aggregations.
7. Blood type A.
8. Viral and toxic myopathies.
9. Diet high in refined sugar and low in fiber.
10. Exposure to carbon dioxide and carbon monoxide.
11. Occupation.
12. Rapid resting heart rate.
13. Selenium or zinc deficiency.
14. Excessive heat or excessive cold.
15. Soft drinking water.
16. Ratio of estradiol and testosterone blood levels.

Patients should begin participating in the program 4 to 6 weeks after myocardial infarction and 4 weeks after cardiovascular surgery unless they have any of the following contraindications:

1. Recent myocardial infarction (less than 4 weeks ago).
2. Recent cardiac surgery (less than 4 weeks ago).
3. Active or recent myocarditis or pericarditis.
4. Recent pulmonary embolism.
5. Uncontrolled congestive heart failure.
6. Third degree A–V heart block.

TABLE 14–1. *Major cardiac risk factors*

Risk factor	Association with cardiac disease
Middle to old age	Atherosclerosis begins very early in life, but disease is not clinically apparent until fourth, fifth, and sixth decades
Hypertension	Triples chance of myocardial infarction
Male sex	Women have 4:1 lower prevalence until menopause, when chances are same as for men
Diabetes mellitus	Strong association, even in subclinical cases
Blood lipids	Reduced if serum cholesterol level is kept below 225 mg/100 ml and serum triglycerides level under 150 mg/100 ml
Obesity	Weight 15% above median ideal weight
Smoking	Mechanism of association unknown
Personality	Associated with chronic restlessness, achievement orientation, underlying passivity, and suppressed hostility
Severe emotional stress	Stresses tend to peak during middle age; emotions can produce serious arrhythmias, venous pressure alterations, cardiac output changes, abnormal pulse and blood pressure, altered peripheral resistance, electrocardiographic changes mimicking ischemic heart disease due to sympathetic stimulation, altered blood viscosity

7. Congenital heart disease with cyanosis.
8. Cardiac arrhythmias: uncontrolled atrial fibrillation, paroxysmal ventricular tachycardia, multifocal premature ventricular contraction (more than 15/100 cardiac cycle).

Cardiac Exercise Tests

The purpose of a cardiac exercise stress test is to monitor the patient and electrocardiogram (ECG) continuously for signs and symptoms that indicate tolerance for physical work. Specific findings include the presence or absence of myocardial ischemia, cardiac rhythm or conduction disturbances, circulatory disturbances, and respiratory embarrassment. Indications for cardiac exercise testing are known cardiac disease, possession of three or more major cardiac risk factors, and age over 40 before beginning a strenuous physical activity program.

The two most frequently used types of cardiac exercise tests are the standard two-step test and the stress test using the multistage treadmill or bicycle ergometer. The first type is limited to patients who have a normal resting ECG and requires only a 12-lead ECG machine and a two-step stair. If the standard two-step test is normal, a "double two-step test" is repeated in 2 hr. In the most widely used treadmill test, walking speeds are increased and uphill grades elevated every 3 min. The patient's ECG and blood pressure are monitored during exertion (Fig. 14–1) and for 5 min after recovery. Exercise is stopped if any of the following symptoms occur: angina, excessive dyspnea, abnormal ECG signs (such as three or more consecutive premature beats), hypotension (below resting level), or ataxia.

As the referring physician, you will receive a report from the cardiac exercise stress test laboratory that typically includes:

1. The patient's heart rate at rest.
2. The predicted heart rate.
3. Heart rate at different working loads.
4. ECG findings during resting periods.
5. Maximum work capacity.
6. Target heart rate (70% to 80% of maximum allowable rate for patient).

This report will provide you with enough information to write a prescription for the exercise therapist. In the prescription, designate the target heart rate, duration of each exercise session, number of sessions per week, and the threshold workload in metabolic units (METs), as indicated in the two sample exercise prescriptions in Table 14–2. (One MET is the amount of oxygen required at rest, approximately 3.5 cc per kilogram of body weight per minute.) Also recommend activities of daily living and various types of exercise that are consistent with the patient's energy expenditure limitations. The New York Heart Association has tabulated the energy level that can be comfortably attained by cardiac patients with activity limitations (Table 14–3). The amount of energy expended during various activities is outlined in Table 14–4.

Although death during cardiac exercise testing is rare, 10% to 30% of patients develop premature ventricular contractions (PVCs), 1% to 10% develop unstable blood pressure, and 0.01% to 0.1% may develop a myocardial infarction. Because of these possible complications, the supervising physician and therapist should have training in cardiopulmonary resuscitation techniques and a defibrillator should be readily available.

As an additional test of cardiac function during everyday activities, the patient may wear a Holter monitor for continuous ECG recording during normal work and recreational activities. Three or five electrodes are attached to the chest and to a small portable tape recorder that the client wears over the shoulder or around the waist (Fig. 14–2). Study of the tape recording suggests which activities the patient should limit.

After evaluation, the patient who has had a myocardial infarction is managed in one or more of four phases in a cardiac rehabilitation program: hospital, home, outpatient, and work.

HOSPITAL MANAGEMENT

An early bedside cardiac rehabilitation program usually is started within 48 to 72 hr after

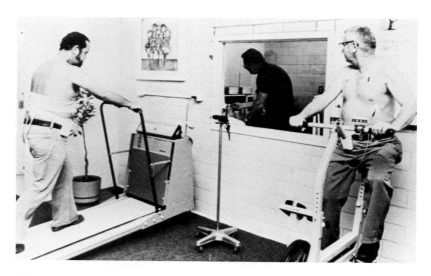

FIG. 14–1. Patient's blood pressure and heart rate are monitored during cardiac stress test on motor-driven treadmill. [From Naughton, J. (1977): Exercise prescription. In: *Coronary Heart Disease, Exercise Testing, and Cardiac Rehabilitation*. Symposia Specialists Medical Books, Miami, Florida.]

myocardial infarction, as soon as there is no chest pain, unstable blood pressure, serious arrhythmia, or signs of acute heart failure. For the first 3 days, the bed is rolled up to 45° and patients are allowed to wash their faces, brush their teeth, feed themselves, and use the bedside commode.

The physical therapist begins a supervised exercise program that includes:

1. Diaphragmatic breathing exercises to prevent hypostatic pneumonia (see Chapter 13).
2. Five repetitions of raising and straightening the legs to decrease the risk of thrombophlebitis.
3. Five repetitions of dorsiflexion and plantar flexion of the ankles.
4. Three repetitions of placing the hands behind the head and abducting the arms to

TABLE 14–2. *Two sample exercise prescriptions*

Threshold	Patient A[a]	Patient B[b]
Workload	4 METs	6 METs
Heart rate	120/min	140/min
Intensity (training heart rate prescription)	84–102/min	98–119/min
Duration	15–25 min/day	15–25 min/day
Frequency	3 days/week	3 days/week
Recommended activities	Slow walking; relaxation exercises	Fast walking; relaxation exercises; interval training with games such as volleyball

[a]A 67-year-old man with a history of diabetes mellitus and mild hypertension; myocardial infarction 6 weeks ago.

[b]A 48-year-old man with moderate obesity (20 lb overweight), Type A personality traits, and a 2-year history of arrhythmias.

TABLE 14–3. *Comfortable energy level limits for patients with heart disease*

Functional class	Activity limitation	METs
I	No limitations; no symptoms with ordinary activity	7+
II	Slight limitation; comfortable at rest; symptoms with ordinary activity	5–6
III	Marked limitation; comfortable at rest; symptoms with less than ordinary activity	3–4
IV	Discomfort with any activity; may have symptoms at rest	1–2

TABLE 14–4. *Energy expenditure for selected exercises and activities of daily living*

Activity	Cal/min	METs
Activities of Daily Living		
Resting, supine	1.0	1.0
Sitting at ease	1.2	1.0
Talking	1.4	1.0
Eating	1.44	1.0
Calculating	1.78	1.5
Writing	1.9	1.7
Listening to radio	1.97	1.7
Reading	1.98	1.7
Standing	1.98	1.7
Playing piano	2.0	1.5
Brushing clothes	2.57	2.3
Washing face, hands and brushing hair	2.74	2.4
Driving car	2.8	2.5
Showering	3.31	2.9
Cleaning shoes	3.49	3.0
Shaving	3.56	3.3
Using bedside commode	3.6	3.0
Using bed pan	4.7	4.0
Sexual activity	6.46	5.5
Physical Exercise		
Walking, 2 mph	3.1	2.7
Stationary bicycle, no resistance, 5 mph	3.0	2.5
Motorized treadmill, 0% grade, 2 mph	3.6	3.3
Walking 2.5 mph	3.8	3.4
Walking 3.0 mph	4.4	3.7
Stationary bicycle, no resistance, 6 mph	4.5	3.8

lessen the chances of a shoulder-hand syndrome developing (see Chapter 9).

On the fourth through seventh days of the cardiac rehabilitation program, the patient is able to perform additional exercises three times a day while sitting up in bed:

1. Two repetitions of moving the shoulders through the full range of motion.
2. Five repetitions of isometric contractions of the quadriceps without holding breath.
3. Two repetitions of extending the hands over the head.
4. Five repetitions of extending each leg.
5. Ten repetitions of flexing the knees to 90° by sliding the feet over the bed surface.

During the second week of rehabilitation, the patient is helped into a high-backed arm chair at the bedside. All exercises are increased to 10 repetitions three times a day and gluteal muscle contractions are added. The occupational therapist begins a supervised program of activities such as leather lacing and copper tooling.

From the 13th to 16th days, sitting in a chair may be increased from 30 min to 1 hr four times daily and all previous exercises are continued. A walking program is begun with 50 yards two to three times daily. The distance is increased to 100 yards and 300 yards by the 21st day, providing the patient does not experience any serious cardiac symptoms. These activities should be diminished in intensity any time the pulse rate elevates 20 beats over the resting pulse. If the patient also develops chest pain, dizziness, or severe dyspnea, reduce activities by 25% and give nitroglycerine at the onset of chest pain.

HOME MANAGEMENT AFTER HOSPITAL DISCHARGE

Patients are usually allowed to go home on the 14th to 21st day after an uncomplicated myocardial infarction. Each patient should receive instructions for a walking exercise program, which may begin as early as 3 to 4 weeks after a heart attack, as well as written guidelines for home activities, such as the following:

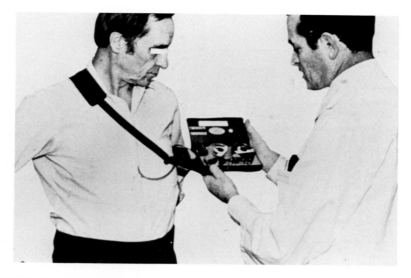

FIG. 14–2. Patient wearing Holter portable electrocardiogram recorder with battery-powered ECG tape deck and 24-hr monitoring capacity. [From Blocker, W. P. (1982): Electrocardiographic and blood pressure ambulatory monitoring. In: *Rehabilitation in Ischemic Heart Disease*, edited by W. P. Blocker and D. Cardus. SP Medical and Scientific, Jamaica, New York.]

1. Get 6 to 10 hr of sleep each night, take 20- to 30-min naps twice a day, and rest after each meal and whenever tired.
2. Plan each day's activities, space the hard tasks, and don't rush.
3. Sit down to work whenever possible and eliminate unnecessary tasks.
4. Don't hold your breath and tense your body, such as when straining with a bowel movement, lifting heavy objects, or opening a stuck window.
5. Don't work with your arms over your head.
6. Avoid performing activities under very hot or cold conditions.
7. If angina occurs, try to stop, rest, and lie down; if angina recurs during a certain activity, slow the pace or reduce the level of the activity.
8. Avoid letting your heart rate exceed 110 beats per minute or increase over 25 beats from the resting rate.
9. If you become short of breath, stop and rest; if you become severely short of breath for no apparent reason, call your physician.

On the first day of the walking program, the patient should try walking about ¹⁄₁₀ mile, or one average city block, in 5 or 6 min. After 3 to 4 days, the distance can be increased to ¼ mile, or two long blocks. This longer distance should take 8 to 10 min and be continued twice each day for 2 weeks before increasing the distance to ½ mile.

From then on, patients stay at a given walking level for about 2 weeks, then increase either the distance or the speed of walking. A reasonable objective would be 1 mile in 15 min by the 14th week after discharge from the hospital. Patients should check their pulse before increasing to a higher level, and if the heart rate increases by more than 25 beats per minute or exceeds 100 beats per minute, postpone advancing until the next check-up. Exercise should be discontinued altogether if new or more severe chest discomfort or shortness of breath develops at any stage of the walking program.

OUTPATIENT MANAGEMENT OF HIGH-RISK PATIENTS

The outpatient cardiac rehabilitation program begins 6 to 8 weeks after a patient's myocardial infarction, or after the ability to walk 2 miles at a comfortable rate has been attained. Each exercise period begins with 15 min of "warm up" calisthenics (Fig. 14–3). A typical warm-up program is described in Table 14–5. This is followed by a 20- to 30-min aerobic exercise period of walking, jogging, swimming, bicycling, or treadmill of sufficient intensity to generate the patient's target heart rate. If expense is not a factor, the treadmill is preferred because walking is a more natural activity than riding a bicycle or swimming. The exercise period ends with a cool down period of slow walking or bicycling for at least 10 min. Then the patient lies down on an exercise pad and listens to tapes instructing in relaxation techniques.

As the patient exercises on the treadmill or bicycle ergometer at the predetermined workload and within the limits of the target heart rate, monitoring by ECG is continuous and blood pressure is checked every 5 min. After 3 to 6 weeks, the patient is taught to monitor his or her own heart rate during bicycling, walking, or jogging. At no time should the pulse rate of a middle-aged or elderly patient exceed 130 beats per minute, nor should the initial workload exceed 2 or 3 METs for high-risk patients. Adjust the workload every 2 weeks to achieve the target heart rate, but no more than 1 MET per step of increased work.

The purpose of the relaxation period is relief of muscle tension that may result not only in painful muscles and joints after exercise but also in altered blood pressure, heart rate, and rhythm and inadequate oxygenation of the heart, lungs, and skeletal muscles. First, the patient tries to stretch the upper extremities, neck and face, trunk, and lower extremities separately and for as long as possible. The difference between tightness and relaxation is then learned by flexing and relaxing the extremities while breathing slowly. As the last step, the patient mentally relaxes the ankles, knees, thighs, wrists, forearms, shoulders, and head.

After 8 to 12 weeks in a supervised cardiac exercise program, patients can continue their cardiac rehabilitation program at home, at the local YMCA, or health club. Regular office visits for evaluation by the primary care physician, however, are essential to detect indications for further cardiac evaluation and temporary discontinuance of the exercise program, such as the following:

1. PVCs in pairs or with increasing frequency, ventricular tachycardia (runs of three or more PVCs).

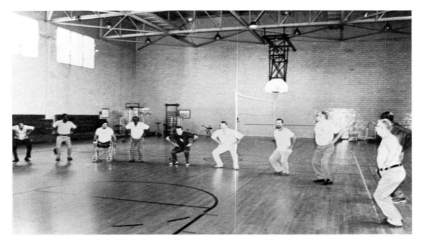

FIG. 14–3. Warm-up period of calisthenics preceding cardiac rehabilitation exercise program. [From Hartung, G. H. (1982): Stage IV cardiac rehabilitation recovery and outpatient follow-up program. In: *Rehabilitation in Ischemic Heart Disease*, edited by W. P. Blocker and D. Cardus. SP Medical and Scientific, Jamaica, New York.]

TABLE 14–5. *Flexibility and warm-up calisthenics*

Exercise (3×/week)	Repetitions		
	Starting	Increase/week	Final
Circle both arms forward in full circle together	5	5	50
Circle both arms backward simultaneously	5	5	50
Swing both arms forward in full circle alternately, simulating crawl stroke	5	5	50
Leaning forward slightly, swing arm forward and backward in half circle, starting with one arm back and the other forward	5	5	50
Swing arms horizontally, rotating at waist, left to right and right to left; allow arms to bend at end of swing	5	5	50
Swing arms between legs, return and "pump" arms backward three times at top of swing	5	5	50
Swing arms between legs, then up overhead to side; bend body alternately left and right	5	5	50

From Hartung, G. H. (1982): Stage IV cardiac rehabilitation recovery and outpatient follow-up program. In: *Rehabilitation in Ischemic Heart Disease*, edited by W. P. Blocker and D. Cardus. SP Medical and Scientific, Jamaica, NY.

2. Atrial tachycardia or atrial fibrillation.
3. Onset of heart block, either second or third degree.
4. Increasing anginal pain with ECG changes.
5. Unusual fatigue.
6. Claudication or pain.
7. Dizziness.
8. Cyanosis or pallor.
9. Dyspnea.
10. Fall in systolic blood pressure (10 mm Hg) with increasing workload.
11. Extreme rise in systolic (above 220 mm Hg) or diastolic (110 mm Hg) blood pressure.
12. S–T segment displacement of 1.0 mm above or below the baseline.
13. Cool skin.
14. Cessation of sweating.

Success will be maximized by participating in activities that emphasize aerobic or low-intensity isotonic exercise rather than isometric and intense isotonic exercise. The latter increase systolic and diastolic blood pressure, a hypertensive response that greatly increases the demand of the heart muscle for oxygen and that may produce angina.

PSYCHOSOCIAL ADJUSTMENT

Adverse emotional reactions to myocardial infarction and cardiac surgery can be expected. Depression, anxiety, irritability, and exhaustion are typically noted for at least 3 months after the infarction. Six months to 1 year later, 88% of patients are still feeling anxious or depressed, 83% complain of weakness, 55% have disturbed sleep, and 38% are unable to return to work for psychological reasons. How the patient overcomes these reactions is not related to the severity of attack but to his or her premorbid personality, preparation for resuming normal activities by the physician and other members of the rehabilitation team, and accurate medical instruction about fitness and work.

Two personality types are highly susceptible to maladjustment during convalescence: the "supermale" and "cardiac invalid." The supermale verbally and nonverbally discounts medical recommendations about physical activity, work, medications, and sexual activity. Disregarding symptoms, this patient typically embarks on a seriously self-destructive course by continuing to smoke, failing to keep appointments, refusing to take prescribed medications, and overindulging in physical activity. The cardiac invalid plays a helpless, dependent role and exhibits excessive somatic preoccupation. Typically, this patient interprets tachycardia, orthostatic hypotension, shortness of breath, and weakness caused by physical inactivity (see Chapter 22 for a detailed explanation of this immobilization syndrome) as evidence of cardiac impairment and becomes even more inactive.

Evaluation

Do not expect the patient to volunteer information about his or her emotional status. During routine office visits, most patients will not complain about fears of death, pain, dyspnea, or further attacks unless directly questioned about what bothers them. A useful evaluation tool, known as BASIC ID, identifies:

B —Behavioral excesses or deficits that represent ineffective coping.

A —Affect such as depression, anxiety, or the lack of appropriate emotional response typical of denial.

S —Sensory distortions, neurological impairment, and somatic complaints.

I —Imagery, dreams, and other symbolic representations of self-concept.

C —Cognitive factors, such as fallacious thinking and attentional deficits.

I —Interpersonal relations, social awareness, and maturity.

D —Drug-induced behavior and propensity to adhere to risk reduction programs, including compliance with the medication regimen.

Role of the Spouse

It is recommended that the cardiac patient's spouse undergo brief, outpatient psychotherapy to help modify methods of dealing with the patient. The spouse may inadvertently support maladaption to myocardial infarction or cardiac surgery by extremes of behavior: acting punitive, overprotective, and oversolicitous or, at the other extreme, being unsympathetic and nonsupportive. Participation in therapeutic groups with other spouses may help alleviate feelings of guilt and enable him or her to benefit from their experiences. The wife, for example, may believe that she somehow contributed to her husband's heart attack and, as a result, inhibit the expression of any strong feelings toward him. Her emotional withdrawal only intensifies his humiliation and depression.

Education of Patient and Family

Emotional conflicts are often precipitated by inconsistent medical instructions for convalescence from the physician at different times or from different members of the rehabilitation team. To reduce confusion and discourage conflicts between the patient and spouse, avoid vague, generalized statements about treatment and permissible activities. Give the patient specific written instructions about what should and should not be done during the progressive phases of recovery and adapt these instructions to the patient's condition after each follow-up office visit. Being specific about the patient's medical progress will also help alleviate anxiety and foster hope.

Because stress hampers the ability to absorb information, verbal and written instructions should be reinforced and repeated frequently. Modifications in the patient's lifestyle that will reduce cardiac risk factors cannot be emphasized too often. The following are the recommended components of a cardiac education plan:

1. General medical information: nature of myocardial infarction heart function, healing process.
2. Rehabilitation plan: goals, introduction to team members and their roles, progression of activity.
3. Psychosocial: understanding of reactions to myocardial infarction, financial and vocational problems, family expectations.
4. Risk factors and need to modify lifestyle.
5. Medication regimen and side effects.
6. Recommended diet.
7. Exercise.
8. Recognition of warning symptoms during work, sex, driving.

These topics are often scheduled as weekly lectures or question and answer periods in an outpatient cardiac rehabilitation program.

Encouraging Compliance and Discouraging Recidivism

A cardiac rehabilitation program is unlikely to benefit the patient who does not regularly attend:

1. Cardiac exercise program to maintain cardiopulmonary fitness, develop a better self-image, and increase work tolerance.
2. Behavioral modification program to learn to cope with emotional stress.
3. Lectures by the dietician to maintain optimum body weight and, when indicated, lower blood glucose and blood lipid levels.

Telephone any patient who has missed 2 or more days and encourage regular participation.

Resuming Sexual Activity

Following a myocardial infarction, patients are frequently reticent about asking questions regarding their future sexual activity. Other patients who have had a heart attack are under the misconception that sexual intercourse may lead to death. They may refrain from sex, or have intercourse only with a great deal of anxiety; 10% to 30% of patients become impotent after myocardial infarction.

Despite such misgivings, it is usually safe to resume sexual intercourse 6 to 12 weeks after a heart attack, depending on the individual's rate of recovery. In terms of energy expenditure, intercourse is comparable to climbing one or two flights of stairs or taking a brisk walk. The heart rate may increase up to 120 heart beats per minute and systolic blood pressure by 30 to 40 mm Hg. The ECG during intercourse may show some ectopic beats and ischemic S–T changes that would be seen during moderate exercise. The following are guidelines to give your patients about sexual activity during recovery from a heart attack:

1. Avoid intercourse after a heavy meal, when intoxicated, or fatigued.
2. Avoid intercourse in unfamiliar surroundings or when it is uncomfortably hot or cold.
3. Select positions that do not require prolonged body support by the arms and legs, such as side by side or lying on the back.
4. Notify your physician if rapid breathing or a rapid heart rate persists longer than 15 min after intercourse.
5. If you experience chest pain during intercourse, take your nitroglycerine when prescribed, before you again engage in intercourse. If chest pain persists, notify your physician.
6. Any temporary absence of spontaneous erections following myocardial infarction is probably due to the physical strain and emotional exhaustion that accompany a heart attack. You can expect this problem to resolve as your overall level of activity increases.
7. Discuss with your physician openly any questions you may have concerning sexual activity.

Returning to Work

Approximately 80% of persons who have experienced a myocardial infarction are capable of returning to work. Of those returning to work, 80% will return to their former jobs and 20% to less strenuous work duties. Of the blue collar group of workers, 25% will not return to work, while only 2% of the executives will fail to return to work. Of those patients who have had a coronary bypass operation, 11% of the younger patients will retire, while 26% of the older patients will no longer work. Among those returning to work, 30% will change their occupation. Patients who attend a cardiac rehabilitation program after myocardial infarction or coronary bypass surgery are more apt to return to work, have a higher work tolerance, and enjoy better physical and mental health.

PROGNOSIS

The survival of the patient early after myocardial infarction has improved greatly during the past decade. A less favorable prognosis for survival is associated with complaints of dyspnea, cyanosis, shock, arrhythmias such as auricular fibrillation, frequent ventricular premature systoles, ventricular tachycardia, pericardial friction rub, and systolic arterial pressure persistently less than 90 mm Hg after infarction. Other signs associated with increased mortality rate are persistent fever of 103°F or higher, leukocytosis with white blood cell count >15,000/cu mm, and ECG evidence of an auriculoventricular or intraventricular block. Pulmonary, cerebral, renal, or peripheral thromboembolic complications may also be life-threatening.

Of patients who survive the early postinfarct period, 95% will eventually succumb to cardiac death, and 10% to 15% will be totally incapacitated for the rest of their lives. Although 30% will not need to restrict their activities at all, partial restriction of activity will be necessary in 60% of patients.

One-fourth of patients, particularly those over age 50, will be rehospitalized within the first year of the initial infarct. The more primary cardiac risk factors a patient has, the more prone he or she will be to having a future heart attack. The factors that most frequently precipitate a heart attack include unusual fatigue resulting from travel or prolonged or violent physical exertion, overeating, emotional strain, excessive intake of alcoholic beverages, exposure to cold, and smoking.

It is well established that a high percentage of patients with coronary heart disease who have coronary bypass surgery experience relief from angina, increased work tolerance, and an improved sense of well-being. However, the value of cardiac surgery in prolonging life remains undecided. These patients appear to have less postsurgical graft occlusion if they participate in a cardiac exercise program than do their sedentary counterparts.

The degree of recovery from myocardial infarction and extent of disability 1 year later are often unrelated to prognostic indicators. As demonstrated in the following case reports, it is not uncommon for one patient to remain a cardiac invalid after a relatively mild attack while another completely leaves the sick role to resume

full-time employment, only slightly reducing his former activity level.

ADJUSTMENT TO MYOCARDIAL INFARCTION

Report of Two Cases

PATIENT 1. Mr. H., a successful executive in a competitive, sales-oriented business, had a myocardial infarction at age 49. After 3 weeks of hospitalization with no complications, he was discharged home to join his wife and five children. In his interview with a social worker during hospitalization, he expressed an optimistic attitude about his future. Expressing the belief that a man is better off working than retiring after a heart attack, he expected eventually to return to work full-time. His judgment of the severity of the attack was realistic; he agreed with his physician that it had been moderate.

Six weeks after discharge, he was not working yet, but had been out driving and had been following his physician's advice about resuming former activities. He was able to return to work part-time 3 months after the infarction and full-time in 10 months. In an interview 1 year later, he stated that he continued to see his physician every 4 months, but was not especially concerned about his condition and was taking no medications. However, some degree of anxiety was revealed by macabre humor as he joked about his condition. Despite his apparent calm in the hospital, he admitted that he had worried that he might not pull through and had expected to die after the attack.

Although he continued to "slow down" 1½ years after the infarction, he considered himself fully recovered. In response to questioning about what he enjoyed doing most, he did not mention specific diversions, but simply stated that what he really enjoyed was "the pleasure of being here." His physician confirmed that Mr. H. was performing at his full level of capacity and was physically able to perform all activities.

PATIENT 2. Mr. D., 50 years old and in good health, rated his mild myocardial infarction as moderately severe despite his 4-week hospitalization without complications and his normal recovery. In his hospital interview with the social worker, he expressed the belief that he would have to slow down almost to a complete stop. Also unlike Mr. H., he believed that a man should not return to work or try to do anything strenuous after a heart attack. Mr. D. was a blue-collar jewelry worker who was under pressure to produce quickly, yet he blamed his illness on family troubles and weekend drinking. Living with his in-laws, he pronounced his mother-in-law as the head of his family, which consisted of his wife and teenage son.

Six months after discharge, Mr. D. had not returned to work, yet continued to say that he needed to. He had applied for a total disability pension and complained of terrible headaches and feeling weak. His feelings of helplessness had increased with the death of the head of the household, his mother-in-law. He began taking medication for depression and "nervousness" and nitroglycerine for angina. Although his complaints about his heart trouble were vague and unsubstantiated by his physician, Mr. D. believed that he had a strong chance of having a second attack that would kill him, as his brother had died from a heart attack. He also felt that his family and friends expected him to die like his brother had.

One year after the infarction, Mr. D. was still spending his days quietly, watching television and taking naps. He reported few social contacts and felt he had nothing to look forward to. He had ignored his physician's advice to take longer walks. His physician felt that Mr. D. was spending most of his time thinking about his heart and was capable of returning to work and functioning at a much higher level. His physical symptoms were due to inactivity rather than to the infarction, which had left little residual damage.

SUGGESTED READINGS

American College of Sports Medicine (1978): *Guidelines for Graded Exercise Testing and Exercise Presciptions.* Lea and Febiger, Philadelphia.

Blocker, W. P., and Cardus, D. (1982): *Rehabilitation in Ischemic Heart Disease.* Spectrum Medical Publications, New York.

Bruce, E. H., Fredrick, R., Bruce, R. A., et al. (1976): Comparison of active participation and drop outs in CAPRI cardiopulmonary rehabilitation programs. *Am. J. Cardiol.*, 37:53–59.

Cousins, N. (1983): *The Healing Heart: Antidotes to Panic and Helplessness.* Norton, New York.

Gentry, W. D., and Williams, R. B., Jr. (1979): *Psychological Aspects of Myocardial Infarction and Coronary Care.* C. V. Mosby, St. Louis.

James, W. E., and Amsterdam, E. A., editors (1977): *Coronary Heart Disease, Exercise Testing, and Cardiac Rehabilitation.* Symposia Specialists Medical Books, Miami, FL.

Kaplan, N. M., and Stamler, J. (1983): *Prevention of Coronary Heart Disease: Practical Management of the Risk Factors.* W. B. Saunders, Philadelphia.

Monteiro, L. A. (1979): *Cardiac Patient Rehabilitation: Social Aspects of Recovery.* Springer, New York.

Pollock, M. C., Wilmore, J. H., and Fox, S. M. (1984): *Exercise in Health and Disease.* W. B. Saunders, Philadelphia.

Wenger, N. K., and Hellerstein, H. K. (1978): *Rehabilitation of the Coronary Patient.* John Wiley and Sons, New York.

Wilde, S. W., Miles, D. S., Durbin, R. J., et al. (1981): Evaluation of myocardial performance during wheelchair ergometer exercise. *Am. J. Phys. Med. Rehabil.*, 60:277–291.

Medical Rehabilitation,
edited by L. S. Halstead et al.
Raven Press, New York © 1985.

CHAPTER 15

Stroke

Shelly E. Liss

Department of Physical Medicine, Memorial Hospital and Baylor College of Medicine, and Department of Family Practice, University of Texas Medical School, Houston, Texas 77030

With approximately 500,000 new stroke victims annually, including 250,000 survivors, the United States now has an estimated 2.5 million disabled survivors of stroke. When cost of care and the loss of earnings are considered, the economic impact of stroke in this country totals an estimated $9.5 billion annually in 1982 dollars.

Because of its high incidence, especially in populations over 55 years of age, most physicians are aware of current developments in stroke prophylaxis, diagnosis, and management. The focus of this chapter is the rehabilitation techniques recommended for the treatment of residual stroke-induced disabilities. With proper rehabilitation services, approximately 80% of those who survive a stroke can walk without assistance, 70% can master self-care activities, and 30% can return to work.

EVALUATION

The purpose of the rehabilitation evaluation is to identify deficits and problem areas resulting from the stroke so that a rehabilitation treatment program can be developed to help the stroke patient reach realistic functional goals. Whether performed by individual members of a rehabilitation team or the primary care physician alone, the examination includes assessments of medical status, extent of neurological deficit, functional performance, psychosocial factors, and family support.

Medical Status

The presence of other medical problems often influences the course of rehabilitation for the stroke patient, making evaluation of the cardiovascular, pulmonary, and genitourinary systems vital. The decrease in energy level and endurance caused by cardiac and pulmonary disease often requires a modification and limitation of rehabilitation activities. An estimated 12% of stroke patients have associated symptomatic heart disease, and as many as 75% have one or more signs of cardiac failure, atrial fibrillation, or an enlarged heart demonstrated by radiography or the electrocardiogram (ECG). Urinary incontinence secondary to neurogenic bladder or urinary retention secondary to an enlarged prostate is common. If hypertension or diabetes is present, proper control of these diseases is necessary to avoid medical complications that will retard the rehabilitation program. Osteoarthritis, particularly in the knee or hip of the uninvolved side, can impede successful ambulation unless special precautions are taken to protect these joints during the rehabilitation process.

Neurological Deficit

The neuromusculoskeletal evaluation includes an assessment of cerebral and cerebellar function, sensation, vision, cognition, muscle tone and strength, and range of motion. A detailed discussion of neuromusculoskeletal evaluation techniques is presented in Chapter 3.

One simple test for basic awareness of the environment is to offer your hand and observe whether the patient reaches out unassisted with the uninvolved arm to touch or shake it. A bedside assessment for neurogenic communicative disorders can be made by noting the patient's spontaneous speech. If nonfluency is noted in the presence of good comprehension, suspect a motor dysphasia (Broca frontal lobe type). Fluency in the presence of poor comprehension suggests sensory dysphasia (Wernicke parieto-temporal lobe type). Dysarthria is probable if speech is slurred due to oral-facial weakness but comprehension is normal. If verbal deficits are significant enough to impair function, further evaluation and treatment by a speech pathologist is recommended.

Stroke-induced disabilities often involve intellectual deficits specific to left or right hemisphere involvement. To evaluate judgment, memory, intelligence, and orientation, ask the patient to perform simple bedside skills. Table 15–1 shows common cognitive dysfunctions often seen after a stroke. If such deficits are noted upon initial examination, further evaluation by specialized members of the rehabilitation team is recommended.

Functional Performance

Many patients, because of lack of stimulation, opportunity, or motivation to become in-dependent, may function at a much lower level than their neurological abilities warrant. The cause behind a patient's inability to perform a specific functional skill must be determined. Functional skills usually evaluated are activities of daily living (eating, washing, dressing, personal hygiene), transfers, and ambulation. A detailed discussion of functional evaluation techniques is presented in Chapter 3. The degree of independence in each of these areas is noted, along with the need for assistive devices.

Psychosocial Factors and Family Support

Psychosocial factors such as motivation to achieve independent function and family involvement are often the best predictors of post-rehabilitation outcome. A thorough assessment of family relationships, economic resources, vocational and recreational activities, and environmental resources provides indispensable information to aid in counseling the family and setting realistic goals. Family members may experience a great deal of anxiety regarding the health and longevity of the stroke patient and their own ability to make the adjustments that

TABLE 15–1. *Common mentation/cognitive intellectual dysfunctions in stroke patients*

Core intellectual abilities	Right cerebral vascular accident with left hemiplegia	Left cerebral vascular accident with right hemiplegia
Verbal skills	Usually no deficit in the ability to understand and express language; a dysarthria may be present	Impaired ability to receive and/or express verbal information commonly present; aphasia
Perceptual skills	Impaired ability to assess own position in space and to safely interact with environment; driving and kitchen activities unwise; neglect of left side may be present	Usually unimpaired
Memory skills	Verbal memory is usually intact; perceptual memory impairments usually accompany perceptual deficits	May display impaired ability to retain recent verbal information; remote memory is likely to be impaired
Quality control	Tendency to be careless and oblivious of mistakes; impulsive with decreased ability to anticipate the consequences of behavior	Usually unimpaired
Emotional appropriateness	May display inappropriate emotion, such as unexplained weeping	Emotional expression usually appropriate
Alertness	Impairment in alertness during early phases common; condition usually improves rapidly unless brain stem is involved	Impairment in alertness during early phases common; condition usually improves rapidly unless brain stem is involved

may be required. Financial concerns, including mounting medical expenses and temporary or permanent loss of income, are often considerable. Knowing how these concerns affect the individual patient and his family will enable you to provide appropriate counseling while mobilizing family support during the rehabilitation process. As the patient progresses, ongoing assessment is important to meet the evolving needs of the individual and his family.

REHABILITATION PROGRAM

Acute Phase

Basic elements of rehabilitation that emphasize good nursing care start as soon after the stroke as possible, even while life-saving medical management is the primary concern. Three nursing orders that can be implemented on admission are positioning, frequent turning, and range of motion exercises to prevent contractures and to preserve function.

Proper positioning in the supine, side-lying (on the involved side to allow the good arm to be free), or prone positions can prevent contractures that would restrict function as neurological recovery occurs (Fig. 15–1). Without correct placement, the patient can quickly develop adduction contractures of the shoulder, flexion contractures of the hand, external rotation contractures of the hip, and plantar flexion contractures of the ankle. A resting splint on the hand or ankle may be necessary to ensure maintenance of proper positioning. A detailed discussion of positioning and splinting is presented in Chapter 6.

Alternating the positions every 2 hr increases the patient's comfort while helping to prevent pulmonary complications and decubitus ulcers. You should also consider ordering special mattresses, sheep skins, and boots with foam inserts (such as those made by Stryker Company).

Full passive range of motion exercises for the involved extremities are completed from one to three times a day by a nurse or physical therapist to prevent contractures and maintain muscle tone. These exercises are described in Chapter 4.

When there are no complications, medical stability usually is achieved in 1 to 2 days, at which time the patient can participate in an active mobilization program.

Mobilization

In most stroke patients, mobilization consists of four phases. It begins with bed activities and progresses to sitting, standing, and ambulation with the ultimate goal of obtaining functional independence. Early mobilization not only helps prevent orthostatic postural hypotension, venous stasis in the paralyzed leg and severe weakness, but also improves the patient's sense of well-being. You can bolster the patient's sense of accomplishment and self-confidence in his ability by proceeding sequentially and never asking the patient to attempt a new task until he has mastered the preceding tasks.

Bed Phase

When the patient is medically stable, he can begin to participate actively in the rehabilitation program. A gradual progression from passive to active range of motion is undertaken as motor function returns. Strengthening exercises of the involved and uninvolved sides are introduced, usually by a physical therapist, with special attention to those muscles used in transfer and ambulation.

The first elements of mobility learned by the patient are moving up and down in bed, turning from side to side, pulling up to a sitting position, and sitting on the edge of the bed. To move up and down, the patient grasps the headboard with his good hand, bends his knees and hips, places his feet flat on the bed, then pulls with his good arm while pushing with his good leg. Rolling over is accomplished by using the good arm to pull on the side rails on both the involved and uninvolved sides. The good foot is crossed under the bad ankle to shift the buttocks into the roll. The patient rolls onto his uninvolved side to sit up, pushing his body up on his uninvolved arm and slowly extending his elbow while dropping his legs off the bed (Fig. 15–2). Through practice and proper body positioning, good un-

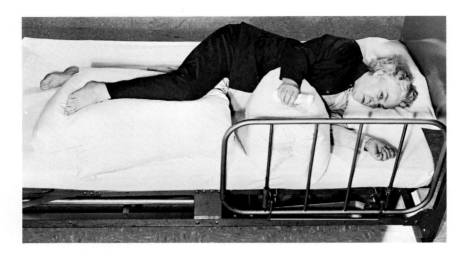

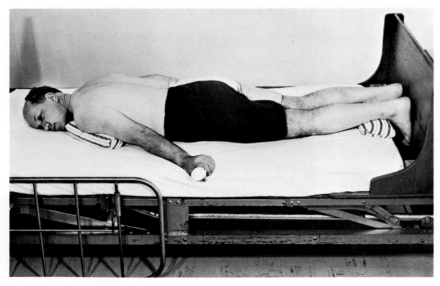

FIG. 15–1. Proper positioning. **Top:** Side-lying position *(black side of clothing indicates involved side).* **Bottom:** Prone position. [From Ellwood, P. M. (1982): Bed positioning. In *Krusen's Handbook of Physical Medicine and Rehabilitation,* 3rd edit, edited by F. J. Kottke, et al. W. B. Saunders, Philadelphia.]

supported sitting balance can be attained. When these maneuvers have been mastered, the patient is ready for standing and transfers.

Stand-Up Phase

Before standing transfers and walking can be undertaken, the stroke patient must strengthen the uninvolved leg and obtain maximum standing balance and tolerance. If the knee of the involved leg does not maintain full extension, a temporary, long leg brace or knee splint provides stable support, enabling the musculature of the trunk and leg of the uninvolved side to perform the bulk of the motion and momentum of the exercise.

The equipment required includes a stable chair with some mechanism for altering the level of the seat height. This can be accomplished easily by placing risers or lifts on the chair at 2-inch

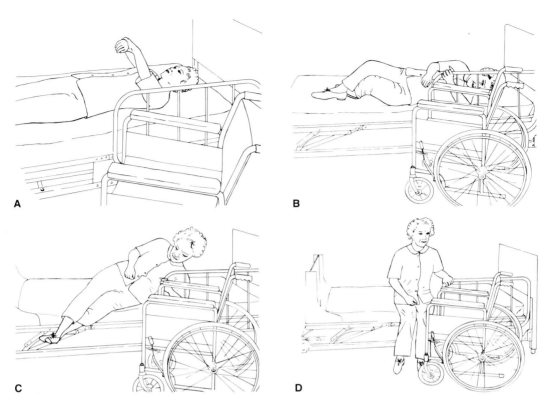

FIG. 15–2. Sitting up. **A:** The patient moves her involved arm. **B:** She crosses her good foot under the bad ankle, grasps the side rail, and turns onto her normal side. **C:** She drops her legs off the bed and swings into a sitting position. **D:** She is prepared to transfer into a wheelchair. [From Ellwood, P. M. (1982), see Fig. 15–1 for complete ref.]

increments. The seat height is adjusted to approximately one-and-a-half times the patient's leg length from knee to foot. To assist the patient in maintaining balance, a stable object such as the foot of the bed, the back of a heavy chair, or a parallel bar is needed (Fig. 15–3).

Minimal assistance is provided by the therapist or nurse during the exercise when the patient is requested to stand up. Since most of the work should be done by the legs, not the arms, the patient should be discouraged from using his arm to pull up or from pushing up by leaning forward over his good arm and extending his elbow. The entire weight of the body must be lifted by the uninvolved leg if strengthening and hypertrophy of the antigravity musculature are to occur. When the patient is able to complete 10 stand-ups with little or no assistance, the level of the chair is lowered 2 inches and the process

repeated until he is able to stand up independently from a standard chair. As strength increases, standing balance is improved by leaning forward, backward, and from side to side.

The standing transfer (Fig. 15–4) only requires mastering a pivot technique if introduced after the stand-up phase. The patient starts by sitting on the side of the bed with a wheelchair parallel to the bed on his uninvolved side. He then stands up using the uninvolved leg and places his normal hand on the far arm of the wheelchair. To complete the transfer, he pivots 90° on his normal foot so that the wheelchair is directly behind him and lowers himself into the chair. To get back into bed, the patient reverses the process, placing the chair again so that he would be moving toward his good side. He approaches the bed, locks the chair, and swings the footrest out of the way. Leaning forward

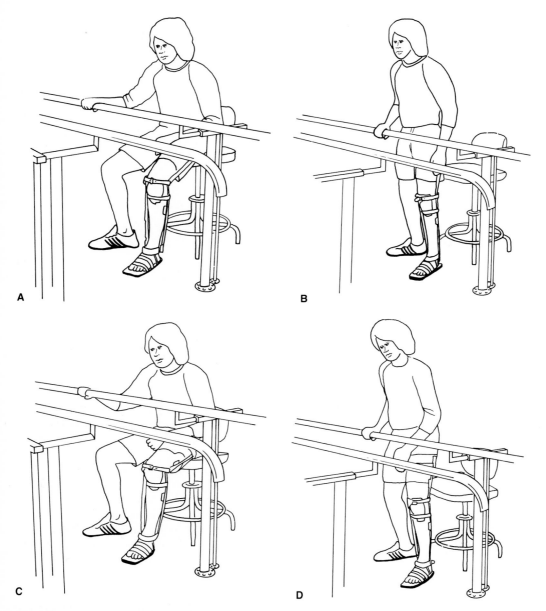

FIG. 15–3. Stand-up with assistance of parallel bars and adjustable chair.   **A:** The patient begins his standing exercise in a high sitting position.   **B:** The patient grasps the parallel bar with his good hand to maintain balance as he stands up.   **C:** The chair is lowered as the patient progresses.   **D:** He learns to stand from the lowered position. Note the maintenance of knee extension by the long leg brace.

toward the edge of the seat, he grasps the arm rest and pushes himself into a standing position. Grasping the side rail of the bed, he pivots and lowers himself to sit on the bed.

The ability to perform a standing transfer gives the patient a great deal of mobility and independence. The hemiplegic patient can propel himself in a standard wheelchair by using the

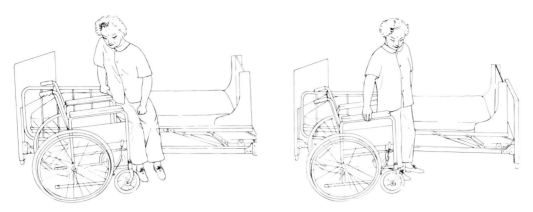

FIG. 15–4. Standing transfer into wheelchair. **Left:** Grasping the side rail with her good arm, the patient stands. **Right:** Grasping the far arm of the wheelchair, she pivots and prepares to sit down. [From Ellwood, P. M. (1982), see Fig. 15–1 for complete ref.]

uninvolved hand to provide forward motion and the uninvolved foot to maintain the proper direction. In most cases, the wheelchair is considered a temporary assistive device until ambulation is achieved. A patient should not purchase a wheelchair until the rehabilitation team determines that walking will not progress to an independent, safe level.

Step-Up Phase

The step-up phase is initiated prior to ambulation so that the patient can lift his feet, lead, and continue to strengthen the uninvolved foot. Temporary bracing may be necessary to stabilize the involved extremity during this activity or to allow adequate clearance of the foot during the swing phase of gait. In approximately 30% of hemiplegic patients, recovery of the foot dorsiflexors is inadequate to allow the foot to swing through, causing the drop foot to catch on the floor. In addition, spasticity can cause equinovarus deformity of the foot, which impairs proper foot placement.

If no significant spasticity is present, a simple elastic strap running from the toes to the lower leg may be sufficient to maintain the foot at a 90° angle. Minimum to moderate spasticity calls for a plastic ankle-foot orthosis. A metal short leg brace, which has an ankle joint and a durable aluminum upright and calf band, may be nec-

essary when spasticity is moderate to severe for preventing mediolateral instability and possible injury to the unstable ankle. A permanent long leg brace or knee splint is rarely necessary and is reserved only for when the quadriceps function is very poor and knee control cannot be achieved with a short leg brace. Surgery is indicated only to correct very severe spasticity.

Once the patient has mastered the stand-up phase and is adequately braced, stair climbing is not difficult and has greater exercise value than walking on a level surface. The only equipment required is a series of 2-inch, 4-inch, and 6-inch stairs with handrails. The patient is instructed to climb the 2-inch stairs by stabilizing himself with the normal hand on the handrail and the extended or braced involved leg on the lower step or floor. The patient then lifts his uninvolved leg to the next step (Fig. 15–5A), extending his knee and lifting the involved leg to the same level (Fig. 15–5B). To descend the stairs (Fig. 15–5C), he leads with the involved foot, placing it on the step below and bending the normal knee until the involved foot is firmly placed on the step (Fig. 15–5D). After mastering the 2-inch steps, the patient progresses to the 4-inch and then the 6-inch staircases.

Ambulation Phase

After mastering the step-up phase, the hemiplegic patient can progress to walking with a

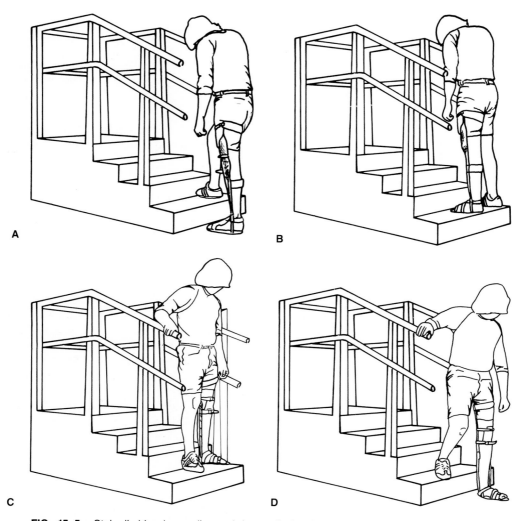

FIG. 15–5. Stair climbing (ascending and descending) using 6-inch stairs with handrails (see text).

minimum of training. You should provide him with a hemiwalker (one-sided walker) or a quad cane. Problems that may impede successful ambulation (Table 15–2) include leaning to the involved side, the inability to clear the involved foot during the swing phase, or uncoordinated hip, knee, and ankle motion. More intensive training may be necessary to teach the patient to lean toward the good side so that the uninvolved arm can bear the bulk of the total body weight during walking. Also, leaning toward the uninvolved side will assist in clearing the in-

volved leg during the swing phase. In some patients, a heel and sole lift added to the bottom of the shoe of the normal foot corrects the problem.

As strength, coordination, and balance improve, the patient may progress from a hemiwalker to a large-base quad cane, to a small-base quad cane, and finally to a standard cane (Table 15–3). Many patients eventually are able to walk without any type of aid. It is important to discharge the patient with the minimum equipment needed for safe ambulation.

TABLE 15–2. *Gait training*

Phase	Normal movement	Common movement errors	Causes	Correction recommended
Stance				
Heel strike	Hit floor heel first, with foot dorsiflexed	Toes touch first		Instruct patient to stand very straight, shoulders back and pelvis forward; bracing to provide support for unstable ankle and knee; exercise to strengthen weak muscles
Stance	Bend 15° at knee; fully extend knee and stand straight; trunk is upright	Trunk falls forward; knee buckles	Weak gluteus maximus muscle; weak quadriceps muscle	
Push off	Push off with toes and ball of foot; bend knee slightly while bending hips slightly			
Swing	Other leg is in stance phase; ankle and foot are at 90° angle; body weight shifts to other leg; leg swings forward	Unable to perform one or all of these functions; leg feels glued to floor	Stiff knee joint; weak ankles; weak hip flexors; plantar flexion; contractures	Short leg brace; attach lift to bottom of shoe on uninvolved leg to equalize functional longer length of involved leg; exercise to strengthen weak muscles; serial splints to correct contractures
	Leg swings past other leg; hamstrings control speed, and quadriceps fully extend knee	Knee not fully extended; leg doesn't clear other leg; knee pops back into hyperextension (genu recurvatum)	Nonfunctioning quadriceps and hamstrings	
	With knee straight, foot dorsiflexes beyond 90° angle and patient's leg is again in position for heel strike. Gait pattern repeats			

TABLE 15–3. *Walking aids*

Type of cane	Problem	Comments
Walkcane or hemiwalker (4 legs, rubber tips, adjustable)	Hemiplegia One good arm only Lateral instability, with falling to one side, primarily hemiplegia Take weight off of involved foot General balance problems	Provides much more stability than regular cane; recommended as first device used in progress toward independence without cane; use in hand opposite involved leg
Walkcane with glider tips (same as above except metal plates on tips instead of rubber)	All the above Inability to lift cane without falling backward	Even better with balance problems
Quad cane	Same problems listed under walkcanes, but less severe	Gives less support than walkcane; used as second device in progress toward independence without cane
Standard curved-top cane	Same as above, but even less severe	Most stable of all standard canes; gives less support than quad cane; use as third device to independence

Activities of Daily Living

Even when neurological return is incomplete, the majority of patients achieve independence in activities of daily living (ADL). You should encourage the patient to begin immediate therapy of the involved arm as well as training to learn independent one-handed ADL activities so that he will not adopt an attitude of dependence while waiting for full neurological recovery. If possible, ADL skills should be introduced and mastered under the guidance and supervision of an occupational therapist.

Therapy is first directed toward developing gross function of proximal muscles and then proceeds distally. As neurological function returns, grasp, placement, and release of the hand are stressed before the patient advances to fine coordination exercises. Biofeedback techniques can be used to improve individual muscle control in the arms and legs as well as to alleviate spasticity.

With appropriate adaptive equipment, one-handed self-care can be accomplished more easily than most patients anticipate. Even when the dominant upper extremity is involved, the patient can master the necessary skills with the nondominant hand through practice.

Eating is usually one of the first activities mastered. To prevent the plate from moving while the patient is learning to eat, place a wet wash cloth, suction cup, or suction holder under the plate. A plate guard or deep dish will facilitate getting the food on the utensil and prevent the food from falling on the table. Limit food to that which can be cut with the edge of a fork or serve it to the patient already cut. Built-up handle eating utensils, a rocker knife, or sharp-edged fork are useful. A straw is helpful for drinking liquids.

Personal hygiene independence is facilitated by grab bars in the patient's bathroom for tub and toilet transfers (Fig. 15–6), bathtub seats, nonskid tape on slippery surfaces, and an elevated toilet seat if necessary.

Dressing independence is enhanced by using clothes slightly larger than normal with front openings. When dressing, the involved extremity is always placed in the clothing first. Shaving with an electric razor and wearing easy-care, short hairstyles are examples of other useful modifications.

Communication

If a language deficit is noted, a speech pathologist should be consulted and therapy ini-

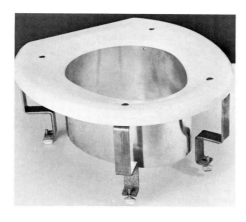

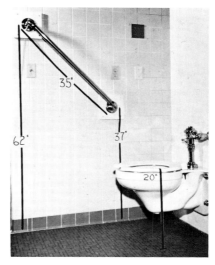

FIG. 15–6. Adaptive equipment for hemiplegic's bathroom. **Left:** A raised toilet seat attached to the toilet facilitates transfer. **Right:** Position of the 45° angle handrail at the toilet for transfers. [From Ellwood, P. M. (1982), see Fig. 15–1 for complete ref.]

tiated. Patients with left hemisphere involvement (right hemiplegia) respond best to silent gestures, pantomime, and pictures. They communicate more readily if encouraged to use pantomime initially instead of attempting speech. Although the prestroke level of speech in significantly aphasic patients is difficult to achieve, early treatment and the patient's efforts to communicate as fully as possible decrease frustration and foster better communication skills. Patients with right hemisphere involvement (left hemiplegia) usually respond well to verbal and written cues. In communities where speech pathologists are not available, the physician and team, including nursing staff and family, can assist the patient by following these guidelines:

1. Speak clearly and simply.
2. Repeat or re-word if the patient does not understand, but do not shout.

3. Use pantomime if the patient does not appear to understand verbal communication.
4. Accept the patient's best efforts to communicate.
5. Give positive reinforcement rather than merely correct errors.

Psychosocial Adjustment

Misunderstandings by the patient and his family about the severity, prognosis, and recovery process of the stroke can lead to unnecessarily high anxiety that may impede recovery. Frank discussions about all facets of the illness and treatment in lay terminology foster realistic adjustment. Maintaining a reasonably optimistic attitude within the context of the medical probabilities positively influences outcome. Most stroke patients progress through the psychological stages of disability of shock, denial, depression, anger, adjustment, and accommodation. Members of the health care team must be aware of this phenomenon so that appropriate support and encouragement can be provided for the patient as he works through the various stages. Depression, anger, and apathy are normal emotional responses often related to the patient's feelings of being overwhelmed by the disabilities and the amount of work required. As function returns and the patient experiences successes and rewards, these emotions usually begin to resolve.

Adjustment is usually facilitated if family members are involved in the rehabilitation program from the onset, including goal setting, participation in all types of therapy and counseling, and evaluation. An accurate estimate of expected recovery may not be possible early in the treatment. Once a prognosis is ascertained, however, you should prepare the family for the eventual outcome and for possible family difficulties related to the following:

1. Role reversal.
2. Discipline of children.
3. Change in sexual relationships.
4. Employment potential.
5. Behavioral changes.

When the left hemisphere is involved (right hemiplegia), frustrations often are attributed to the patient's difficulty with communicating. Because the patient may retain comprehension of visual cues, gestures, and intonation patterns, the family rarely appreciates the frustration produced by the auditory comprehension deficits. With right hemisphere involvement (left hemiplegia), frustrations usually are related to perceptual deficits, impaired quality control, and emotional lability.

Some patients and families benefit from counseling with a psychologist or social worker. Additional information and support are available through local stroke clubs, which provide a forum for sharing experiences and discussing solutions to common problems.

When discharged home, the patient should adapt daily routines that are as much like pre-stroke schedules as the impairment will allow.

A balance between periods of stimulation and rest is desirable. The needs of the patient may be so demanding that other family members are placed under great stress, making some time spent apart essential and beneficial. If the patient and family accept the importance of continuing the independence initiated during rehabilitation, the patient's self-image will be maintained.

The following are some guidelines for maximizing the functional independence of the stroke patient with hemiplegia:

1. Teach the patient one-handed techniques, with the assistance of special self-help devices.
2. Train the patient to use the affected arm to assist the unaffected arm in stabilizing objects and performing tasks requiring gross dexterity.
3. Teach the patient to walk again assisted by a walkcane.
4. Show the patient with homonymous hemianopia how to compensate for visual loss by moving the head to see objects outside the visual field.
6. Help the patient return to work and find other rewarding activities.
7. Teach the patient and family how to balance energy conservation with progressive activity.
8. Accommodate the home environment to the patient's disability, referring the family to local agencies that could recommend practical alternatives.

COMPLICATIONS

Spasticity

Spasticity is a normal part of neurological return. During the recovery process, a progressive increase in tone from flaccidity to spasticity results in the development of motor synergy patterns and individual muscle function. In complete neurological recovery, spasticity develops and then diminishes as normal motor function returns. While a minimal-to-moderate degree of spasticity may compensate for weak muscles, severe spasticity can present the following complications and impede recovery:

1. Mask voluntary efforts.
2. Lead to contracture formation.
3. Interfere with ADL and ambulation.
4. Cause painful muscle spasms.

In the arms, spasticity causes adduction and internal rotation of the shoulder and flexion of the elbow, wrist, and fingers. In the legs, spasticity causes external rotation of the hip, extension of the hip and knee, plantar flexion, and inversion of the foot. With proper bracing of the foot and ankle to prevent plantar flexion and inversion, extension of the hip and knee can successfully stabilize the hemiplegic leg. Occasionally, a withdrawal response will occur when the foot touches the floor, causing flexion at the hip and knee and making ambulation difficult. You may want to attempt knee and ankle bracing (see section on Mobilization) to decrease this flexion withdrawal.

Daily range of motion exercises help prevent contractures and must be performed daily. Spasticity that does not interfere with function is seldom treated due to the numerous side effects of antispasticity drugs. If indicated, medications such as diazepam, dantrolene sodium, and baclofen can reduce spasticity but must be monitored closely. A detailed discussion of spasticity is presented in Chapter 24.

Weakness

Generalized weakness frequently occurs in older or previously inactive stroke patients. If, before the stroke, an individual was only functioning at the minimal level of physical activity necessary to perform ADL, significant disuse atrophy can occur in the unaffected extremities after the patient rests in bed for just 1 to 2 weeks. Strength in the uninvolved side is extremely important in gaining maximum function. A progressive mobilization program should be designed to overcome weakness (see section on Mobilization). The immobilization syndrome is discussed in detail in Chapter 22.

Painful Shoulder

The absence of normal tone in paralyzed shoulder muscles allows stretching of the soft tissues that hold the humerus in the glenoid cavity. A painful shoulder often results from this subluxation and the subsequent stretching of the joint capsule. Trauma to the paralyzed arm during transfers or positioning can also cause or intensify painful shoulder. Care by the nursing staff and others when using the involved arm to turn the patient and a well-fitted sling, designed to hang from the shoulder rather than the neck can help prevent this complication.

Once a shoulder has become painful, hot packs, short-wave diathermy, ultrasound, range of motion exercises, and shoulder support may reduce the inflammation and pain (see Chapter 4). Transcutaneous electrical nerve stimulation (TENS) over the shoulder combined with active movements during or immediately following the application of the TENS is often helpful. Occasionally, local infiltration of steroids and anesthetic in the shoulder joint or bicipital tendon may be required. Vigorous treatment must be continued until symptoms are controlled to prevent the development of the shoulder-hand syndrome, a vicious cycle of intensified pain, contracture, and osteoporosis. If the shoulder-hand syndrome does occur, a short-term trial with oral steroids may be necessary. If edema is present, the extremity is elevated and treated with Jobst stockings.

Homonymous Hemianopia

Homonymous hemianopia is a visual defect experienced by many stroke patients that leads to perceptual and learning disorders. If your patient has this deficit, you should tell the patient, family, and hospital staff how to modify their behavior and the environment to compensate. Adjustment of habits, such as rotating the head and visualizing objects in the intact visual fields, is appropriate. Furniture placement that positions significant objects in the patient's field of vision also facilitates the adjustment.

Neurogenic Bladder and Bowel

The loss of central inhibitory influences usually results in a neurogenic bladder or bowel, manifested by increased uninhibited contractions and incontinence. The use of an indwelling catheter is discouraged because it leads to urinary tract infections, interferes with mobilization, and often requires extensive bladder retraining when removed. Although men can use an external catheter, women may have to use diapers or an indwelling or intermittent catheter until satisfactory bladder control can be regained. A program of timed voiding every 2 hr can usually improve bladder control. Add an anticholinergic such as propantheline, if necessary, to reduce the uninhibited contractions. The bowel training program involves a stool softener twice a day, prune juice in the morning, a glycerin suppository after breakfast, and placement on the commode. For more details on the management of bowel and bladder, see Chapter 25.

Decubitus Ulcers

Decubitus ulcer complications and treatment delay the rehabilitation process unnecessarily while adding as much as 25% to the hospital bill. With good nursing care, decubitus ulcers almost always can be avoided in stroke patients. The various methods used to prevent bedsores by decreasing pressure include proper positioning, frequent turning (every 2 hr), and the use of assistive devices such as egg crate mattresses, sheep skins, and boots made with foam inserts. A detailed discussion of the prevention and treatment of decubitus ulcers is presented in Chapter 23.

Thrombophlebitis

Studies have shown an occurrence of thrombophlebitis as high as 30% in stroke patients due to prolonged bed rest and resultant inefficient venous "muscle pump" that leads to venous stasis in the paralyzed leg. Careful attention to mobilizing the patient as soon as possible, the use of elastic stockings, and elevation of the extremities significantly reduce this problem.

ALTERNATIVE LEVELS OF CARE

The availability of rehabilitation services has a direct bearing on the management of the stroke patient's recovery. The various alternatives available throughout the country consist of inpatient and outpatient services. Inpatient services provide acute, rehabilitative, and/or long-term care. Outpatient services, although more varied, generally provide continued rehabilitative care or general homemaking-related services to the recovering stroke patient living at home.

Inpatient Services

Acute care in a general hospital focuses primarily on life support measures until the patient is stabilized. Some hospitals have found that centralizing the care of stroke victims in one unit, rather than dispersing them throughout the hospital, offers the following benefits:

1. Decreased mortality and morbidity.
2. Improved functional outcome.
3. Increased staff interest and expertise by dealing mainly with one disability.
4. A more consistent approach to problem solving.
5. Improved communication between the various members of the multidisciplinary team.
6. Better patient interaction with others suffering from similar disabilities.

In most communities, inpatient rehabilitative care is provided exclusively by the general hospital as a continuation of acute care. The rehabilitation services normally provided include nursing care, physical therapy, occupational therapy, speech therapy, and psychosocial counseling. The rehabilitation program is continued until the patient's progress plateaus, at which time he or she is referred to another institution or discharged home. If a specialized rehabilitation center is available, patients with severe residual deficits who cannot be home may benefit from the more intensive therapy usually available at such centers.

Patients who cannot walk, who are incontinent, or who are so confused or perceptually unaware that they cannot be left unattended usually cannot be managed in a home setting and constitute the group most frequently referred for long-term care in health-related facilities or nursing homes.

Outpatient Services

A variety of hospital-based programs that bring patients to the hospital for care as an alternative to prolonged inpatient stays are available in many communities. Patients may attend from 1 to 5 days a week and remain in the program as long as they continue to make functional gains.

Independent and hospital-based programs, such as visiting nurse services which send personnel out to the patient's home to render care, offer a desirable alternative for many individuals. Services vary from certified therapists in all specialties to routine nursing care and homemaker services.

The relatively new concept of day care programs for individuals with a stable deficit offer a much needed alternative for working families. No formal therapy is provided, so specific orders from the individual's physician are not required. Primarily a resocialization program staffed by volunteers or a small number of paid staff, a typical day might include arts and crafts, games, discussions, group exercises, and a meal provided by the participants. Individuals may attend up to 5 days a week from several hours to a full day.

COMPLETED STROKE WITH RIGHT HEMIPLEGIA

Report of a Case

HISTORY. For one day preceding admission to a large community hospital, this 59-year-old, right-handed, white woman experienced slurred speech and mild, right-handed weakness. She had a history of hypertension controlled by diuretics and a beta blocker, but prior to the stroke had enjoyed good health. She had been a teacher for 30 years and lived with her husband in a two-story house. Since hospitalization she has required an indwelling catheter and has had occasional bowel incontinence.

PHYSICAL EXAMINATION AND LABORATORY RESULTS. There was a mild receptive and expressive aphasia with right homonymous hemianopia and right seventh nerve central palsy. Deep tendon reflexes were increased on the right compared with the left side, with right Babinski reflex. The right upper extremity had a 1 + shoulder subluxation, decreased range of motion at the shoulder, mild spasticity, and a flexor synergy pattern. Mild spasticity with fair proximal muscle power and poor distal muscle power were noted in the right lower extremity. The ECG revealed borderline cardiomegaly and nonspecific ST–T wave changes. She was dependent in all activities of daily living except feeding herself with her left hand.

REHABILITATION MANAGEMENT. During the initial 2 days, the nurses changed the patient's position every 2 hr (side-back-side) and her bed was positioned so that the door, bedside stand, and other key furniture were within her field of vision on the left side. When she started sitting, her right arm was placed in a sling to relieve shoulder pain and prevent further subluxation.

When she was able to go to physical therapy, hot packs were applied to her right shoulder for 20 min, followed by active assisted range of motion exercise of the right arm. Active assisted ROM was also initiated to the right leg to prevent contracture and to facilitate later ambulation training. Progressive resistive exercises to strengthen and limber the left side were especially important because before the stroke, the patient had led a sedentary lifestyle, with no regular exercise program to maintain muscular strength. Neuromuscular training emphasized reeducating motor control of the right side. The patient also learned to turn herself from side to side and to sit up in bed. This program of early mobilization prevented the development of thrombophlebitis and decubiti. More active exercise was undertaken with caution to avoid overstressing the heart.

Using the spasticity in her right leg, the patient was able to start practicing transfers, balancing, and eventually standing with the aid of parallel bars. By the end of the second week, she had successfully learned the standing transfer into a wheelchair, and learned how to operate the wheelchair with her left hand and foot. She was able to propel herself to the physical therapy room to practice step-ups. A foot-ankle plastic orthosis sufficiently compensated for her mild spasticity to support step-ups.

A timed voiding program supplemented by propantheline to reduce contractions of the bladder enabled removal of the indwelling catheter. A simple schedule of using the commode 30 min after the evening meal gradually eliminated bowel incontinence.

The goal of occupational therapy was independence in self-care activities. Self-feeding was aided by using a plate suction holder, plate guard, and built-up handle utensils. She also was taught about aids such as a utility cart with casters and utensils clamped to the counter, as well as energy conservation principles for eliminating unnecessary motions in homemaking. Her husband made these adaptations in the kitchen at home. Using a long-handled shoe horn, button hook, and loose-fitting clothes, she learned one-handed dressing and brace application.

In speech therapy, the patient was encouraged to practice reciting favorite poems and songs and to practice reading and writing familiar material, with the aid of a book holder, cut-out window, clipboard, and large felt-tipped pen. She was enrolled in group therapy to practice speaking and listening to other post-stroke patients. Regular meetings were scheduled with the patient's husband and daughter to discuss her progress and suggest ways to improve communication with her. Simple sign language, a backup communication mode, was taught to her husband and daughter, as well as to the patient.

The patient was prepared for eventual discharge by making overnight and weekend visits home. The two-story home was adapted to the patient's limited ambulation by converting the family room downstairs into a bedroom to replace her upstairs bedroom. A bath specially equipped with support bars on the shower and toilet was installed adjacent to the downstairs bedroom. Her family was taught to take her pulse so that overexertion leading to cardiac distress could be avoided.

After discharge, a rehabilitation-trained nurse in her area visited once a week to assess her progress and she was referred to a speech therapist in her community to continue daily therapy. Follow-up included visits to her family physician three or four times a year for reevaluation of physical, mental, and functional status.

SUGGESTED READINGS

Ahlsio, B., Britton, M., Murray, V., and Theorell, T. (1984): Displacement and quality of life after stroke. *Stroke*, 15:886–890.

Delia, J. A., Mikulic, M. A., Melnick, R. R., and Miller, R. M. (1982): Stroke rehabilitation: Part II. Recovery and complications. *Am. Fam. Physician*, 26:143–151.

Dove, H. G., Schneider, K. C., and Wallace, J. D. (1984): Evaluating and predicting outcome of acute cerebral vascular accident. *Stroke*, 15:858–864.

Grabois, M. (1982): Rehabilitation of patients with completed stroke. In: *Diagnosis and Management of Stroke and TIAs*, edited by J. S. Meyer and T. Shaw. Addison-Wesley, Menlo Park, CA.

Hirschberg, G. G., Lewis, L., and Vaughn, P. (1976): *Rehabilitation*. J. B. Lippincott Co., Philadelphia.

Johnston, M. V., and Keister, M. (1984): Early rehabilitation for stroke patients: A new look. *Arch. Phys. Med. Rehabil.*, 65:437–441.

Johnstone, M. (1982): *The Stroke Patient: Principles of Rehabilitation*, 2nd edit. Churchill Livingstone, Edinburgh, NY.

Johnstone, M. (1983): *Restoration of Motor Function in the Stroke Patient: A Physiotherapist's Approach*. Churchill Livingstone, New York.

Lehmann, J. F., Delateur, B. J., Fowler, Jr., R. S., et al. (1975): Stroke rehabilitation: Outcome and prediction. *Arch. Phys. Med. Rehabil.*, 56:383–387.

Liss, S. E. (1973): Rehabilitating a stroke patient. *Texas Med.*, 69:84–90.

Lubic, L. G., and Palkovitz, H. P. (1983): *Stroke*, 2nd edit. Medical Examination Publication Co., Garden City, NY.

Ruskin, A. P. (1983): Understanding stroke and its rehabilitation. *Stroke*, 14:438–442.

Sahs, A. L., Hartman, E. C., and Aronson, S. M. (1979): *Stroke: Cause, Prevention, Treatment, and Rehabilitation*. Castle House Publishers, London.

Schuchmann, J. A. (1983): Stroke rehabilitation. Minimizing the functional deficits. *Postgrad. Med.*, 74:101–111.

Sine, R. D., Liss, S. E., Roush, R. E., et al. (1981): *Basic Rehabilitation Techniques—A Self Instructional Guide*, 2nd edit. Aspen Systems, Rockville, MD.

Medical Rehabilitation,
edited by L. S. Halstead et al.
Raven Press, New York © 1985.

CHAPTER 16

Head Injury

Laxman Kewalramani

Louisiana State University, New Orleans, Louisiana 70112

About 4 million accidental injuries per year involve the head, with over half a million of them caused by motor vehicle collisions. Additional causes include falls from heights, industrial accidents, blows to the skull, penetration by objects, such as weapons and firearms, sports and recreational activities, and birth trauma.

The major causes of head injury in children under the age of 10 years are pedestrian accidents and falls. The incidence of head injuries reaches its maximum between the ages of 20 and 30 years. At all ages, the incidence of head injury among males is much greater than that of females.

Because of the complexity of these injuries, they are best treated initially in neurotrauma centers, where a coordinated team of physicians and allied health therapists can provide optimal care and minimize the sequelae.

MANAGEMENT OF ACUTE CONDITIONS

Damage to the Brain

Effective management of head injury depends on the prevention of secondary insults to the traumatized brain. Depending on the magnitude of forces applied, head injury may produce widespread hemorrhaging, bruising, contusion, and laceration of the brain. There is often a rise in intracranial pressure, as well as compression of vital centers, vascular channels, and cranial nerves. Neurological deficit can result from the irritation of neurons, ischemia, or cellular death.

The pathological mechanisms in head injury may be described as follows:

1. Intracranial pressure rises.
2. Brain flattens and shortens on its axis in line of applied force.
3. Transmitted impulses of force damages structures along course of transmission.
4. Shearing forces produce contusions of the brain.
5. Intracranial bleeding and edema compress vital centers, vascular channels, and cranial nerves.
6. Localized tissue dies.

Seizures during the first few hours after the injury almost always indicate a cortical contusion or laceration. Occasionally, seizure activity may be due to the presence of blood in the subarachnoid space or to a tear of the meningeal vessels.

Hemiparesis or hemiplegia indicates either a local cerebral contusion involving the motor strip, or posttraumatic thrombosis of the internal carotid or middle cerebral arteries. Hemianesthesia may be due to a contusion of the sensory cortex; however, the sensory defect, either cortical or subcortical, needs to be precisely defined.

Defects in the visual field indicate lesions of the optic chiasm, optic radiations, or occipital lobe. Anosmia is the result of trauma to the olfactory nerve or olfactory lobe, along with fractures of the cribiform plate. Common pathological syndromes produced by head injury and their possible effects on the brain are outlined in Table 16–1.

TABLE 16–1. *Pathological syndromes produced by head injury*

Syndrome	Definition	Findings
Concussion	Transient, reversible loss of awareness and responsiveness immediately following injury, lasting minutes to several hours	Posttraumatic amnesia, both retrograde and antegrade; no changes in cerebral or cerebellar cells; no local edema, hemorrhage, inflammation, or glial reaction; minimal cellular changes in large ganglion cells of brainstem reticular formation, retro-olivary cells of medulla, cells in vestibular nuclei, and scattered cells of midbrain
Contusion and laceration	Bruising and tearing of cerebral tissue, frequently associated with parenchymal hemorrhage, usually directly under site of impact but often also contrecoup (opposite side)	Upper cranial nerve dysfunction; changes in level of consciousness; sensory or motor disturbances; visual and auditory aberrations
Epidural and subdural hematoma	Compressive forces cause bleeding, forming a hematoma, frequently associated with fracture	Hematoma pressing on vital areas of brain produces neurological deficits, including progressive dementia, gait disturbance, incontinence, or communicating hydrocephalus; symptoms and signs of cerebral compression from epidural hematoma develop more rapidly than those from subdural hematoma
Skull fracture	Associated with any of above syndromes	Epidural hemorrhage resulting from laceration of middle meningeal artery in fractures of temporal bone; leakage of cerebrospinal fluid in basilar fractures; pituitary trauma, resulting in diabetes insipidus, in basal skull fractures; acute respiratory failure as result of direct trauma to brainstem in basal fracture extending to foramen magnum

When to Hospitalize

All patients with a history of head injury should be carefully observed and examined for any neurological abnormalities for a period of at least 24 hr. This is especially true for individuals with a history of unconsciousness, posttraumatic amnesia, nausea, vomiting, and convulsions. If a patient is conscious, cooperative, and without any neurological deficit, if there is no history of unconsciousness, nausea, vomiting, bowel or bladder incontinence, or convulsions, and if appropriate X-ray films of the skull and other affected regions are normal, he or she should be sent home with clear instructions to contact the physician if any of the abnormalities appear. Make sure that a family member or friend who is aware of dangerous signs will be staying with the patient.

Although patients with minor head injuries occasionally require hospitalization for observation, patients with any of the following characteristics have moderate to severe head injuries and must be tended in a neurosurgical intensive care unit:

1. Closed or compound skull fractures.
2. History of unconsciousness lasting longer than 60 min.
3. Posttraumatic amnesia lasting longer than 24 hr.
4. Localizing or lateralizing signs suggesting intracranial lesions, such as sensory, motor, or reflex abnormalities.

These patients commonly require emergency surgical intervention for depressed skull fractures, epidural and subdural hematoma, or intracerebral hematoma.

REHABILITATION MANAGEMENT OF SEQUELAE

Clinical studies have shown that rapid, timely, and continuous rehabilitation leads to improved functional recovery in patients with damage to the central nervous system. The rehabilitation program, whether inpatient or outpatient, should include 1 to 2 hr per day each of occupational, speech, and physical therapy supplemented by appropriate psychological and vocational counseling. Failure to initiate rehabilition of head-injured patients during the first month postinjury can significantly delay recovery. Patients, especially the severely injured, who are admitted late for rehabilitation intervention may require twice as much acute rehabilitation as those admitted to a program soon after injury. Neurological retraining may be greatly impaired if delayed past the specific time interval after injury when brain plasticity is optimal. Furthermore, cost savings to the patient and family are impressive with early intervention, primarily due to improved functional outcome or to prevention of secondary complications.

Prevention of Secondary Complications

Secondary respiratory, cardiovascular, renal, and metabolic disturbances should be prevented and treated aggressively because they can seriously impede neurological recovery and compromise functional restoration. These disturbances typically impair stamina, exercise tolerance, general vigor, and peripheral vascular supply. In addition, biochemical equilibrium in general is disturbed. These complications, in turn, delay rehabilitation and the resumption of preinjury activities.

Respiratory problems are the most common causes of death in patients surviving 48 hr after severe head injury. They may compound cerebral damage by elevating intracranial pressure (cerebral vasodilatation) and by inducing hypoxia. Adequate oxygenation, careful intravenous fluid therapy without excessive loading of fluids, and diuresis help control these complications.

Following head injury, systemic blood pressure rises while the heart rate slows, due to increased intracranial pressure. Placement of a central venous pressure line will help prevent overloading of the heart with parenteral fluids.

The most common gastrointestinal complications in head injured patients are malnutrition and neurogenic gastroduodenal ulceration and bleeding. Hyperalimentation may help prevent these complications.

Immobilized patients with head injury are susceptible to urinary tract infection, reflux, hydronephrosis, and urolithiasis. Careful progression from indwelling to intermittent catheterization can help minimize the development of these complications.

Musculoskeletal Weakness, Contractures, and Spasticity

Steps to prevent and manage weakness, contractures, and spasticity must be implemented early in the postinjury period because these conditions are the most serious impediments to gaining functional independence. Most head-injured patients, regardless of the severity of the injury, can benefit from some rehabilitation measures. Without early rehabilitation, the potential functional recovery of the comatose patient is severely curtailed when full consciousness returns. Functional goals, which vary from one patient to another, must be revised periodically according to changes in the patient's condition and in prognosis. These goals include optimal independence in dressing, eating, transfers and ambulation, working, and recreation (see Chapter 5).

Progressive Mobilization and Exercise

A four-phase program of progressive mobilization—bed activities, sitting, standing, and ambulation—should be implemented as soon as the immediate danger to the patient's life has been overcome. Progressive mobilization is mandatory to prevent characteristic contractures of head injury that result from disuse, gravity, postural attitude, spasticity, and superimposed peripheral nerve impairment.

To prevent contractures that would prohibit future mobilization, a nurse or physical therapist should provide even comatose patients with at least passive range of motion (ROM) exercises once or twice a day. Patients lying supine in bed tend to keep the upper limbs adducted and internally rotated at the shoulders, with pronated forearms, flexed wrists, and flexed metacarpophalangeal and interphalangeal joints. This position favors the development of adduction internal rotation contracture at the shoulder, flexion contracture of the wrist joints, and tightness of the long flexors of the fingers. Therefore, when placing the comatose patient in a supine position, an attempt should be made to keep the shoulders abducted and externally rotated, elbows flexed, wrists extended, and forearms pronated.

In the lower limbs, hip flexion and abduction with external rotation (Fig. 16–1), flexion contracture at the knee, and tendoachilles contracture are very common. All joints of the lower extremities must receive ROM exercises at least once a day (preferably twice a day) to prevent these contractures. In addition to preventing contractures and deformities, the main objectives of exercising comatose patients are to preserve functional ROM, minimize muscle atrophy, and generally counteract the detrimental effects of prolonged bed rest (see Chapter 22).

Conscious patients require, besides ROM, active and assistive exercises (see Chapter 4) to strengthen muscles weakened by disuse and to improve endurance. Bimanual exercises and eye-hand coordination exercises are also prerequisites for functional training. Occupational therapy is especially suited to developing dexterity of the fingers and hands while improving strength, coordination, and endurance (Fig. 16–2).

After bed activities, the next step in progressive mobilization is practice sitting, standing, and walking with assistance in parallel bars, on stairs, and with appropriate supportive braces (see Chapters 5, 6, and 15). Repetitive sitting and standing exercises also prepare the bedridden patient for independent transfers from bed to

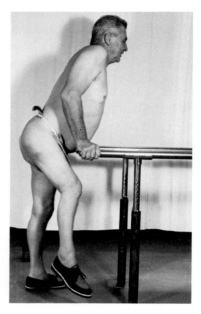

FIG. 16–1. Typical postural deformity of flexion, abduction, and external rotation of the hip due to flexion contractures of the hip. [From Kottke, F. J. (1982): Therapeutic exercise to maintain mobility. In: *Krusen's Handbook of Physical Medicine and Rehabilitation*, edited by F. J. Kottke, G. K. Stillwell, and J. F. Lehmann. W. B. Saunders, Philadelphia.]

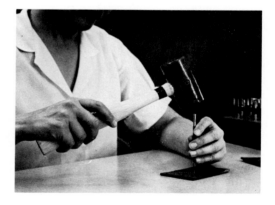

FIG. 16–2. Leather stamping in occupational therapy to help improve finger dexterity and strength. [From Kottke, F. J. (1982): Therapeutic exercise to develop neuromuscular coordination. In: *Krusen's Handbook of Physical Medicine and Rehabilitation*, edited by F. J. Kottke, G. K. Stillwell, and J. F. Lehmann. W. B. Saunders, Philadelphia.]

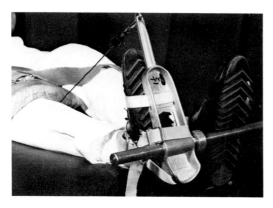

FIG. 16–3. Stretching of gastrocnemius and soleus on exercise table using toe extension boot. Weight of 10-30 lb applied for 20 min helps control spasticity. [From Kottke, F. J. (1982): Therapeutic exercise to maintain mobility. In: *Krusen's Handbook of Physical Medicine and Rehabilitation*, edited by F. J. Kottke, G. K. Stillwell, and J. F. Lehmann. W. B. Saunders, Philadelphia.]

wheelchair. Approximately 60% of severely injured patients are unable to walk because of weakness, loss of coordination, and spasticity; these patients require a wheelchair as their means of ambulation. (For information on the selection and purchase of wheelchairs, see Chapter 6 and the Appendix.)

Control of Spasticity

In the control of spasticity, drugs such as baclofen and dantrolene (sodium) are usually insufficient without supplementary stretching (Fig. 16–3), exercise, and cold therapy. Severe, intractable spasticity may require motor point phenol or alcohol blocks, peripheral nerve blocks, or rhizotomy to reduce spasticity to a level enabling participation in activities of daily living and some ambulation.

Cold produces long-term reduction of spasticity through vasoconstriction prolonged by insulation from the patient's fat layer. These processes interact to delay the rewarming of muscle tissue from both inside and outside the body. Depending on the patient's weight and proportion of body fat, muscles should be cooled for 10 to 30 min.

Two popular techniques of cold application that are readily adaptable to home use are ice baths and ice towels. To prepare an ice bath, add ice chips or ice cubes to cold water, maintaining a temperature of 15.5°C, and soak the involved body part. Ice bath immersion can reduce clonus in spastic patients for 4 to 6 hr after treatment. Ice towels are made by soaking a Turkish towel in water, dipping it in crushed ice, which will stick to the towel, then wrapping the towel around the body part.

Progressive mobilization and control of spasticity are necessary not only to prevent contractures but also to enable the patient to resume social and leisure activities and, if possible, return to work. Posttraumatic epilepsy and mental sequelae, however, are much more prevasive impediments to resuming preinjury activities than are physical disabilities.

Posttraumatic Epilepsy

Most posttraumatic seizures occur during the first year after injury. These seizures often can be prevented by the administration of anticonvulsant medication for 12 to 18 months after injury. At high risk of acquiring epilepsy are children under the age of 5 years and patients with gunshot wounds, amnesia lasting longer than 24 hr, or depressed skull fracture (Table 16–2). Following moderate to severe head injury, the most common types of epilepsy are minor motor seizures, focal motor seizures, and aura. By contrast, grand mal seizures are less common. Seizure activity should be diagnosed by an electroencephalogram (EEG) during sleep and wakefulness and skull X-rays for evidence of fracture, old intracranial calcification, and asymmetry, supplemented by CT scan.

The epileptic patient's lifestyle should be altered to exclude hazardous activities such as driving a car, working on a ladder or scaffolding, or operating machinery with exposed parts and to avoid alcohol consumption. Posttraumatic seizures are most effectively controlled by barbiturates (phenobarbital, mephobarbital), hydantoins (Dilantin®, Mesantoin®), mysoline (Primidone®) and, if severe, phenacemide (Phenurone®). Effective control of very frequent seizures may require intravenous regi-

TABLE 16–2. Long-term risk of posttraumatic epilepsy in head-injured patients with selected characteristics

Characteristic	Percentage with epilepsy	
	Characteristic present	Characteristic absent
Epilepsy during first week of injury	70	5
Intracranial hematoma	30	5
Depressed skull fracture, intact dura	50+	5
Posttraumatic amnesia >24 hr	50+	—
Depressed skull fracture, tear in dura, combined with amnesia >24 hr	80	—

mens of phenytoin (Dilantin®), diazepam (Valium®), or amobarbital sodium (Amytal® sodium). Selective surgical excision of the focal lesion producing seizure activity is usually successful if medical therapy fails.

Posttraumatic Mental Sequelae

The postconcussion syndrome, including dizziness, headache, poor memory, and poor concentration, is the most common sequela of minor to moderate head injury. Most of these bothersome, nonspecific symptoms resolve within days to months. Fewer symptoms are likely to be reported when the physician provides information about the type of injury, explains the symptoms, and encourages the resumption of pretraumatic activities. About 33% of patients with severe head injuries develop significant mental disturbances, primarily affecting drive, social restraint and judgment, memory, and emotional stability. Elderly people with arteriosclerotic changes of the intracranial blood vessels are at the highest risk.

Drive is typically reduced, resulting in apathy, social withdrawal, and decreased sexual interest. The patient may appear euphoric, emotionally labile, less aggressive, and passive. In addition to being tactless, overly talkative, and hurtful in speech, some patients exhibit sudden, unprovoked outbursts of rage. The expression of any combination of these traits is often related to the site of injury, as shown in Table 16–3, and the hemisphere involved (see Chapter 15, Table 15–1).

Speech ability remains intact in patients with right hemispheric involvement, but intellectual, perceptual, and comprehension functions are severely impaired. Memory impairment may be for both verbal and nonverbal material. Patients with mild to moderate head injury can expect some recovery from such cognitive deficits over a 2-year period. Motor skill and speed and language skill are usually the first functions to improve, while complex problem solving and mental stamina are recovered much later during the rehabilitation process (Table 16–4).

PROGNOSIS

Predicting the outcome of head injury is impossible until the patient has successfully survived the first 24 hr after injury. Mortality during this period is associated with trauma to the brainstem region, fractures of the foramen magnum, intracerebral hematoma, and severe lacerations of the brain. An appreciable degree of mortality and morbidity accepted as the inevitable aftermath of head injury is potentially preventable through careful early diagnosis and treatment. Intracranial infection, for example, often results from unsatisfactory treatment of scalp lacerations and failure to diagnose underlying depressed fractures of the vault, while meningitis may result if a fracture of the base is overlooked. The detection of skull fractures is particularly important because they predispose to the development of intracranial hematoma.

Recovery of Lost Function

A major obstacle to assessing outcome of head injury has been the lack of a standardized, quantitative measure of severity. Over the past decade, however, assessments have been developed

TABLE 16–3. *Mental conditions related to type of brain damage*

Injury	Clinical findings
Frontal lobe	Loss of inhibition; lack of drive; lack of productive thinking and perseverance; euphoria; indifference; incapacity for decision making; demanding, aggressive, criminal behavior; increased libido with disregard for sexual partner; sexual deviations or offenses
Parietal lobe	Abnormal spatial perception; indifference to deficits and lack of awareness of disability; occasionally, impairment of intelligence and schizophreniform personality
Basilar fracture (midbrain, hypothalamus, orbital part of frontal lobe)	Disturbances of appetite, thirst, and sleep; sluggishness and apathy
Temporal lobe	Intense emotions such as anxiety and fear; aberrant sensations of vision, sound, taste, and smell; profound memory loss of recent events; disturbances of spatial and temporal relations; depersonalization
Minimal brain damage syndrome in children	Hyperkinesis; decreased attention span; temper tantrums and impulsive acts; poor frustration tolerance; intellectual deficits; difficulties in memory, speech, and comprehension; occasionally, below-normal IQ

TABLE 16–4. *Recovery from cognitive deficits with mild to moderate head injury*

Deficit	Postinjury time for recovery (months)
Motor skill and speed	0–3
Language skill	3–6
Attention/concentration	6–12
Memory/learning	6–24
Complex problem solving	6–24
Mental stamina	6–24

TABLE 16–5. *Glasgow Coma Scale*

Best eye-opening response	
Spontaneously	4
To voice	3
To pain	2
None	1
Best motor response	
Follows commands	6
Localizes pain	5
Complex arm movement	4
Reflex flexor posturing	3
Reflex extensor posturing	2
Flaccid	1
Best verbal response	
Oriented, converses	5
Confused, converses	4
Inappropriate words	3
Incomprehensible sounds	2
None	1

1, poor prognosis–6, good prognosis. Total possible score: 3(poorest)–18(best) prognosis.

that base severity on not only level of consciousness but also clinical history, neurological response to various stimuli, or extent of disability. The clinically based approach is the most general, least quantitative, and best suited for acute assessment of outcome. By contrast, evaluating neurological response allows repetitive assessment of severity over the course of recovery. Assessment of disability, while the most predictive of functional outcome, is rarely adequate when performed only once during recuperation.

In one clinically based system, head injury is considered severe when the following are present: unconsciousness lasting more than 6 hr, fractured skull, and intracranial hemorrhage or need for neurosurgery. In the absence of this history, patients who are hospitalized for more than 3 days and unconscious from 30 min to 6

hr have a moderate head injury, while those hospitalized for less than 3 days and unconscious less than 30 min have a mild injury.

Most trauma centers use the Glasgow Coma Scale (Table 16–5), in which the patient's best responses to verbal and painful stimuli are rated and recorded as indicative of level of consciousness. Total scores can range from 3 to 15, with a score below 7 designating severe injury in which patients are unable to open their eyes, follow commands, move their extremities appropriately, or speak recognizable words.

A useful diagnostic tool for predicting future recovery from disability at various times during the course of treatment is the Glasgow Outcome Scale:

1. Vegetative state—comatose.
2. Severe disability—conscious, but dependent.
3. Moderate disability—independent, but disabled.
4. Good recovery—independent, not disabled.

No single prognostic indicator, however, can reliably predict neurological and functional outcome. The most important factors that determine recovery and mortality rate are age, duration and other aspects of coma, duration of posttraumatic amnesia, episodic hypertension, and intracranial pressure. Less strongly related to outcome are abnormalities of respiration, cardiovascular function, and body temperature control. These indicators of brainstem dysfunction occur in a minority of even severely injured patients.

Age

Capacity for recovery markedly diminishes with increasing age. Children demonstrate a remarkable capacity for recovery, even with substantial neurological disturbances. Reduced neuronal reserve, the limited availability of alternative structural pathways, reduced capacity to learn, and less responsive vascular system limit the recovery of older adults. Children with atypical decerebrate rigidity and abnormal motion patterns have a poor functional outcome that worsens with age. Head injured patients up to 20 years old with atypical rigidity, and up to 30 years old with coma and normal motor pattern, have experienced good recovery.

Coma

In an international survey using the Glasgow Outcome Scale, no patients who were still vegetative 6 months after injury survived. No patients diagnosed as vegetative 3 months after injury gained independence; 60% of these patients, compared to 50% of those comatose after 1 month, died within a year. Satisfactory functional outcome can be expected in about two-thirds of comatose patients who regain consciousness within 4 weeks. Aspects of coma designating poor functional outcome include abnormal pupil response, absent eye movements, abnormal motor response patterns, and limitation of motor response in the best extremity to extensor response. The outcome at 1 month postinjury of patients with various types of injuries and resulting dysfunctions is summarized in Table 16–6.

Social and Vocational Recovery

Recovery of most cognitive functions can be expected within the first year for the majority of patients with minor to moderate head injuries. By contrast, patients with severe injuries typically report that they still have not regained their full working capacity 2 years after injury, despite having returned to work.

Social life appears to suffer greater decrements, especially for patients who had posttraumatic amnesia for more than a week. Possibly, lingering memory deficits make these patients socially inept and due to a general lack of motivation, they seek social contact less frequently than do noninjured people.

Although personality changes after injury occasionally affect social and occupational recovery, premorbid personality appears to have a more pervasive effect on resumption of activities and personal relationships. Preaccident nervousness hinders resumption of both work and leisure activities, while verbal expansiveness, or brashness, promotes early activity. Patients who played a helpless role before injury tend to have poor family relationships or few social contacts after injury.

Rehabilitation toward physical capacity does help the head-injured patient return to work, but does not help social recovery. In several studies, patients complained about loneliness and social isolation, which in turn provide little motivation for active participation in rehabilitation. After injury, patients often lack a close friend or confidante, which is associated with heightened anxiety and depression. Family cohesion is also disrupted more by mental decline than by physical disability.

TABLE 16–6. *Recovery from brain injuries*

	Mild concussion	Cerebral concussion	Diffuse injury	Shearing injury
Dysfunction				
Loss of consciousness	None	Immediate	Immediate	Immediate
Length of unconsciousness	None	<24 hr	>24 hr	Days to weeks
Decerebrate posturing	None	None	Occasional	Present
Posttraumatic amnesia	Minutes	Minutes to hours	Days	Weeks
Memory deficit	None	Minutes	Mild to moderate	Severe
Motor deficits	None	None	Mild	Severe
Outcome at 1 month				
Good recovery	100%	95%	21%	0
Moderate deficit	0	2%	21%	0
Severe deficit	0	2%	29%	9%
Vegetative	0	0	21%	36%
Death	0	0	7%	55%

Adapted from Cooper, P. R., editor (1982): *Head Injury.* Williams and Wilkins, Baltimore.

It is recommended, therefore, that the physician pay close attention to family support and encourage the maintenance of relationships with family and friends, as well as the development of new relationships. Most resocialization should occur during the early posthospitalization period. Community outings can be introduced, beginning with nonthreatening, anonymous public places and progressing to private parties and restaurants from which leaving abruptly is more difficult. You should encourage the patient to maintain contact with vocational and other rehabilitation counselors, even if there does not seem to be much progress. Counseling and social skills training may shorten the duration and improve the results of resocialization.

When referring the head-injured patient for vocational counseling, emphasize that although the counselor will provide guidance, instruction, technical resources, and some psychological support, virtually all of the motivation to obtain employment must come from the patient. This may be particularly difficult when the patient's lack of motivation can be traced directly to the site of central nervous system injury. The physician may need to appoint a family member constantly to remind the patient, as well as provide close supervision.

Ultimately, the patient is responsible for the outcome of vocational counseling. He should not be reassured unrealistically that the counselor will help him get a job. Rather, suggest that the counselor will help him make some plans or determine what he would like to do. Inaccurate expectations for counseling may perpetuate disappointment and failure.

The physician should note that the patient who responds well to medical treatment is not necessarily a good candidate for employment. You can expect, however, to receive a report of the anticipated outcome of vocational rehabilitation and the steps and timetable needed to achieve that goal. For some severely head injured patients, employment outside the home is not feasible. These patients may, nevertheless, welcome the opportunity to spend more time with their family and may contribute significant emotional support and well-being to the family members. The person who is encouraged to cultivate some interests and activities despite the severity of physical or mental disability is likely to maintain better mental and physical health and to be less burdensome to others.

SEVERE HEAD INJURY WITH MENTAL SEQUELAE

Report of a Case

HISTORY. This single, 28-year-old man sustained a severe head injury when his car overturned. He was unconscious for 8 hr and suffered from posttraumatic amnesia for 4 months. Right hemiplegia and dysphasia resulted from a left frontal cerebral hematoma. The hemiplegia disappeared when the hematoma was aspirated, but left residual speech hesitation. He resumed talking 6 weeks after the accident and was transferred to a major rehabilitation center. Perception, quality control, alertness, and remote memory were unimpaired. Retention of recent verbal information and mental concentration, however, remained mildly impaired.

The patient had been working as a police detective for a large south central state. He was living alone in a condominium and was engaged to be married in 6 months at the time of the accident.

REHABILITATION MANAGEMENT. The patient was discharged to his parent's home 4 months after the accident. He continued to see the vocational counselor and social worker who had been handling his case in the rehabilitation center. All physical abilities had been restored.

Although the patient had been very ambitious before the injury, he now lacked drive and enthusiasm. He demonstrated indifference to his fiancee's visits and expressed no interest in returning to work. She broke off the engagement indefinitely but continued to visit him as a friend. He did not exhibit aggressive behavior that would disrupt the work place.

Six months after injury, the patient's recovery from mild cognitive deficits was considered adequate to enable him to return to work. Due to the patient's premorbid exemplary work on the police force, his employer agreed to accept him back. He was restricted to office work in the intelligence division, however, to avoid jeopardizing his life or that of his partner in dangerous situations that would require quick decisions and reactions. His social life remained limited, and he was still living in his parent's home 2 years after injury.

Considering the severity of his head injury, this patient demonstrated good recovery by the second postinjury year. Some memory deficit can be expected after recovery from amnesia. If he had returned to his job earlier than 6 months after injury, he may have experienced unexpected and atypical difficulty and failure due to his cognitive deficits. The alteration of his job responsibilities enabled the avoidance of failure at previously well-managed tasks, which might have produced increasing anxiety, loss of self-esteem, and depression. These responsibilities compensated for his memory problem by emphasizing the meeting of long-term investigative goals rather than the day-to-day productivity required on the streets.

SUGGESTED READINGS

Bond, M. R. (1976): Assessment of the psychosocial outcome of severe head injury. *Acta Neurochir.* (Wien), 34:57–70.

Brooks, N., editor (1984): *Closed Head Injury: Psychological, Social, and Family Consequences.* Oxford University Press, New York.

Cartlidge, N. E. F., and Shaw, D. A. (1981): *Head Injury.* W. B. Saunders, Philadelphia.

Cooper, P. R., editor (1982): *Head Injury.* Williams & Wilkins, Baltimore.

Cope, D. N., and Hall, K. (1982): Head injury rehabilitation: Benefits of early intervention. *Arch. Phys. Med. Rehabil.*, 63:433–437.

Diller, L., and Gordon, W. A. (1981): Rehabilitation and clinical neuropsychology. In: *Handbook of Clinical Neuropsychology*, edited by S. B. Filskov, and T. J. Boll. John Wiley & Sons, New York.

Edelstein, B. A., and Couture, E. T., editors (1984): *Behavioral Assessment and Rehabilitation of the Traumatically Brain-Damaged.* Plenum, New York.

Jennet, B. J., and Teasdale, G., editors (1981): *Mangement of Head Injuries.* F. A. Davis, Philadelphia.

Pitts, L. H., and Martin, N. (1982): Head injuries. *Surg. Clin. North Am.*, 62:47–60.

Raphaely, R., Swedlow, D., Downes, J., et al. (1980): Management of severe pediatric head trauma. *Ped. Clin. North Am.*, 27:715–727.

Rose, J., Valtonen, S., and Jennett, B. (1977): Avoidable factors contributing to death after head injury. *Br. Med. J.*, 2:615–618.

Rosenthal, M., Griffiths, E. R., Bond, M. R., and Miller, J. D. (1983): *Rehabilitation of the Head-Injured Adult.* F. A. Davis, Philadelphia.

Shapiro, K. editor (1983): Pediatric Head Trauma. Mount Kisco, New York.

Valpolahati, M. (1971): Prognosis for patients with severe brain injuries. *Br. Med. J.*, 3:404–407.

Medical Rehabilitation,
edited by L. S. Halstead et al.
Raven Press, New York © 1985.

CHAPTER 17

Spinal Cord Injury

*, † Lauro S. Halstead and **,†R. Edward Carter

*Departments of *Rehabilitation, Physical Medicine, and Community Medicine, **Rehabilitation and Physical Medicine, Baylor College of Medicine, and †The Institute for Rehabilitation and Research, Houston, Texas 77030*

INCIDENCE AND PREVALENCE

Nationwide, there are an estimated 7,000 to 10,000 new cases of spinal cord injury each year that require medical care and rehabilitation. Of these, approximately 50% are paraplegic and 50% are quadriplegic. More males than females represent new cases of spinal cord injury in a ratio of 8:1.

The prevalence, or number of persons in the United States who are currently paralyzed as a result of traumatic spinal cord injury, is estimated at 150,000. Roughly 70% of the cases of functional and neurological impairment of the spinal cord are due to trauma and 30% are due to localized or systemic diseases such as neoplasms, congenital anomalies, and neurological disorders.

Data from the National Data Research Center show three trends in spinal cord injury over the past few years. First, an increasing number of people have sustained incomplete injuries, so that some motor and/or sensory function remains. Second, a greater number of people have survived high cervical injuries but have been left apneic quadriplegics and ventilator dependent. Third, more people have survived to require rehabilitation despite being over age 60.

ETIOLOGY

Traumatic Causes

Although the causes of traumatic spinal cord injury vary from region to region, the most common causes are:

1. Motor vehicle accidents.
2. Falls from accidents at work or home.
3. Sports injuries, such as diving, football, surfing, gymnastics, and trampoline.
4. Gunshot wounds.

Mechanism of Injury

The three basic mechanisms of injuries are flexion-rotation with dislocation or fracture/dislocation, compression fracture, and hyperextension injuries. The most common type is a forward flexion injury associated with rotation. The most common sites of injury are C5-C6 in the cervical spine and T12–L1 in the thoracolumbar spine (Fig. 1). Regardless of the original mechanism of injury, most damage to the spinal cord probably occurs posttraumatically because of improper handling of the patient at the scene of injury.

Pathophysiology

The types of spinal cord injury are concussion, contusion, and laceration. In concussion of the spinal cord, which is similar to a brain concussion, numbness or paralysis disappears within 72 to 96 hr with no permanent residual neurological or functional impairment. Contusion produces edema, hemorrhage, and ischemia, resulting in an area of permanent injury bounded by an area of transient damage. Occurring in the majority of patients who ultimately require rehabilitation, contusion can result clinically in either a "complete" or an "incom-

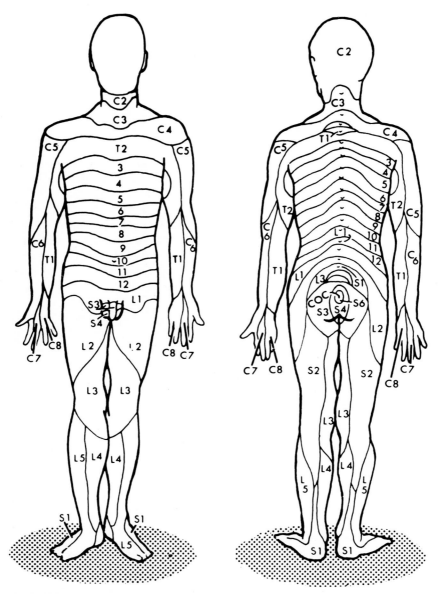

FIG. 17–1. Distribution of sensory (dorsal) roots of spinal cord segment innervating surface regions of body. [From Tedeschi, L. (1977): *Forensic Medicine: A Study in Trauma and Environmental Hazards.* W.B. Saunders, Philadelphia.]

plete" lesion. Laceration is physical transection of the cord with complete loss of motor and sensory function below the level of injury. Relatively rare, a complete transection is usually associated with a gunshot or stab wound.

Atraumatic Causes

Atraumatic spinal cord injuries are much less common than traumatic ones. Generally, the frequency parallels the occurrence of the underlying condition in the population, and the mechanism of injury and pathophysiology depend on the underlying cause. Some of the common atraumatic causes are:

1. Vascular surgery for removal of thoracic or abdominal aneurysms.
2. Idiopathic transverse myelitis.
3. Primary or metastatic tumors involving the spinal cord.
4. Connective tissue diseases, such as lupus erythematosus.
5. Orthopedic surgery for spinal fusion or diskectomy.
6. Infectious diseases, such as tuberculosis.

FUNCTIONAL ASSESSMENT

Classification

Based on clinical findings from the routine bedside neurological examination, spinal cord injuries are classified as complete or incomplete. Incomplete lesions show preservation of some motor and/or sensory function below the injury, while complete lesions show none. Occasionally, the only indication of an incomplete injury is sensation in the sacral and perianal pathways, which lie more peripherally in the cord.

Common Syndromes

Transverse myelopathy is the most common syndrome. Others include anterior cord, central cord, Brown-Sequard, and cauda equina injuries. Central cord injury is particularly distinctive because it is commonly seen in elderly people with osteoarthritic changes in the neck who sustain a hyperextension injury but frequently without a fracture. Impairment from these syndromes is described in Table 17–1.

Neurological-Functional Correlation

A careful neurological examination is important not only to establish a precise level of injury but also to forecast functional recovery. Al-though the motor, sensory, and reflex examinations are considered in localizing a lesion, the level of preserved muscle function is generally the most helpful in predicting long-term outcome and the eventual degree of independence in performing routine activities. Because of the importance of motor function, the level of injury is usually classified in terms of the lowest intact and normally functioning motor unit. Thus, a patient who has normal motor power down to and including the C5 myotome level is diagnosed as a C5 quadriplegic. When the exact location of myotome involvement is difficult to establish in a routine bedside examination, then the lowest intact sensory level is generally used to determine the diagnostic classification.

Table 17–2 lists the critical levels of preserved muscle groups and related functional expectations. Patients with intact motor-nerve roots down through C4 (C4 quadriplegia) will be totally dependent except for tasks they can perform with their head and neck, such as mouthstick activities. With preservation of the C5 motor nerve roots, patients usually have good shoulder control and elbow flexion, which allows them to be semi-independent in eating, facial hygiene, typing, and similar activities. Patients with lesions below this level begin to acquire increasing degrees of independence in a wide variety of activities, which are often sufficient to allow them to live on their own. Limited ambulation is frequently possible with lesions in the mid- to lower-thoracic region, and walking independently outside the home is generally practical with injuries to the lower lumbar and upper sacral nerves.

The achievement of these functional goals, however, can be enhanced or impaired by a number of factors. For example, in many instances, the performance of certain activities is enabled or facilitated by the use of various assistive devices, such as orthoses (see Chapter 6). At the same time, conditions such as spasticity, contractures, or obesity may make the functional expectations listed in Table 17–2 impossible to achieve despite good strength and appropriate adaptive equipment.

TABLE 17–1. *Common syndromes of spinal cord injury*

Syndrome	Anatomical sites of injury	Impairment
Transverse myelopathy	Anterior and posterior portions of cord	Symmetrical loss of motor and sensory function below level of injury
Anterior cord	Anterior tracts of cord	Paralysis below level of injury; variable loss of pain, temperature, light touch, and pressure; deep touch and proprioception intact
Central cord	Central portion of cord	Major motor and sensory changes occur in arms; legs and bladder are less involved; frequently no bony fractures
Brown-Sequard	One side of cord only	Ipsilateral motor involvement, contralateral sensory loss below level of injury; limbs with best motor power have poorest sensation and vice versa
Cauda equina	At or below L1, involving conus medullaris and/or cauda equina, resulting in lower motor neuron lesion	Variable loss of motor and sensory function below level of injury; decreased muscle tone, muscle wasting, decreased or absent reflexes in lower extremities

Table 17–3 provides a more detailed summary of the close correlation between various neurological levels and the anticipated functional goals for ten activities. While these goals will not be achieved by all patients with the levels of injury indicated, they provide a guide for the degree of independence that is possible with good rehabilitation techniques and if no major complications are present.

PRINCIPLES OF MANAGEMENT

Initial Stage: 1 to 10 Days

There is probably no disability that can cause such serious and widespread disruption of bodily functions as does spinal cord injury. Paralysis is only one manifestation of the injury and its aftermath. While many complications stem from the loss of normal neural control, often

TABLE 17–2. *Critical levels of preserved muscles and related functional expectations*

Nerve roots intact[a]	Preserved muscles	Functional expectation
C3	Diaphragm	Totally dependent
C4	Neck muscles, levator scapulae	Totally dependent
C5	Deltoid, biceps	Semi-independent
C6	Latissimus dorsi, serratus anterior, pronator teres, extensor carpi radialis longus	Independent from wheelchair
C7	Triceps	Independent from wheelchair
C8, T1	Hand intrinsics, extensor carpi ulnaris	Independent from wheelchair
T1–T6	Upper intercostals, upper back	Independent from wheelchair
T6–T12	Abdominals, thoracic extensors	Limited ambulation
L3, L4	Quadriceps	Community ambulation
L4, L5	Anterior tibialis	Community ambulation
S1, S2	Gastrocnemius, soleus	Community ambulation

[a]These levels represent common segmental origins.

TABLE 17–3. *Functional goals in spinal cord injury for various levels*

Activities	Functional significance of spinal cord lesion level								
	C1–C3	C4	C5	C6	C7	T1	T6	T12	L4
Mouthstick	±	±	NA	NA	NA	NA	NA	NA	NA
Eating	−	+	+	+	+	+	+	+	+
Sitting	−	−	+	+	+	+	+	+	+
Transfers	−	−	−	+	+	+	+	+	+
Dressing	−	−	−	+	+	+	+	+	+
Bathing	−	−	−	+	+	+	+	+	+
Toileting	−	−	−	−	+	+	+	+	+
Driving	−	−	+	+	+	+	+	+	+
Walking	−	−	−	−	−	−	+	+	+
Using public transportation	−	−	−	−	−	−	−	+	+
Major assistive devices	Environmental control	Ballbearing feeder	Powered reciprocal	Wrist driven reciprocal	W/C	W/C	W/C	Long leg braces	Short leg braces

(−) = dependent; (±) = semi-independent; (+) = independent; NA = not applicable; W/C = wheelchair.

just as many complications are the result of improper treatment and/or neglect. Unfortunately, initial treatment of spinal injured patients is all too often directed only at maintaining life supporting functions while other aspects of their care are ignored, resulting in avoidable, short- and long-term complications that prolong hospitalization, increase the cost of care, and frequently compromise functional outcome. For this reason, comprehensive management of the early spinal injured person should always include a number of simple, basic preventive measures in addition to the life-supporting interventions. Most of these measures, described in Table 17–4, can

be started during the first 1 to 10 days of injury and then continued throughout the rehabilitation program.

Acute Stage: 11 Days to 3 Months

The acute period, 11 days to 3 months after injury, covers the crucial stage of in-hospital rehabilitation. Although many of the treatment procedures required during this time can be carried out at a general hospital, referral to a rehabilitation facility experienced in the management of spinal injured persons is desirable whenever possible. The cost and length of hospitalization in regional centers that specialize in

TABLE 17–4. *Stages of management of spinal cord injury*

Stage	Goals	Therapeutic interventions
Initial: 1–10 days	Maintain life support functions Prevent short-term and long-term complications	Daily skin checks of entire body surface and frequent turns Intermittent catheterization every 4 hr when patient is medically stable Daily bowel evacuation using stool softeners, suppositories, digital stimulation and, if necessary, enemas Daily pulmonary therapy with IPPB four times a day until vital capacity is 1,800 to 2,000 cc, then incentive respirometry twice a day Daily mobilization in wheelchair or on standing table Regular diet with no restrictions unless patient has history of calcium stone formation requiring limitation of calcium to 300 mg/day Hyperalimentation for patients who remain anorectic and catabolic, with continuous weight loss for more than 3 weeks
Acute: 11 days–3 months	Achieve early mobilization Initiate program of tasks patient can perform independently	Gradual performance of self-care, such as eating, bathing, transfers, dressing Education and adjustment of patient and family Regular bowel program with predictable evacuations daily or every other day Withdrawal from indwelling catheter Training in use of assistive devices Completion of architectural changes in home Day and weekend passes to ease transition from hospital to home
Intermediate: 3 months–3 years	Adapt patient to community Resume school, work, or vocational training Conclude any pending litigation	Close medical follow-up, with periodic reevaluations scheduled Anticipatory treatment
Long-term: >3 years	Maintain health through annual comprehensive check-ups	Routine blood tests, spinal roentgenograms, evaluation of renal function by urinalysis, urine culture, intravenous pyelogram, and 24-hr urine observation for creatinine clearance Reassessment of equipment and assistive devices

the care of spinal injured patients has been shown to run 20% to 30% lower than in general medical facilities, yet with the same or better outcome.

Intermediate Stage: 3 Months to 3 Years

The intermediate phase, 3 months to 3 years after injury, is crucial for achieving a healthy adaptation to the community and resumption of self-responsibility. As most morbidity and mortality occur during the first 3 years following spinal injury, close medical follow-up is desirable. In general, but especially for quadriplegics, full metabolic as well as psychosocial adaptation is not achieved until 2 to 3 years after injury.

Long-Term Stage: Greater Than 3 Years

After 3 years, health maintenance is the major long-term goal. The establishment of good rapport between patient and family practitioner is extremely helpful so that psychosocial problems and crises within the family can be identified and dealt with as early as possible. In our experience, these problems frequently precede a preventable medical complication such as a pressure sore.

MANAGEMENT OF SPECIFIC PROBLEMS

Neurological Assessment

During the first few days following injury, a neurological examination should be performed several times a day, especially to detect ascending motor and sensory loss, which is almost always an indication for prompt surgical intervention. In cervical or high thoracic injuries, respiratory function should be monitored several times a day and the patient should be placed on a cardiac monitor because of the frequent occurrence of severe bradycardia.

Spinal Stability

Initial evaluation should include X-ray films of the entire spine, skull, and long bones, as well as evaluation for intraabdominal trauma, because noncontiguous spinal fractures occur at two or more sites in 20% of cases.

Cervical Fractures

Contrary to the widespread practice of several decades ago, most paraplegists now recommend conservative management of cervical fractures. Following reduction of the fracture, the patient is placed in traction for 4 to 6 weeks to maintain bony alignment. Some centers use a Halo apparatus attached to a modified body jacket (Fig. 17–2), which permits early mobilization. If satisfactory healing is occurring, the patient is placed in a hard cervical collar such as a SOMI (sternal—occipital—mandibular—immobilization, Fig. 17–3) for another 4 to 6 weeks, and a soft collar for the final 4 to 6 weeks. Although the issue is still controversial, most neurosurgeons and orthopedists who work in spinal injury centers agree on the following principal indications for surgical treatment of cervical fractures:

1. A deterioration in neurological function.
2. Gunshot and stab wounds, to remove debris and devitalized tissue.
3. Incomplete lesions associated with a burst fracture, which results in the displacement of portions of the vertebral body and disk against the anterior aspect of the cord.
4. Any fracture that remains unstable after at least 3 months of conservative treatment.

Thoracic and Lumbar Fractures

If the spine is stable, as in many uncomplicated compression fractures, it is treated conservatively with an external support such as a Jewett brace or a molded body jacket (Fig. 17–4) for 3 to 6 months. If the spine is unstable, as in most flexion-rotation dislocation and hyperextension injuries, spinal fusion with Harrington distraction rods is generally indicated. Following surgery, patients are placed in a body jacket to permit early mobilization.

Cardiovascular Complications

Cardiovascular complications from spinal cord injury include bradycardia, autonomic dysre-

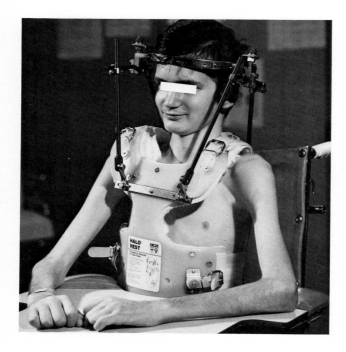

FIG. 17–2. Halo apparatus attached to modified body jacket permits early mobilization. (Photo by Gordon Stanley.)

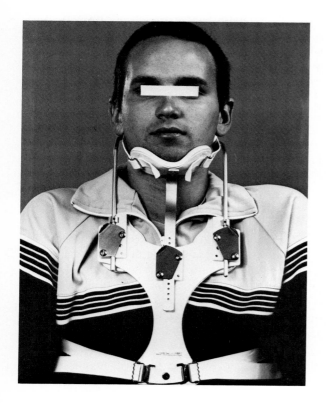

FIG. 17–3. SOMI hard cervical orthosis immobilizes head and neck.

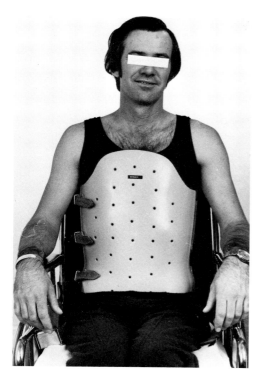

FIG. 17–4. Molded body jacket supports lumbar fracture. (Photo by Gordon Stanley.)

flexia or hyperreflexia, orthostatic hypotension, and thrombophlebitis. With the exception of orthostatic hypotension, these conditions are common causes of death in the early postinjury period. Effective treatments are suggested in Table 17–5.

Gastrointestinal Tract Complications

Common gastrointestinal complications of spinal cord injury include acute gastric dilatation and paralytic ileus, peptic ulceration in the acute abdomen, and neurogenic bowel. Patients who develop an acute abdomen due to appendicitis, intestinal perforation, or renal stones are particularly difficult to diagnose because the severity of these lesions are often unrelated to the clinical findings. In addition, the historical features and clinical signs commonly present in able-bodied persons are usually altered or absent in spinal injured patients. Not only are symptoms ill-defined and poorly localized, but spas-

ticity of the abdominal wall makes examination of the abdominal wall and its contents difficult. Therefore, diagnosis must be based on the results of laboratory tests and X-ray examinations. Neurogenic bowel can be the most serious gastrointestinal complication from spinal cord injury not only because stool incontinence can limit social interaction, but also because it can cause severe illness. Impactions may cause diarrhea or intestinal obstruction. The pathophysiology and management of neurogenic bowel are discussed thoroughly in Chapter 25. Guidelines for treating these gastrointestinal complications are presented in Table 17–6.

Genitourinary Tract

Complications of the genitourinary tract usually begin early after injury, but may also remain potential problems throughout the life of the patient. Genitourinary complications are the second most common source of morbidity after skin problems and are the leading cause of mortality. These problems, including neurogenic bladder, bladder calculi, reflux, and hydronephrosis, are described in Table 17–6. The pathology, evaluation, diagnosis and treatment of the neurogenic bladder are detailed in Chapter 25. In general, treatment of genitourinary complications should emphasize prevention throughout the life of the spinal injured patient.

Spasticity

After the period of initial spinal shock, most patients with upper motor neuron lesions experience involuntary muscular contractions as uninhibited segmental reflexes below the level of injury gradually return. Muscular spasms range in intensity from mild hypertonicity and increased stretch reflexes to clonus and flexion or extension contractions severe enough to throw a patient out of a bed or wheelchair. As a rule, spasticity is more severe in incomplete than complete injuries. Generally, the higher the level of injury, the more likely spasticity will occur.

The patients and family often mistake the appearance of spasticity for the recovery of spinal cord function. While spasticity can help main-

TABLE 17–5. *Cardiovascular problems associated with spinal cord injury*

Condition	Causes	Findings	Treatment
Bradycardia	Interruption in cardiac sympathetic accelerator fibers supplied by first five segments of thoracic cord	Generally occurs during first few days or weeks after injury; heart rate 40–60/min; worsened by conditions that stimulate vagus nerve or produce hypoxemia	Continuous cardiac monitoring until resting heart rate is consistently above 65–70/min; atropine 0.3–0.5 mg s.c. for heart rate below 50/min
Autonomic dysreflexia or hyperreflexia	Noxious afferent impulses arising from below lesion; bladder distention or sphincter dyssynergia; rectal or colon distention from gas or feces; ejaculation; gravid uterus contraction	Occurs after spinal shock, only with injury above T6; sudden onset of hypertension, sweating above injury level, reflex bradycardia; can lead to seizures, cerebral vascular accident, or death if untreated	Decompress distended bladder; elevate head of bed to enhance venous pooling and decrease cardiac output; give hydralazine, 5–10 mg, or diazoxide, 300 mg i.v.; if recurrent give maintenance dose of guanethidine, 10–20 mg, phenoxybenzamine, 20–30 mg, or propranolol, 20–80 mg, daily divided doses
Orthostatic hypotension	Reduction in normal sympathetic tone; failure of renin-angiotensin system to respond to upright position	Generally occurs during early mobilization; systolic blood pressure drops precipitously; patient becomes pale and dizzy; syncopy	Readapt to vertical position using reclining wheelchair or tilt table; corset and thigh-length elastic hose to enhance venous return; no wheelchair sitting after meals or early in morning; if persistent, give ephedrine, 25 mg p.o., 30 min prior to sitting; sodium chloride 1g q.i.d.
Thrombophlebitis	Coagulation abnormalities; immobilization; paralysis of muscle pump in lower extremities; dehydration; decreased respiratory function	Clinically apparent in up to 40%, silent in another 30%; pulmonary embolism is leading cause of death in early postinjury period; fever; increased spasticity; local warmth, redness, and fullness of thigh with pedal edema	Restrict patient to bed; elevate affected extremity 15° and maintain knee slightly flexed to avoid hyperextension and pressure on popliteal vein; anticoagulant with heparin 10–14 days, then oral agent for additional 8–12 weeks; continue oral anticoagulant 16–24 weeks if pulmonary embolism

tain muscle bulk, improve lower limb circulation, and possibly retard osteoporosis, the difficulty in positioning and maintaining personal hygiene can contribute to contractures, pain, and the development of pressure sores. Nevertheless, the potential for some patients to use their spasticity to compensate for poor strength in performing transfers or ambulating should always be considered when planning medical or surgical treatment.

Conservative management of spasticity includes physical and pharmacological therapy. As a general rule, patients with chronic injuries (more than 6 months), incomplete lesions, or complications require more medication and are harder to manage than those without these characteristics. Passive range of motion during bathing and dressing reduce spasticity by fatiguing the stretch reflex. More severe spasticity is alleviated by prone lying and the use of a standing frame, both of which also stretch contractures of the hips, knees, and ankles. Hydrotherapy, cold or hot packs, and functional electrical stimulation (see Chapter 4) can supplement these treatments. Pharmacological treatment is often effective for mild spasticity but relatively ineffective for moderate to severe spasms. The three major drugs currently used are diazepam (Valium®), dantrolene sodium (Dantrium®) and baclofen (Lioresal®). Combining two of these drugs is usually more effective than using only one. Taking all three drugs simultaneously, however, generally is not well tolerated.

If physical therapy and medications are ineffective, try peripheral nerve blocks, motor point blocks, and subarachnoid blocks. Surgical procedures, including neurectomy, rhizotomy, and myelotomy, can be extremely effective, but are irreversible and produce a lower motor neuron-type lesion.

Heterotopic Ossification

Thirty to forty percent of spinal injured patients develop heterotopic ossification (HO), the formation of cancellous bone outside the long bones. Heterotopic ossification occurs only below the level of injury, usually adjacent to the hip and the knee joints. Early symptoms are local swelling, increased warmth, redness, and decreased range of motion, resembling thrombophlebitis, cellulitis, or an articular abscess. A hard, irregular, palpable mass later replaces these features. The sedimentation rate, alkaline phosphatase, and creatine phosphokinase are frequently elevated, but other laboratory test results are normal. Radionuclear bone scans are reliable in confirming the diagnosis and in indicating when the bone has matured.

To maintain range of motion, gentle, passive exercises should be started once the acute symptoms have subsided. The only medical treatment available at the present time is a diphosphonate (Didronel®), administered prophylactically immediately after injury and after surgical removal of the extraskeletal bone. However, diphosphonate cannot stop the growth of new bone formation once it has started or cause it to regress. Surgical removal of HO is indicated when the bone is implicated in recurrent pressure sores or when it impedes joint function. Surgery should be postponed until the bone has matured because the extraskeletal bone is more likely to regrow if surgery is performed too early. The administration of diphosphonate substantially reduces the recurrence rate.

Metabolic and Endocrine Changes

In general, metabolic and endocrine changes are more severe in quadriplegics than paraplegics and in patients with recent rather than longstanding injuries. Metabolic and endocrine adaptation to spinal cord injury evolves gradually over many months. In the absence of persistent complications or major medical problems, a new homeostasis is usually achieved between 12 and 18 months after injury. Metabolic and endocrine conditions commonly associated with spinal cord injury are described in Table 17–7.

Respiratory Complications

The majority of respiratory complications in patients with spinal cord injury are due to the loss of function of intercostal and abdominal wall muscles. In cervical injury, approximately 30% of inspiratory capacity is lost to intercostal paralysis, with an additional 30% lost for each diaphragm involved. In quadriplegics, intercostal paralysis as well as abdominal muscle paralysis leads to ineffective sneezing and coughing. Initial vital capacities in quadriplegics range from 1,000 to 1,300 cc and usually improve by discharge to 2,500 to 3,000 cc.

Respiratory infections must be treated vigorously not only with antibiotics to eradicate bacterial infection but also with mucolytic and bronchodilating agents administered with an intermittent positive pressure breathing machine followed by postural drainage and assistive coughing. To assist coughing, apply pressure

TABLE 17–6. *Gastrointestinal and genitourinary problems associated with spinal cord injury*

Condition	Causes	Findings	Treatment
Acute gastric dilatation, paralytic ileus	Spinal shock; metabolic factors	Complete atony or diminished peristaltic activity during first 1–2 weeks after injury; distended abdomen; nausea and vomiting; dyspnea secondary to elevation of diaphragm; dehydration secondary to vomiting and trapped fluids in gut	Nasogastric tube with intermittent suction; intravenous fluids; discontinue or reduce dosage of drugs with anticholinergic effects (pain medications, tranquilizers, sedatives)
Peptic ulceration in acute abdomen	Stress of depleted body reserves; steroids; surgery	Affects 3–5% in acute phase; up to 50% may have gastric or duodenal lesions after acute phase; diagnosis difficult due to vague, nonspecific symptoms and unremarkable physical examination; localized warmth on rectal or vaginal examination provides clues	Avoid surgery 4–10 days postinjury; spasticity, cardiovascular instability, altered thermoregulation, and decreased pulmonary function make treatment difficult
Neurogenic bowel	Irregular bowel habits; lack of normal peristaltic activity	Anorexia, nausea, and general malaise as early symptoms of constipation; clinical symptoms of intestinal obstruction—abdominal distention, nausea and vomiting, fever, dyspnea, low blood pressure, dehydration; stool incontinence, diarrhea	Develop routine schedule for regular evacuation, preferably after a meal, sitting on commode to increase intraabdominal pressure; stool softeners, suppository or rectal stimulation to initiate evacuation reflex; for impaction, oral cathartics, increase fluids, retention enemas
Neurogenic bladder	Upper motor neuron lesion produces reflex bladder; lower motor neuron lesion produces autonomous or mixed type bladder	Areflexic bladder immediately following injury; absent bulbocavernosus and anal wink reflexes during spinal shock, negative bladder ice water test; may be sphincter dyssynergia	Foley catheter taped to midline of abdomen for initial bladder drainage; clean meatus three times a day with Betadine® or pHisoHex® to discourage infection; intermittent catheterization when patient is medically stable, every 4 hr; urecholine® to improve detrusor tone; Ditropan® or Pro-Banthine® for irritable or hypertonic bladder; Dibenzyline® to decrease internal sphincter tone; Dantrium® to decrease external sphincter tone; urine culture every 3–6 months and annual IVP to detect complications

TABLE 17–6. *(continued)*

Condition	Causes	Findings	Treatment
Bladder calculi	Infection, especially *Proteus* or *Klebsiella*, caused by indwelling catheter, high residual volume; urinary stasis, low output, or alkaline urine	Asymptomatic or history of recurrent febrile episodes, increased spasticity or leaking around Foley catheter due to obstruction or bladder irritation; radiopaque calcium phosphate on routine KUB film	Keep urine sterile, bladder drained and urinary output high; give 3,000 cc of fluid a day; avoid unnecessary immobilization, give Mandelamine® and ascorbic acid, 1 g q.i.d. or trimethoprim/ sulfamethoxazole; transurethral crushing and removal of stones
Reflux and hydronephrosis	Strong bladder contractions against high outlet resistance leading to vesicourethral reflux	Often asymptomatic with no infection until late stage	Reverse reflux with catheter draining; reimplant ureters or create ileal loop for nonreversible reflux

over the chest cage after the patient has taken a full inspiration and attempted to cough. See Chapter 13 for a more detailed discussion of these procedures.

Pressure Ulcers

Pressure ulcers, easily acquired but difficult to heal, are one of the most common and ex-

TABLE 17–7. *Metabolic and endocrine changes after spinal cord injury*

Condition	Duration postinjury	Treatment
Increased catabolic rates, with decreased hemoglobin, low serum iron and iron binding capacity, reduced total serum proteins, decreased albumin	First month	High protein, high calorie diet
Hypercalcuria; normal serum calcium	Up to 18 months	Upright activity; progressive exercise; high urinary output; acidification of urine; sterilization of urine when catheter is removed
Poikilothermia	Chronic	Regulate environmental temperature at comfortable level; keep patient appropriately clothed
Low fasting blood sugar and glucose tolerance levels; decreasing tolerance of sitting and standing	Chronic	Give rapidly absorbed carbohydrates
Progressive weight loss with increased proportion of body fat	Several months to a year	Restrict caloric intake; increase activity
Elevated uric acid in urine; normal serum uric acid levels	Chronic	No treatment necessary

pensive complications in spinal injured patients. Caused by prolonged pressure exceeding capillary pressure and compounded by shearing forces, they surprisingly occur more commonly in paraplegics than in quadriplegics. The most effective treatment is prevention, chiefly by frequent changing of position. The pathophysiology, classification, and treatment of pressure ulcers is described in Chapter 23.

Sexuality

Despite the major alterations of normal neural control that occurs after spinal injury, the achievement of pleasurable and fulfilling sexual expression is a realistic goal for most patients. The physician's role in helping the patients realize this goal is twofold: (1) providing medical sanction and permission to become sexually active, and (2) providing medical information about specific questions and problems.

Recovery of sexual function in spinal cord injured patients is very different for men and women. In spinal cord injured women, sexual function and fertility appear to be relatively unimpaired. Although precautions should be taken to avoid an unwanted pregnancy, spinal injured women should use oral contraceptives only with extreme caution, since the risk of thromboembolic phenomenon appears to be greater than in able-bodied persons. Pregnancy, labor, and delivery usually present no special problems, but patients with lesions above T6 should always be considered at risk for developing autonomic dysreflexia.

Sexual function in spinal injured men depends primarily on the level of injury and completeness of the lesion. For example, erections, ejaculation, and coital success are all more likely to be preserved in patients with incomplete lesions than in those with complete injuries. Patients with injuries in the cervical or thoracic regions with the sacral segments intact are more likely to have reflex erections, mediated in the sacral reflex arc at S2–S4, than patients with injuries in the lumbar or sacral areas. Regardless of the level or completeness of the injury, fertility is markedly impaired in spinal injured men and only 1% to 10% ever father children. In addition to problems with erections and anterior grade ejaculation, changes in the testes and epididymis may alter spermatogenesis.

For a more comprehensive discussion of the management of specific problems that interfere with sexual functioning in spinal injured persons, see Chapter 26.

Psychological Consequences

Spinal cord injury, because it occurs unexpectedly and leaves its victims permanently altered, is one of the most psychologically traumatic of all disabilities. The primary care physician can play a crucial role in helping the patient and his family cope with the devastating emotional consequences of spinal injury. Patients tend to cope with spinal injury much the way they cope with other stresses in their life. Thus, an important determinant in adjustment is the premorbid personality, which varies from one patient to another.

Patterns of adaptation are somewhat predictable, however; most patients exhibit denial and depression at some time during rehabilitation. The initial response to injury of many patients is disbelief or denial. Denial expressed in terms of hope persists indefinitely in many patients. For example, a patient with a cervical injury may unrealistically expect to walk again if only he tries hard enough. As long as patients continue to work at improving their skills and self-reliance and take the necessary precautions to avoid medical complications, their beliefs about eventual recovery should not be discounted or discouraged.

At some point in recovery, most patients demonstrate a degree of depression, often accompanied by anxiety, frustration, and anger. This depression, considered a natural response to catastrophic loss, seldom needs to be treated with drugs. Tricyclic antidepressants should be prescribed only if the patient has a prior history of depression, develops chronic, severe depression, or fails to respond to conservative therapy. In the absence of previous depression, formal and informal counseling, together with behavioral therapy, are probably the most effective management techniques to overcome depression. The patient's feelings should be acknowledged and validated as the patient is encouraged to become more active and regain as much initiative and independence as the disability will allow.

A few patients seem to experience no depression. Although the absence of depression in the face of serious disability may be disconcerting, there is no evidence that a period of depression is necessary for healthy adjustment. The most important determinant of successful adjustment and rehabilitation outcome is behavior, what the patient actually does to cope with disability, rather than the feelings the patient should or should not have.

PROGNOSIS

Functional Outcome

In general, the more motor and sensory function that returns early, the greater the total neurological recovery. An estimated 90% to 95% of neurological return occurs by the end of the first year. Even after 2 years, functional ability often continues to improve significantly through better education of the muscles to perform new tasks even though no neurological changes have occurred.

Vocational Adjustment

One of the major goals of a rehabilitation program for spinal cord injured patients is to help them enter the competitive labor market. At the present time, approximately 20% of all spinal patients become gainfully employed 3 years after injury. Another 20% are able to function as students or homemakers. As with most other outcomes, the level and extent of the injury have a strong influence on becoming employed, as does the psychosocial support system and premorbid level of education. In general, paraplegics do better than quadriplegics, and patients with incomplete injuries do better than those with complete lesions.

LONG-TERM COMPLICATIONS FROM THORACIC SPINAL INJURY

Report of a Case

HISTORY. This 22-year-old college student presented to his family physician with a 3-day history of progressive shortness of breath, anorexia, constipation, febrile spikes up to 101°F, and dark urine. He denied nausea, vomiting, cough, or unusual urinary odor.

At the age of 18, he sustained a spinal injury in a motor vehicle accident, resulting in T6 paraplegia. He had no major complications during his rehabilitation program at a regional spinal cord center, where he eventually became independent at a wheelchair level in all activities of daily living. Since discharge from the center, he has enjoyed generally good health. He lived with his family for a year and a half until he started college, where he continues to room with an able-bodied student.

PHYSICAL EXAMINATION AND LABORATORY RESULTS. The patient's temperature was 100.5°F and there was tachypnea, but the chest was clear to auscultation and percussion. Head, neck, and extremities were unremarkable, an external catheter was in place, and the genitalia were normal. The abdomen was moderately protruberant and mildly high-pitched bowel sounds were audible. The neurological examination was compatible with complete motor and sensory deficit at T6 with increased spasticity in the lower extremities.

On X-ray film, the chest was clear with mildly elevated diaphragms. Flat plate of the abdomen showed increased gas and a large amount of stool. The throat and sputum culture were negative, and white blood cell count was slightly elevated, and hemoglobin was normal. Urinalysis revealed numerous white blood cells, and the urine culture showed > 100,000/ml of *E. coli*.

DIAGNOSIS AND TREATMENT. The physical examination and laboratory results were consistent with a diagnosis of acute lower urinary tract infection and secondary intestinal ileus. The patient was put on a 10-day course of ampicillin and was encouraged to increase fluid intake. He was given 2 ounces of milk of magnesia and an enema that evacuated the bowel thoroughly. He then resumed his regular daily bowel program.

Urinary tract infection accompanied by ileus is a typical complication with spinal cord injury, even in the long-term stage. These patients often present with symptoms that suggest pulmonary complication, but that can be readily differentiated by the physical examination and laboratory testing in the primary care physician's office. Ileus should be suspected as a secondary complication whenever a patient develops a urinary tract infection.

SUGGESTED READINGS

Bedbrook, G. (1981): *The Care and Management of Spinal Cord Injuries*. Springer-Verlag, New York.

Burke, D. C., and Murray, D. D. (1975): *Handbook of Spinal Cord Medicine*. Raven Press, New York.

Boyarsky, S., Labay, P., Hanick, P., et al. (1979): *Care of the Patient with Neurogenic Bladder*. Little, Brown and Co., Boston.

Chantraine, A., Crielaard, J. M. Onkelinx, A., and Pirnay, F. (1984): Energy expenditure of ambulation in paraplegics: Effects of long-term use of bracins. *Paraplegia*, 22:173–181.

Corbet, B. (1980): *Options: Spinal Cord Injury and the Future*. Hirschfeld Press.

Hanak, M. and Scott, A. (1983): *Spinal Cord Injury: An Illustrated Guide for the Health Care Professional*. Springer, New York.

Haney, M., and Rabin, B. (1984): Modifying attitude toward disabled persons while resocializing spinal cord injured patients. *Arch. Phys. Med. Rehabil.*, 65:431–436.

Jocheim, K. A. (1983): Psychological aspects of spinal cord injuries—an important point in the outcome of rehabilitation. *Ann. Acad. Med. Singapore*, 12:377–379.

Trieschmann, R. B. (1980): *Spinal Cord Injuries: Psychological, Social and Vocational Adjustment*. Pergamon Press, New York.

Wu, Y.-C. (1983): Total bladder care for the spinal cord injured patient. *Ann. Acad. Med. Singapore*, 12:387–399.

Young, R. F., and Feldman, R. A. (1981): *Spinal Cord Injuries: Case Studies*. Medical Examination Publishing Co., Garden City, NY.

Medical Rehabilitation,
edited by L. S. Halstead et al.
Raven Press, New York © 1985.

CHAPTER 18

Peripheral Nerve Injuries and Neuromuscular Disorders

Randall L. Braddom

Department of Physical Medicine and Rehabilitation, University of Cincinnati Medical Center, Cincinnati, Ohio 45230

PATHOPHYSIOLOGY OF NERVE INJURIES

Most causes of neuropathy are divided into two types—segmental demyelination and axonal degeneration—based on whether the initial insult to the nerve is to the myelin or to the axon. Localized nerve injuries—axonotmesis, neurapraxia, and axonostenosis—are classified according to the nature of the injury and whether it was produced by compression or trauma.

Segmental Demyelination

Neuropathies initially produced by injury to the myelin covering the nerve are often called Gombault demyelination or segmental demyelination. Such conditions as Guillain-Barré syndrome, diabetic peripheral neuropathy, and Dejerine-Sottas neuropathy begin with segmental demyelination. Since the myelin disturbance has a major impact on nerve conduction, decreases in nerve conduction velocity as measured by electrodiagnostic techniques are usually obvious in these conditions.

Axonal Degeneration

Nerve injury to the axon only secondarily affects the myelin coating. Axonal degeneration is caused primarily by toxins such as alcohol, vincristine, arsenic, and thalium. Since the myelin coating of the nerve tends to remain intact, its nerve conduction will be close to normal if the axon is still capable of function. Therefore, additional clinical and electrodiagnostic techniques must be used in evaluation.

Axonotmesis

Complete transection of a nerve is called axonotmesis. The nerve undergoes wallerian degeneration, a process of axon dissolution distal to the transection. This degeneration of the nerve usually does not move proximally beyond the first node of Ranvier. Wallerian degeneration is reversible if the nerve sheath is intact or has been reattached. The axon will grow across the site of transection and down the nerve sheath at the rate of approximately 2 cm per month.

Neurapraxia

In neurapraxia, nerve conduction is interrupted across the site of the injury, but the compression is insufficient to produce wallerian degeneration. This conduction block is usually rapidly reversible when the compression or injury is relieved.

Axonostenosis

Axonostenosis occurs when a nerve has been clinically compressed until a localized segment of the nerve is contracted in diameter. It is often accompanied by intraneural scarring. In addition to decompression, this condition may require a careful teasing apart of the nerve fibers under a surgical microscope.

ASSESSMENT OF PERIPHERAL NERVE INJURIES

Sensory Evaluation

Many peripheral neuropathies and most peripheral nerve injuries produce a loss of one or more modalities of sensation. An adequate sensory examination can be performed in minutes, although interpreting the findings will involve subjective judgments by both the patient and the examiner. If pinprick, vibration, light touch, and position sensation are present in the feet, and if the patient can recognize numbers written on the palms of the hands while the eyes are closed, a major sensory deficit is unlikely.

Comparing a single pinprick proximally to a single pinprick distally will help localize peripheral neuropathy (Fig. 18–1). Try to quantitate the difference between the proximal and distal stimulation sites. Ask the patient, "If this pinprick on your chest is worth $100, how much is this pinprick on your foot worth?" The difference is significant if the patient's answer is less than $75.

Summation is another useful, objective sign of sensory loss. If the patient has a toxic or metabolic peripheral neuropathy such as diabetes, pinpricks of the same intensity quickly repeated will suddenly become very painful and the patient will grimace and withdraw the extremity. Ordinarily, pain does not increase with repeated pricking.

The most potentially dangerous sensory problem from peripheral nerve deficits is loss of protective sensation, the pain and temperature sensation necessary to prevent injury to the affected area. A simple bedside test of gross temperature sensation is to have the patient determine which feels colder, the plastic barrel of a ballpoint pen or the metal handle of a reflex hammer. These objects should feel different because metal has much higher thermal conductivity. Protective pain sensation can be grossly tested by the patient's ability to differentiate sharp and dull.

Motor Evaluation

Loss of Joint Range of Motion

Most neuropathies involve some type of motor weakness. Always look carefully for muscle weakness when a patient shows reduced joint range of motion (ROM). Loss of ROM is apt to occur when there is an imbalance in muscle strength of an agonist and antagonist. For example, a radial nerve injury with paralysis of the triceps, but with normal strength in the elbow flexors, tends to produce an elbow flexion contracture.

Muscle Tightness

Muscle weakness in peripheral nerve injuries may also cause tightness due to muscle shortening, especially in muscles that cross two or more joints. For example, peroneal nerve injury often results in a foot drop caused by shortening of the gastrocnemius muscle. Two-joint muscle

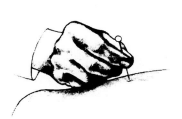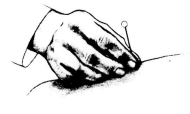

FIG. 18–1. Testing sensation of pain. Grasp pin shaft and allow pin to slide through fingers after pin contacts skin. Compare normal area (e.g., chest) with suspected area of involvement (e.g., foot). [From Olson, W. H., Brumbach, R. A., Gascon, G., and Christoferson, L. A. (1981): *Practical Neurology for the Primary Care Physician.* Charles C Thomas, Springfield, Illinois.]

shortening is a very serious problem because it can lead to serious gait disturbances.

Muscle Strength Testing

A simple technique for muscle strength testing is the make-and-break system. The patient is asked to make a muscle do what it normally does and then the examiner attempts to break this position. For example, in testing the elbow flexor muscles, the patient is asked to flex the elbow and to hold it in this position. The examiner places one hand above the patient's elbow and one hand below the elbow and then attempts to extend the elbow against the patient's maximum resistance. Groups of similarly acting muscles are usually tested together. For example, the elbow flexor muscles that are tested together include the biceps, brachialis, and coracobrachialis. More advanced special techniques can be used to isolate specific muscles for make-and-break testing, if necessary. The most commonly used system for grading muscle strength is described in Chapter 3 (Table 3–6).

Since patients vary widely in natural strength levels, and complaints of weakness often reflect depression or fatigue, determining whether muscles are abnormally weak may be difficult. Practice grading the muscle strength of both male and female patients of various ages and body builds will help overcome this difficulty. Furthermore, patients who are emotionally upset or who have a reduced mental status may not be cooperative enough for accurate strength testing. Patients in pain often appear to be weak when discomfort prevents them from exerting full muscle force, reflecting the pain inhibition of function. The following are some nonneurological reasons for complaints of weakness:

1. Deficient natural strength level.
2. Depression.
3. Fatigue.
4. Chronic insomnia.
5. Pain.
6. Hysterical conversion reaction.

Muscle strength grading and testing are more reliable in patients with lower motor neuron weakness or intrinsic muscle abnormalities than in those with upper motor neuron weakness. The flaccid weakness of motor abnormalities below and including the anterior horn cell level is objectively consistent regardless of the position of the patient or the time of day. Strength level does vary, however, in upper motor neuron weakness. For example, a patient with a stroke-induced hemiplegia who is unable to activate the quadriceps muscle in the sitting position may be able to use this muscle while walking in an upright position.

Hysterical Weakness

Patients under severe psychological stress may undergo a conversion reaction in which their psychological problems are suddenly converted into a physical problem, usually a form of paralysis that the patient has observed in a friend or relative. The typical hysterical patient has relatively poor insight into personal problems and is somewhat socioculturally primitive, but not necessarily unintelligent. A conversion reaction can involve any neurological system. Some examples are "globus hystericus" (feeling of a lump in the throat), sudden inability to talk above a whisper, numbness or weakness of all or part of the body, and tunnel vision.

These patients usually appear indifferent to their physical problem, an affect referred to as "la belle indifference." Clinicians should always consider the diagnosis of a hysterical conversion reaction when a patient is seen with an acute neurological syndrome that is unusual or unlikely and the patient does not seem very concerned about it. The patient with hysterical weakness will usually show one or more of the following signs:

1. A rachety response to muscle testing, in which the joint is allowed unconsciously to be pulled out of position a few degrees at a time.
2. Marked slow motion, in which tasks are done very slowly and laboriously.
3. Inconsistencies between muscle strength grade and functional strength evident during walking or other motor activity.

4. Bizzare gait ("astasia abasia"), which may require marked strength to accomplish without falling, and frequent falling without injury.

Some useful tests for detecting such inconsistencies are illustrated in Fig. 18–2.

Persons with acute hysterical weakness are usually amenable to the power of suggestion, especially by a medical or religious authority figure. They are often resistant to classic psychotherapy, however, because of their lack of insight into their problems.

Reflex Testing

The simplest way to elicit a reflex response is to strike a tendon, which stretches the muscle. The patient must be relaxed during the reflex examination, since an overly tense muscle will not respond to a tap on its tendon. Patients with very bulky muscles may also appear not to have reflexes because their heavy tendons and mus-

cles are not stretched adequately by the usual hammer-strike technique.

Facilitation Techniques

Reflexes may be made more brisk (greater amplitude of the muscle response) by using facilitation techniques. The classic facilitation technique is the Jendrassik maneuver, in which the fingers are interlocked and pulled against each other to facilitate lower extremity reflexes. Actually, almost any muscle activity away from the muscle being testing can be a facilitation maneuver. When doing upper extremity reflexes, for example, ask the patient to hold the chin on the chest or clench the teeth. The grading of reflexes is described as follows:

0—Reflex not elicited by any maneuver.
1 + —Reflex obtained only with facilitation techniques.
2 + —Reflex within usual range.
3 + —Reflex very brisk, but without clonus.
4 + —Reflex accompanied by clonus.

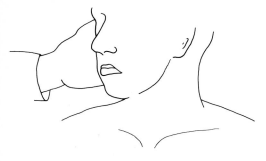

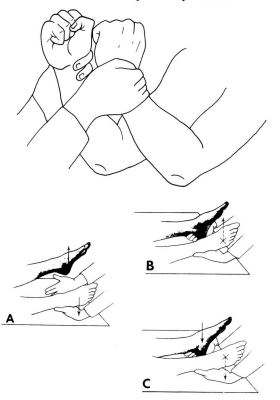

FIG. 18–2. Tests to distinguish true from hysterical weakness. **Left:** Left sternocleidomastoid turns head to right. Patients with psychogenic left-sided weakness often show weakness when turning toward left. **Upper right:** Test comparable muscle strength simultaneously if there is suspicion of nonorganicity. "Giving way" with one muscle while maintaining strength in another is very difficult. **Lower right:** To distinguish true paralysis from hysterical paralysis of leg, place both hands under heels and ask patient to raise good leg. A, Examiner will feel increased downward pressure by paralyzed leg. B, Ask patient to lift paralyzed leg; little or no response is likely. C, Ask patient to bear down with both heels; if same pressure noted in maneuver A cannot be exerted, suspect hysterical paralysis. [From Olson, W.H., Brumbach, R.A., Gascon, G., and Christoferson, L.A. (1981): *Practical Neurology for the Primary Care Physician.* Charles C Thomas, Springfield, Illinois.]

Superficial Reflexes

Superficial reflexes are elicited by stroking the skin or mucous membranes rather than by striking a tendon. A pinwheel is more effective for eliciting plantar, abdominal, and cremasteric reflexes than are other types of stimuli. Other normal reflexes include blinking and gagging. Usually considered abnormal are the Babinski, palmomental, grasp, suck, and glabellar reflexes.

Commonly Used Electrodiagnostic Techniques

Electromyography

Recording the electrical activity of muscle fibers near a needle inserted into the muscle belly is referred to as electromyography (EMG). This technique is most useful for identifying denervated muscle and localizing lesions. The EMG confirms findings in the history and physical examination of a neuropathic or myopathic process. It can also follow the progress of reinnervation of previously injured or destroyed nerves. The five steps in an EMG examination, and what they measure, are described below and in Chapter 3.

1. Observe the muscle at rest for fasciculation and fibrillation potentials.
2. Compare insertional activity to potentials observed after pin movement stops for fasciculations, fibrillations, and positive waves.
3. Observe minimal motor unit activity for motor unit action potentials (MUAPs) as patient voluntarily produces minimal muscle contractions.
4. Observe maximal motor unit activity for the MUAP firing rate and the number of MUAPs as patient maximally contracts muscle.
5. Assess the distribution or pattern of EMG abnormalities found in the light of the history and physical examination.

Clinical deductions are made from the distribution of EMG abnormalities in consideration of the history and physical examinations. For example, a patient whose extremities have distal sensory disturbances and distal weakness, with the EMG changes limited to the distal muscles, would be very likely to have a peripheral neuropathy. This diagnostic impression could be further substantiated by the use of nerve conduction studies.

Nerve Conduction Studies

Nerve conduction studies, the most helpful part of the examination for diagnosing peripheral nerve problems, may be used to determine the conduction velocity of either motor or sensory fibers. Most commonly studied are the large nerves of the extremities, such as the median, ulnar, peroneal, and tibial nerves. Velocity measurement is normal if the myelin sheath is intact. Only injury to the myelin sheath of most of the fast-conducting fibers or total destruction of these fibers results in decreased conduction velocity. Nerve conduction study also helps localize the site of injury to the nerve. However, the age of the patient, as well as the temperature of the extremities, must be considered when interpreting the results, since nerve conduction velocity decreases with both aging and cooling.

Classic Electrodiagnosis

The older techniques of electrodiagnosis are used infrequently now, but they are still useful in differentiating innervated from denervated muscle.

Electrodiagnostic techniques are described in more detail in Chapter 3.

MANAGING COMPLICATIONS OF PERIPHERAL NEUROPATHY

Peripheral nerve injuries commonly result in muscle weakness, which can lead to joint contractures and muscle shortening.

Joint Contractures and Muscle Shortening

These problems can be prevented by daily passive, active, and active-assistive ROM exercises, as well as by muscle stretching, proper postioning during bedrest, and splinting. Patients who have a reduced level of consciousness must be positioned in bed very carefully to avoid injuries to peripheral nerves, which can be compressed easily between bony prominences and the bed. Such complications are commonly seen in comatose patients who develop ulnar nerve injuries in the olecranon groove area of the elbow and peroneal nerve injuries at the head of the fibula. Surgery is seldom required to correct contractures caused by peripheral nerve injury because they are not accompanied by spasticity. Techniques of preserving function are described in detail in Chapter 5.

Loss of Sensation

Patients with skin areas having no protective sensation must examine anesthetic areas daily for evidence of tissue trauma. Some skin areas that lack protective pain sensation are best protected by orthotic devices. The patient with anesthesia of the shin due to peroneal nerve injury may need a plastic shin guard to prevent inadvertent injury. Loss of protective pain sensation of the feet may call for extra-depth shoes and Plastiazote shoe inserts to prevent foot trauma and ulcers. Daily foot soaks followed by application of Alba-3 ointment will help the insensitive foot resist scaling and fissuring.

When large areas of the body lack sensation, susceptibility to pressure sores increases, especially in skin areas over bony prominences. The management of pressure sores is discussed in Chapter 23.

Weakness

Strength Exercises

Patients who are weak from peripheral nerve injury or neuropathy may benefit from muscle strength exercise programs and use of supportive orthotics, as described in Chapter 6. A program of strength-building, isotonic, isometric, isokinetic, progressive resistive, and manual resistive exercise should be individually tailored to improve strength without overworking muscles to the point of paradoxically weakening them further.

MANAGEMENT OF GUILLAIN-BARRÉ SYNDROME

Guillain-Barré (G-B) syndrome or inflammatory polyradiculoneuropathy, a demyelinating disorder, produces an acute or subacute paralysis that often begins in the lower extremities and then ascends.

Although the exact cause of G-B syndrome is unknown, a viral or other infectious process, or immunization, precedes the majority of cases. Therefore, an autoimmune process is suspected. The annual incidence is approximately one case per 10,000 persons. Because G-B syndrome occurs so frequently, physicians must consider it in any case of acute or subacute generalized weakness. Most patients complain of the gradual onset of weakness and of some disturbances in sensation. The weakness may involve peripheral somatic nerves, autonomic nerves, and cranial nerves, and muscle stretch reflexes are generally lost or decreased. The cerebrospinal fluid typically shows an elevated protein level without a pleocytosis, often referred to as cytoalbuminologic disassociation. However, this finding, as well as reduced nerve conduction velocity and motor unit action potentials, may be normal until weeks after clinical onset.

Complete clinical recovery from G-B syndrome takes from 1 to 12 months in the majority of patients. Some patients are left with residual weakness or paralysis, but rarely with residual sensory disturbances. The death rate is approximately 5% to 7%, with the most common causes of death being pneumonia and cardiac arrhythmia. Be sure to alert patients with G-B syndrome that relapses often occur months to years after the initial episode, especially after major surgery.

Medical Treatment

Since there is no known cure for G-B syndrome, medical care is directed toward maintaining the life of the patient until recovery occurs spontaneously. Monitoring respiratory function is essential, as these patients may rapidly lose the ability to breathe normally. Patients whose vital capacity falls acutely under 1,000 cc should be watched very closely and admitted to an intensive care unit. Autonomic function is often abnormal. Therefore, sudden cardiac arrhythmias, changes in blood pressure, circulatory collapse, or reduction in peripheral vascular tone leading to severe orthostatic hypotension are possible. Since most deaths from G-B syndrome are unexpected and sudden, patients should be monitored carefully for quick assistance.

Rehabilitation Methods

Patients with G-B syndrome are particularly susceptible to overwork weakness, which must be considered when planning the exercise program. It is quite common for improving patients to be so excited by the development of new strength that they overwork the muscle and are psychologically devastated by the resulting return of weakness. In these cases, reducing activity and even resting the muscle reinstates strength. Once muscles have progressed beyond the antigravity strength level, they generally can be put through a strength program without further injury.

During the subacute stage of G-B syndrome, the temporary use of assistive devices may be necessary. Rocker feeders are helpful until sufficient strength is regained to lift food to the mouth. Ankle-foot braces, wrist extension splints, long leg braces, clothing adaptations, and dressing assistive devices, as described in Chapter 6, may all be leased for temporary use (see Appendix). In addition, most patients will need a wheelchair at some time during the course of their treatment. The prescription of wheelchairs is covered in Chapter 6.

Gait Retraining

As in other aspects of the rehabilitation program for G-B syndrome, the stages in the gait retraining program should accommodate the temporary nature of the illness. Progressive gait retraining in G-B syndrome involves five steps:

1. Tilt table (see Chap. 22, Fig. 22–4)—Gradual elevation to the upright position until patient overcomes orthostatic hypotension.
2. Standing table (Fig. 18–3)—Standing tolerance increases while preventing falls and

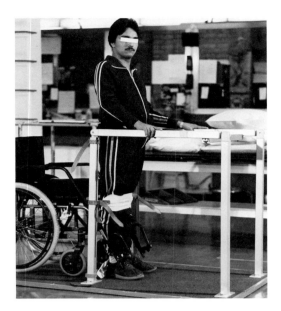

FIG. 18–3. Patient in standing table increases tolerance to the upright position. (Photo by Gordon Stanley.)

allowing work on occupational therapy projects.
3. Parallel bars—Therapist walks with patient between bars to prevent falling to one side or the other.
4. Assistive devices—Walking outside the parallel bars with assistance of walker, crutches, or cane.
5. Without assistance—Walking without supportive devices.

Sensory Loss

Although paresthesias are common in G-B syndrome, occasionally producing an ataxic gait, most patients do not require protective orthotic devices because they maintain adequate protective sensation.

Pulmonary Rehabilitation

Acute Management

Severe respiratory paralysis in G-B syndrome is usually managed in an intensive care unit, where the lack of orienting cues may lead to

"ICU psychosis." Helpful techniques for maintaining orientation are described in Chapter 17.

Subacute Management

Although the return to normal respiratory capacity may be slow, most adult patients can tolerate permanent withdrawal from a mechanical respirator when the vital capacity is 1,000 cc or more. Such a low vital capacity, however, makes it very difficult for the patient to cough or breathe deeply, which predisposes to the development of hypostatic pneumonia. Pulmonary compliance also declines as the chest structures lose normal range of motion. The use of intermittent positive pressure breathing (IPPB) three to four times daily will help preserve the volume of the pulmonary tree (see Chapter 13). Manual abdominal compression may be necessary to assist in coughing. Allow the tracheostomy to close when the vital capacity is greater than 2,000 cc to facilitate the reduction of excessive tracheal secretions.

External devices such as a chest cuirass, pneumobelt, or raincoat device will assist in daytime ventilation, while a rocking bed will facilitate ventilation at night (Fig. 18–4). Postural drainage techniques much like those used for cystic fibrosis patients may also be helpful. In the few patients sustaining a residual loss of respiratory function, such assistance must continue throughout life. In addition, smoking is prohibited and weight should be controlled.

Loss of Joint Range of Motion and Muscle Shortening

Patients with G-B syndrome are more likely to develop shortening of two-joint muscles than actual joint contractures. Depending on the degree of weakness present, they should have passive, active, or active-assistive ROM exercises, as well as stretching of two-joint muscles such as the triceps, gastrocnemius, tensor fascia lata, and the hamstrings.

WEAKNESS IN SEVERE GUILLAIN-BARRÉ SYNDROME

Report of a Case

HISTORY AND PHYSICAL EXAMINATION. One week after the onset of a respiratory infection, this 34-year-old woman reported numbness and tingling in her hands and feet and progressive weakness of her feet and legs. The viral infection had resolved except for residual pharyngitis and a dry cough exacerbated by her smoking habit. Examination revealed symmetrical motor weakness and depressed deep tendon reflexes in all four limbs, but no cranial nerve abnormalities or sensory deficits. The weakness was constant rather than progressive with repetitive movement. Nerve conduction velocities were normal. A lumbar puncture yielded cerebrospinal fluid with an elevated protein content and a low cell count.

Over the next 24 hr, the patient became weaker, somnolent, and developed difficulty breathing. She was subsequently hospitalized, where a tracheostomy was performed and she was placed on a respirator. Extraocular muscle movements, pupillary reactions, and ocular fundi remained intact. Autonomic function was abnormal, with tachycardia, hypotension, and anhidrosis, but sphincter function remained normal. Nerve conduction velocities became abnormally reduced during the third week of hospitalization. The patient began to improve after 2 weeks in the intensive care unit, and she was weaned from the mechanical respirator.

REHABILITATION MANAGEMENT OF WEAKNESS. Abdominal compression to assist coughing and postural drainage was performed daily to clear the lungs and to compensate for the weakened respiratory musculature.

While the patient was on a respirator, her feet were placed flat against a foot board to maintain standing ROM and her joints were moved passively through the normal range of motion twice daily to stimulate proprioceptive pathways and to prevent contractures. Motor reeducation was begun during the third week of hospitalization. Hot moist Hydrocollator packs were applied before each session to relieve pain and facilitate movement. ROM for each joint was performed three times during each session. During the second set, the therapist described the motion and action of the muscles producing the motion and stroked the skin over the area of the prime mover as the patient watched the movement performed. On the third try, the patient attempted to assist the motion as the therapist performed it. The patient's participation gradually increased until she was able to move each joint actively through its normal range without assistance. After one month in the hospital, the patient entered

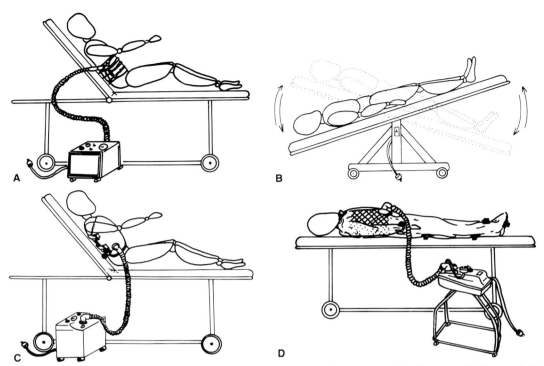

FIG. 18–4. Ventilators that are especially useful for the patient with neuromuscular disease. **A:** Pneumobelt. Corset that contains inflatable bladder is strapped to abdomen. During expiration, bladder is inflated, forcing diaphragm to more cephalad position. **B:** Rocking bed. Bed oscillates in synchronization with breathing, causing augmented diaphragm travel. **C:** Hard shell cuirass. Rigid shell is strapped to chest and negative pressure is generated within shell to cause chest expansion for inspiration. **D:** Wire cage cuirass. Works similarly to hard shell cuirass except that form-fitting shell is not required. Wire cage is placed about chest, creating a chamber. Patient and cage are wrapped in airtight plastic body stocking or raincoat and negative pressure is generated in chamber for inspiration. [From Shapiro, B.J. (1982): Pulmonary rehabilitation of the neuromuscular patient. In: *The Practice of Rehabilitation Medicine*, edited by P.E. Kaplan and R.S. Materson. Charles C Thomas, Springfield, Illinois.]

a progressive program of passive, active, and active-assistive stretching exercises in a heated pool.

Due to orthostatic hypotension, she gained tolerance gradually to the upright position by spending increasing amounts of time on a tilt table, then in a standing frame. With the support of a polypropylene ankle-foot brace, she practiced walking in the parallel bars, then progressed from underarm crutches to forearm crutches, and finally, to a cane.

She was discharged home in the care of her husband when she was able to walk in the parallel bars. As improvement continued, she returned to the rehabilitation center once every 2 weeks.

A rocking bed was rented for use when sleeping because she continued to have some nocturnal respiratory difficulty for 1 month after discharge, despite having given up smoking. She purchased a wrist-supporting extension splint to wear and a rocker feeder to assist eating until her upper extremity muscles reached a strength of at least grade 3.

The patient was able to resume gardening, a former hobby, and returned to her job as a social worker 10 months after the onset of the illness.

The onset of this patient's weakness after a viral illness is typical of G-B syndrome. The physical examination differentiated it from multiple sclerosis (MS), myasthenia gravis, and idiopathic autoimmune phenomena, which are also often triggered by viral infection. Like G-B syndrome, MS often begins with greater weakness in the legs than in the arms. Both MS and myasthenia gravis, however, are more likely to produce abnormal ocular phenomena, which were absent in this patient. Both myasthenia gravis and G-B syndrome compromise respiratory function, but general weakness is constant in G-B rather than progressive with repetitive movement, as in the former. In addition, this patient experienced little genitourinary involvement, which is more frequently an early symptom of MS, and her paralysis was flaccid when it is more likely to be spastic in MS.

This patient was monitored in an intensive care unit because the severity of her illness put her at high risk of pulmonary complication or death from respiratory failure.

The motor reeducation program was similar to that originally developed for patients with poliomyelitis. A graded, resistive exercise program was contraindicated; most physicians agree that such exercise will not improve strength in G-B syndrome, and may actually exacerbate weakness, until nerve function recovers spontaneously. Most ambulation aids and assistive devices were rented for temporary use rather than purchased because complete, or nearly complete, recovery from weakness usually can be expected. Despite essentially complete recovery, this patient should be observed carefully for the possibility of relapses with future occurrences of viral infection or surgery.

MANAGEMENT OF CARPAL TUNNEL SYNDROME

In carpal tunnel syndrome (CTS), the median nerve in the wrist is entrapped within the carpal canal. Carpal tunnel syndrome is very common, especially in women. While most cases are idiopathic, CTS may also be hereditary, posttraumatic (e.g., wrist fractures or after prolonged crutch walking), secondary to rare anatomical variations, due to metabolic disturbances, or caused by rheumatoid arthritis. While CTS occurs in approximately 15% of pregnant women, it usually disappears after delivery.

Diagnosis

You should suspect CTS when any young or middle-aged adult complains of nocturnal paresthesias of the hand, the most common symp-

tom. Many patients report that they can prevent the nocturnal paresthesias by sleeping in an easy chair with the feet on the floor rather than in bed. Pain or numbness usually is felt only in the dominant hand, even when CTS is bilateral. Other common diagnostic signs of CTS are weakness of the opponens muscles, Phalen's sign, and a reproduction of paresthesias by light tapping over the median nerve at the wrist (Tinel's sign). Electrodiagnostic studies are generally indicated, especially motor and sensory conduction studies of the median nerve across the wrists.

Medical and Surgical Treatment

A wrist splint, oral nonsteroidal, anti-inflammatory agents, steroid injection into the carpal canal, and, occasionally, oral diuretic agents provide short-term relief of symptoms. Most cases of CTS, however, are relieved permanently only through surgical decompression of the carpal canal. Due to its high success rate and low morbidity, this procedure is usually considered the conservative treatment for even early CTS. Median nerve injury may not resolve completely if surgery is delayed.

Rehabilitation

Since CTS is usually only curable surgically, only those patients who have very transient conditions, who refuse surgery, or whose CTS may be too severe and chronic to benefit from surgery, will require rehabilitation. Therefore, rehabilitation activities generally focus on overcoming weakness of thumb abduction, pain, and sensory loss in the skin areas covered by the median nerve.

Compensating for Weakness

Weakness of the opponens pollicus and abductor pollicus brevis usually compromises grip strength, causing the patient to accidentally drop things. Severe weakness of thumb opposition may require an opponens splint, which places the thumb in abduction away from the palm so that the thumb touch pad can contact the touch pads of the fingers.

Managing Sensory Loss and Pain

Transcutaneous electrical nerve stimulation (TENS), in which painful skin areas are stimulated by surface electrodes wired to a small battery-powered stimulator, may help alleviate causalgic pain (reflex sympathetic dystrophy) secondary to a permanent partial nerve injury (see Chapter 4). If the patient develops reflex sympathetic dystrophy, TENS of the upper extremity, as well as massage of the hand, contrast baths, and active assistive ROM of the finger and wrist joints, are indicated.

Other Median Nerve Problems

The median nerve may be injured or entrapped anywhere along its course. One of the most common injuries of the median nerve occurs during attempted suicides by wrist-cutting, in which tendons of the flexor digitorum superficialis to the middle and ring fingers are often injured. If the median nerve is injured proximally, weakness of thumb abduction and finger flexion in the index and middle fingers causes the "benediction hand" sign whenever the patient tries to actively flex the fingers. The treatment of these conditions is similar to that of CTS.

The causes, signs and symptoms, and treatment of radial, ulnar, sciatic, femoral, peroneal, and tibial nerve injuries are summarized in Table 18–1.

MANAGEMENT OF DIABETIC PERIPHERAL NEUROPATHY

Peripheral Neuropathy

Injuries to nerves of all types, including myelinated and unmyelinated, somatic and autonomic nerves, are predictable complications of diabetes mellitus. The commonest type of nerve injury is diabetic peripheral neuropathy, in which the longest somatic nerves are affected. Diabetic peripheral neuropathy, present in most persons who have had diabetes for 10 years or longer, gradually increases in severity. The neuropathy is symmetrical and involves both motor and sensory fibers. The sensory abnormalities are greatest for light touch and vibration and least severe for conscious proprioception. You should assume that a patient with peripheral neuropathy also has autonomic neuropathy, since both kinds consistently coexist in diabetic patients.

Diabetic mononeuritis is a condition in which one or more individual nerves may be injured. Painful diabetic neuritis is consistently worse at night, when its burning often interferes with sleeping. Another common form of diabetic neuropathy is the multiple lumbar nerve root syndrome, or diabetic amyotrophy. Its onset may be so rapid that the patient may seem to have an acute cauda equina syndrome. It is accompanied at times by long-tract signs such as Babinski's and by elevated cerebrospinal fluid protein. Since diabetes mellitus predisposes all nerves to injury, there is also a higher incidence of nerve injury from entrapments and trauma. An acute and usually transient form of neuropathy may accompany episodes of diabetic ketoacidosis. Hyperinsulin neuropathy, however, is rarely seen.

With the exception of the transient neuropathy of diabetic ketoacidosis, almost all diabetic neuropathies have a relatively poor prognosis. Good control of diabetes, however, is believed to slow the development or progression of neuropathy.

Clinical Diagnosis

Every diabetic patient should be evaluated for diabetic peripheral neuropathy because few patients are aware of nerve injury in the early stages. When functional deficits do become apparent, complaints range from weakness and fatigue on walking to numbness of the feet. Patients may also complain of autonomic symptoms such as dyspepsia, difficulty swallowing, dry skin, bowel and bladder abnormalities, or impotence. Complaints of impotence are very common, while others, such as nocturnal involuntary bowel movements, are uncommon.

Diabetic neuropathy reduces reflexes, with the Achilles jerk the first one lost in the typical case. Loss of muscle strength distally may be difficult to diagnose in the early cases, but in advanced cases intrinsic atrophy of the hand and foot mus-

TABLE 18–1. *Common peripheral nerve injuries and entrapments*

Nerve	Causes	Signs and symptoms	Treatment
Radial			
Saturday night palsy, honeymoon paralysis	Alcoholism; suppression of normal sleep cycle; sitting for hours with arm across back of park bench; sleeping with bed partner's head on proximal medial arm	Nerve injured around radial groove of humerus; distal to innervation of triceps; active elbow extension maintained; extensors of wrist, fingers, thumb lost; sensory loss in dorsum of forearm and hand in skin innervated by radial nerve	Stop use of alcohol and other drugs; improve overall health of patient; keep wrist and finger joints free of flexion contractures via muscle stretching and joint ROM; apply cock-up splint to wrist
Posterior interosseus nerve syndrome	Trauma	Weakness of ulnar wrist extensors, finger and thumb extensors; intact triceps and extensor carpi radialis muscles; wrist dorsiflexion only in radial direction; no sensory loss; often pain and swelling of ventral aspect of proximal forearm	Usually none needed due to spontaneous resolution; surgical decompression occasionally needed; wrist extension splint seldom necessary
Ulnar			
Injury at olecranon groove	Direct elbow trauma or fracture; placing elbow on hard surface for long time; shallow olecranon groove; dislocation of nerve from groove during flexion and extension of elbow	Sensory disturbance in ulnar aspect of hand, little finger, and ulnar aspect of ring finger; weakness in flexor carpi ulnaris and all intrinsic muscles of hand except median-innervated abductor pollicus brevis and opponens pollicus; benediction hand; Tinel's sign at site of injury in elbow; Froment's sign	Ulnar nerve transposition to position on flexor aspect of forearm; ROM of hand joints; lumbrical bar splint to prevent hyperextension of MP joints of little and ring fingers; strength exercises for hand intrinsics; paraffin bath and ROM for contractures
Tardy ulnar nerve palsy	Insidious development follows elbow trauma; disruption of normal carrying angle of elbow or abnormal movement of ulnar nerve olecranon groove	Same as for olecranon nerve injury	Same as for olecranon nerve injury
Injury at wrist	Trauma or fracture at wrist	Similar to ulnar nerve injury at elbow if in proximal wrist prior to take-off of superficial sensory branch, except normal strength in ulnar-innervated muscles of forearm; injury may be in canal of Guyon, or involve only deep palmar branch distally in palm	Same as for other ulnar nerve injuries
Sciatic			
Injection palsy with injury to lateral division	Injection of medication into or around sciatic nerve, especially in infants	Similar to peroneal nerve injury	Discontinue unnecessary intramuscular injections into buttocks

TABLE 18–1. *(continued)*

Nerve	Causes	Signs and symptoms	Treatment
Medial division injury	Hip fracture or hip surgical procedures	Similar to tibial nerve injury	Reduce hip fracture rapidly; combine any of treatments for complete sciatic nerve injury, depending on extent of medial injury
Complete injury	Same as for medial division injury; entrapment by pyriformus muscle	Weakness of hamstrings and all muscles below knee; sensation reduced below knee except for medial leg	Protective orthotics for feet, e.g., extra-depth shoes with Plastiazote inserts; ROM of knee, ankle, and toe joints; ankle-foot brace
Femoral Injury above or below inguinal ligament	Surgery in which lithotomy position is maintained for long time; hip held in marked extension for long time; venous or arterial catheterization	Quadriceps weakness; complete sensory loss in skin of anterior thigh and medial aspect of leg; partial loss of injury is below ligament	Control of traumatic, infectious, carcinomatous, or other activity producing injury; long leg brace to stabilize knee in extension, short double upright leg brace, or cane; surgical decompression of femoral nerve in region of inguinal ligament; surgical muscle transfer or knee fusion if patient cannot stabilize knee in stance phase of gait
Peroneal Cross leg palsy, other injuries to head of fibula	Chronic crossing of legs; chronic lying in bed with hips in external rotation	Numbness of dorsum of foot and anterior lateral leg; paralysis of ankle dorsiflexors and toe extensors	Remove cause of injury; position comatose or debilitated patient in bed; ankle support to keep foot pointing upward as patient lies supine; surgery to remove site of constriction of nerve; muscle transfer; ankle-foot orthosis for foot drop or quarter-inch heel lift on shoe of unaffected side; ROM of ankle and toe joints; stretching of gastronemius and soleus muscles and Achilles tendon
Tibial Tarsal tunnel syndrome	Ankle fracture or dislocation	Inability to plantarflex foot in complete injury; painful walking long after normal healing interval; weak calf limp; cold, swollen, painful foot and ankle if reflex sympathetic dystrophy; may be patchy osteoporosis of leg and foot bones on X-ray film	Surgical decompression of tibial nerve in tarsal tunnel; ROM of ankle and foot; Plastiazote inserts and extra-depth shoes to prevent injury to sole of foot; TENS if causalgic pain

cles becomes evident. The extensor digitorum brevis muscle of the foot is easily recognized as atrophic or even absent in such cases. The loss of the intrinsic muscles of the hand, especially of the interosseus muscles, leaves depressions between the extensor tendons called guttering.

Electrodiagnostic Procedures

Peripheral neuropathy is relatively easy to diagnose by nerve conduction studies. The neuropathy affects nerves in the following order: lower extremity sensory nerves, upper extremity sensory nerves, lower extremity motor nerves, cranial nerves, and upper extremity motor nerves. Two important exceptions to this pattern are that the median distal motor latency is abnormal as early and as frequently as the median sensory latency and that the ulnar distal motor latency is quite resistant to change in diabetic neuropathy. Considerable care must be taken in interpreting nerve conduction data for the distal median and ulnar nerves, especially since carpal tunnel syndrome may be concurrent.

Controlling Glucose Metabolism

It has been argued for decades that careful and rigid control of diabetic patients results in fewer complications, including less frequent and less severe nerve injuries. Unfortunately, producing normal glucose metabolism is not yet technically possible even with the most stringent regulation of diabetic patients. In the future, when implanted computerized devices can release insulin in a manner more analogous to the normal pancreas, diabetic neuropathy may be preventable, or at least treatable.

Controlling Pain in Diabetic Neuritis

Diabetic peripheral neuropathy is generally resistant to ordinary pain medications except in dosages large enough to produce stupor. Alternative medications include diphenylhydantoin or carbamazepine. The concurrent use of a major tranquilizer (fluphenazine) and an antidepressant (amitriptyline) may help relieve the pain of diabetic neuritis. Whether these medications have

a centrally acting antipain effect of an unspecified nature, or whether they merely treat the patient's pain-induced anxiety and depression, is unknown. Supplementary TENS treatment and comfortable shoes for painful feet may also be helpful.

Controlling Weakness

Treatment of weakness in diabetes depends on what nerves are involved. Diabetic mononeuritis is usually treated like any other injury of that specific nerve. For example, diabetic mononeuritis of the radial nerve is treated with a wrist extension splint and the other methods used for a Saturday night palsy (see Table 18–1).

Compensating for Sensory Loss

Most diabetic patients do not need specific treatment for their sensory loss, as it usually is incomplete until very late in the course. However, when decreased protective sensation is compounded by vascular insufficiency, foot injury and subsequent amputation often result. Patients with diabetic peripheral neuropathy typically have dry skin of the feet because of autonomic neuropathy, which may lead to skin cracking, subsequent infection, and, ultimately, to amputation. Instruct the patient in foot care such as cutting the toenails straight, keeping the feet moist with the use of lanolin creams, and avoiding foot and toe trauma. Warn them to avoid tight shoes and to check their feet daily for injury.

Managing Autonomic Nerve Dysfunction

If the patient develops a neurogenic bowel or bladder, train the patient in the techniques used for paraplegics (see Chapters 17 and 25). The bladder in diabetic neuropathy is typically a flaccid or lower motor neuron type (see Chapter 25). The patient generally will have high residual urine and be unable to empty the bladder completely.

Male diabetics frequently have neuropathy-induced impotence, which can be treated with prosthetic implants such as silicone rods or an inflatable balloon device, or nonsurgically with penile splints. Diabetic males often have retrograde ejaculation, which generally is a problem only when fertility is desired. Chapter 26 discusses specialized techniques to help the diabetic male manage sexual dysfunction.

MANAGEMENT OF ALCOHOLIC NEUROPATHY

The second most common cause of peripheral neuropathy is alcoholism. There is considerable controversy as to whether the neuropathy results from an inadequate diet or from the toxic effects of ethanol. Alcoholics often have a diet consisting only of alcohol, which is deficient in most foodstuffs, particularly the B vitamins. The resulting beriberilike syndrome may well account for the peripheral neuropathy. Alcoholism also involves other neurological syndromes that must be differentiated from the peripheral neuropathy, including localized neuropathy as in Saturday night palsy, alcoholic myositis, and midline cerebellar degeneration with ataxia.

The medical treatment of alcoholic neuropathy includes the cessation of the use of alcohol, maintenance of an adequate diet, large doses of B vitamins (especially thiamine), and supportive medical care as needed. The rehabilitation of alcoholic neuropathy is basically the same as that described for diabetic neuropathies. Alcoholic neuropathy is often reversible if medical treatment is begun before such a late stage ensues as to prevent return of nerve function.

SUGGESTED READINGS

Braddom, R. L., Hollis, J. B., and Castell, D. O. (1977): Diabetic peripheral neuropathy: A correlation of nerve conduction studies and clinical findings. *Arch. Phys. Med. Rehabil.*, 58:308–313.

Dawson, D. M., Hallett, M., and Melinder, L. (1983): *Entrapment Neuropathies*. Little Brown, Boston.

Dyck, P. J., Thomas, P. K., and Lambert, E. H. (1984): *Peripheral Neuropathy*, 2nd edit. W. B. Saunders, Philadelphia.

Illis, L. S., and Glanville, H. J., editors (1982): *Rehabilitation of the Neurological Patient*. Blackwell, Oxford.

Johnson, E. W. (1980): *Practical Electromyography*. Williams and Wilkins, Baltimore.

Keenlyside, R. A., Schonberger, L. B., Bregman, D. J., and Bolyai, J. (1980): Fatal Guillain-Barré syndrome after the national influenza immunization program. *Neurology*, 30:929–933.

Mayo Clinic (1981): *Clinical Examinations in Neurology*, 5th edition. W. B. Saunders, Philadelphia.

Olson, W. H., Brumbach, R. A., Gascon, G., and Christoferson, L. A. (1981): *Practical Neurology for the Primary Care Physician*. Charles C Thomas, Springfield, IL.

Schocet, S. S., and McCormick, W. F. (1979): *Neuropathology Case Studies*, 2nd edit. Medical Examination, New York.

Sunderland, S. (1976): Pain mechanisms in causalgia. *J. Neurol. Psychiatry*, 39:471–480.

Medical Rehabilitation,
edited by L. S. Halstead et al.
Raven Press, New York © 1985.

CHAPTER 19

Degenerative Disorders of the Central Nervous System

Michael A. Krebs

Departments of Physical Medicine and Rehabilitation, Baylor College of Medicine, Houston, Texas 77030

With advancing age, humans are subject to degenerative diseases that attack various parts of the central nervous system. While disease onset is typically middle age or later, a few exceptions, notably multiple sclerosis, begin in young adulthood. Common degenerative diseases such as parkinsonism, amyotrophic lateral sclerosis, and multiple sclerosis are chronic, progressive, idiopathic, and incurable. Therapeutic nihilism, however, has no place in the approach to these diseases, since recent advances in medical treatment and surgical techniques can, in some cases, delay progression and relieve symptoms. Nevertheless, these diseases still produce serious neurological disabilities, the nature of which are dependent on the location of the lesion. The main objectives of the rehabilitation techniques used to manage disability are to maintain physical and psychological function and to limit the effects of disuse.

MANAGEMENT OF DISABILITY IN PARKINSONISM

The clinical syndrome of parkinsonism is marked by the classic triad of tremor, rigidity, and bradykinesia (loss of postural reflexes). Parkinsonism results from degenerative lesions in the basal ganglia, with selective depletion of dopamine in these structures.

Ranking third behind stroke and dementia in frequency, parkinsonism is a leading cause of neurological disability in persons over 60 years of age. Its estimated prevalence is 100 to 150 per 100,000. Although the onset of parkinsonism is insidious, early diagnosis is crucial because prompt treatment can retard loss of function due to rigidity, autonomic dysfunction, gait and postural disturbance, and reactive psychopathology. Life expectancy is normal despite the progressive nature of this condition. Therefore, rehabilitation must aim to preserve maximum function for as long as possible by preventing disability due to inactivity. The comprehensive management of parkinsonism includes not only careful monitoring of medication use but also regulation of activity level, nutritional status, and mental status.

Monitoring Medication Use

The advent of levodopa and its synergist carbidopa has helped individuals with parkinsonism lead more satisfying lives without significant disability. The usual regimen is 600 to 1,200 mg of levodopa with 60 to 120 mg of carbidopa daily. Because levodopa seems to lose its effectiveness with time and adverse effects, especially dyskinesia, become progressively worse, the older anticholinergic drugs or amantadine should be used early in the course of the disease. Levodopa and carbidopa should be administered when disability, particularly that due to rigidity, becomes severe. In levodopa-resistant cases, bromocriptine, 2.5 to 7.5 mg daily, can enhance the therapeutic effect, but may induce psychotic symptoms.

Controlling Autonomic Dysfunction

Complications of parkinsonism resulting from autonomic dysfunction include drooling, difficulty swallowing, excessive perspiration, seborrhea, flushing of the skin, postural hypotension, and constipation. Drooling may result from excessive salivation, poor muscular control of the mouth, or impaired swallowing reflexes. The treatment of choice is anticholinergic drugs such as propantheline, which may be supplemented when necessary by such surgical methods as myotomy, transtympanic neurectomy, parotid duct ligation, enterostoma, or cervical esophagostomy. Facial exercises in front of a mirror and conscious head positioning with the neck extended can improve muscular control and allow drainage of saliva into the pharynx.

Hyperhidrosis may respond to anticholinergics, and careful attention to skin hygiene will help prevent dermatoses. Head-up body tilt at night often improves postural hypotension by reducing renal arterial pressure, promoting renin release, and increasing blood volume. Constipation should be managed by regular exercise, adequate fluid intake, good nutrition, stool softeners, laxatives, and enemas as needed.

Therapeutic Exercises for Rigidity

The major disability of parkinsonism is rigidity, with associated immobility. Regular and frequent exercise is an effective adjunct to pharmacological treatment of rigidity, since movement becomes easier as activity level increases. Although frequent rest periods should be allowed for predictable fatigue, prolonged rest periods can worsen rigidity. Exercise should be gradually increased in intensity and duration. Active and active-assistive exercises can offset the development of disuse atrophy and contracture. An overhead pulley can be rigged at home for active range of motion exercise of the shoulder girdle (Fig. 19–1). Extension exercises in the prone position can also be done at home to stretch hip flexors and extend the spine. Preceding exercise sessions with hydrotherapy and heat (see Chapter 4) helps prevent contractures.

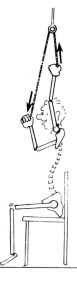

FIG. 19–1. Pulley exercise to maintain shoulder range of motion. [From Cailliet, R. (1968): Rehabilitation in parkinsonism. In: *Rehabilitation and Medicine*, edited by S. Licht. Elizabeth Licht, New Haven.]

In addition to mobility, therapeutic exercise should emphasize the retraining of neuromuscular coordination. Loss of strength usually is not a major problem. Therefore, emphasis should be placed on improving speed, mobility, and well-coordinated motion of the head, trunk, and limbs. Performance of exercises for coordination is improved by gradually increasing the force, speed, and complexity of movements within the patient's capacity to maintain precision. Activities are broken down into movements that are simple enough for the patient to perform them correctly. These movements, or motor patterns, must be repeated frequently to increase the consistency of correct performance and to eliminate errors.

During neuromuscular coordination training, the amount of effort required to execute the movements should be kept low by decreasing both speed and resistance against which the patient must perform. Excessive effort may activate motor neurons that are outside the desired motor pattern, thus producing and reinforcing awkward, uncoordinated movements. To discourage the patient from learning extraneous movements, assistance from the therapist is necessary when the exercise sessions begin and resistance against movement is increased only as the ability develops to contract desired muscles without activating other muscles.

TABLE 19–1. *Frenkel's exercises for coordination retraining*

Supine

Flex one extremity at the hip and knee with the heel held 2 inches above the bed. Bring the heel to rest on the opposite patella.
Successively add patterns so that the heel is touched to the middle of the shin, to the ankle, to the toes of the opposite foot, to the bed on either side of the knee, and to the bed on either side of the leg.
Follow with the toe the movement of the therapist's finger in any combination of lower extremity motions.

Sitting

Mark two cross marks on the floor with chalk. Alternately glide the foot over the marked cross forward, backward, left, and right.

Standing

Practice walking sideways.
Walk forward, placing each foot on a footprint traced on the floor. Footprints should be parallel and 2 inches lateral to the midline. Practice with quarter steps, half steps, three-quarter steps, and full steps.

From Granger, G.B. (1982): *Physical Therapeutic Technique*, J.B. Lippincott, Philadelphia.

Steps should be taken to minimize insecurity and fear, excitement and strong emotions, pain, fatigue, and prolonged periods of inactivity, all factors that promote incoordination. Massage and heat for relaxation and pain relief, supplemented by short rest periods after each two or three repetitions to prevent cumulative fatigue, will help discourage incoordination. Frenkel's exercises are particularly helpful for coordination retraining to offset the cerebellar dysfunction of parkinsonism. A few of these exercises are described in Table 19–1.

Exercise for Gait and Postural Disturbances

The exercise program should include gait retraining exercises. High stepping should be practiced to avoid the shuffling gait. Low hurdles, such as books, may be used to reinforce hip and knee flexion (Fig. 19–2A). A gait using a wider base, with the feet placed 10 to 12 inches apart, will help prevent falling (Fig. 19–2B).

Conscious and active performance of arm swinging will improve balance and loosen the arms and shoulders. Stride lengthening, stopping, starting, and turning must also be practiced.

The stooped posture prevalent in parkinsonism (Fig. 19–3) can be postponed through the regular performance of postural exercises to stretch tight muscles. Scapular adduction exercises are easily performed at home to improve posture and stretch tight pectoral muscles (Fig. 19–4A). Also useful for treating the flexed posture at home is passive hyperextension of the knee joint while sitting with the foot supported (Fig. 19–4B).

Mental Sequelae of Parkinsonism

Although mental deterioration may be related somewhat to basal ganglia dysfunction in parkinsonism, it is generally not directly the result of parkinsonian lesions. Most parkinsonian patients develop either depression or dementia. Personality changes, as well as depression and confusion, may accompany parkinsonism either in reaction to disability or as a result of associated organic disease such as arteriosclerotic infarcts or Alzheimer's disease. In addition, medications used to treat parkinsonism may induce lethargy, confusion, depression, delusions, obsessional behavior, or global dementia.

Mild drug reactions may be alleviated merely by withdrawing amantadine or anticholinergics. If the disturbance is severe, however, and threatens family life or work, all drugs, including levodopa, should be withdrawn temporarily under hospital supervision. If drug withdrawal results in a patient who is rational but immobile, a reasonable compromise is to add a small dose of a neuroleptic such as a thioridazine to the levodopa regimen. Daytime sleepiness that disrupts activity can be alleviated by reducing the levodopa dosage or by occasional "weekend drug holidays."

Although levodopa may provoke depression in patients with a prior psychiatric history, it may alleviate reactive depression in patients who are obtaining relief from the disabling neuro-

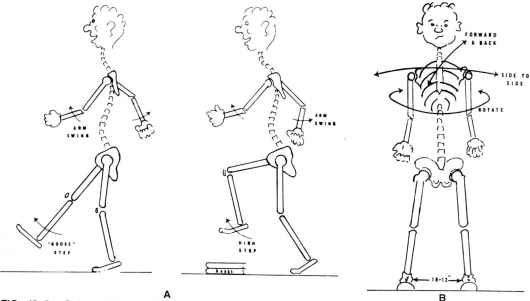

FIG. 19–2. Gait retraining exercises for parkinsonism. **A:** Practice walking over books to discourage "goose step" and increase height of step. **B:** To improve balance, practice trunk movements with a wide base of support. [From Cailliet, R. (1968): Rehabilitation in parkinsonism. In: *Rehabilitation and Medicine*, edited by S. Licht. Elizabeth Licht, New Haven.]

logical symptoms. Tricyclic antidepressants, particularly imipramine and desipramine, may reduce depression and fatigue in parkinsonian patients, as well as improve rigidity and akinesia. As an additional advantage, these drugs can be administered simultaneously with levodopa without producing untoward effects.

In addition to careful drug regulation to control mental sequelae, parkinsonian patients need constant encouragement to continue participation in family, vocational, and social affairs to help them avoid depression and undue dependency. Coping with the unpredictable fluctuations of disability resulting from drug therapy and from the disease process can be frustrating. A patient who is responding well to medication, for example, may suddenly become immobile. Such fluctuations frequently make employment or independent travel outside the home unfeasible. For some patients, exercise classes or parkinsonism groups are effective ways of providing motivation and support. The patient's and family's active cooperation should be obtained by

defining realistic goals and explaining treatment methods and rationale.

Correcting Dysarthria

The speech of parkinsonian patients is typically reduced in intensity, higher and unvarying in pitch, and abnormal in rate. Since these prosodic features of speech typically convey subtle changes of meaning and emotion, defects often produce misunderstandings in interpersonal relationships. Family members may perceive the patient as cold and unfeeling, no longer caring for them. The first impression at social gatherings or work settings may be that the patient is demented, depressed, or apathetic. Embarrassment may lead to social withdrawal or refusal to use the telephone. Under the instruction of a speech-language pathologist, the patient can practice several techniques to monitor the prosodic features of his or her own speech at home. Levodopa therapy also helps reduce speech impairment.

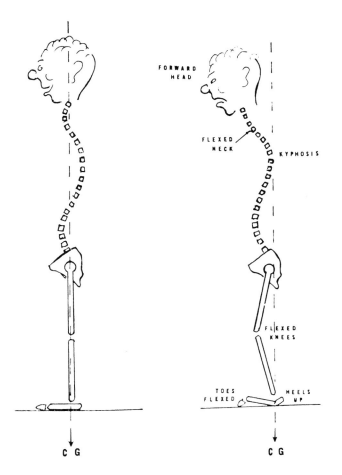

FORWARD HEAD

FLEXED NECK

KYPHOSIS

FLEXED KNEES

TOES FLEXED

HEELS UP

C G

C G

FIG. 19–3. Comparison of normal and parkinsonian postures. **Left:** Normal posture. **Right:** Flexed posture of advanced parkinsonism. CG, Center of gravity, plumb line. [From Cailliet, R. (1968): Rehabilitation in parkinsonism. In: *Rehabilitation and Medicine*, edited by S. Licht. Elizabeth Licht, New Haven.]

SPEECH IMPAIRMENT IN PARKINSON'S DISEASE

Report of a Case

HISTORY. This widowed, 59-year-old man presented to his physician with resting tremor in his hands, mental depression, and insomnia. Because he had a previous history of depression—a major depressive episode occurring after his wife died of cancer 9 years previously—a recurrence of depression was diagnosed and he was put on imipramine, 75 mg/day, taken at bedtime. A follow-up visit 3 months later revealed that his mood had improved, but he was beginning to experience difficulty speaking clearly, as well as tremor. Neurological examination revealed rigidity, mild bradykinesia, and resting tremors at a rate of about 5/sec. He was diagnosed as having Parkinson's disease and he began taking levodopa, 250 mg twice daily with meals, gradually increased to a maintenance dosage of 800 mg daily, with 80 mg carbidopa.

REHABILITATION MANAGEMENT OF SPEECH PROSODY. Although the patient's speech improved on the levodopa regimen, continuing problems with communication were jeopardizing his work as an account executive in computer equipment sales. Embarrassed to contact clients by telephone or meet them face to face due to his high-pitched, soft, monotonous voice, he was relying more and more on his assistant to deal directly with clients. As a result, he lost several important accounts and his supervisor warned him about his declining performance. His secretary frequently complained that she could not decipher his dictation or his handwriting. Consequently, his physician referred him to a speech pathologist, who saw him once a week and encouraged practice sessions at home.

To enable feedback during home practice, the patient purchased a tape recorder and a Vocalite, a voice-operated light source that provides visual re-

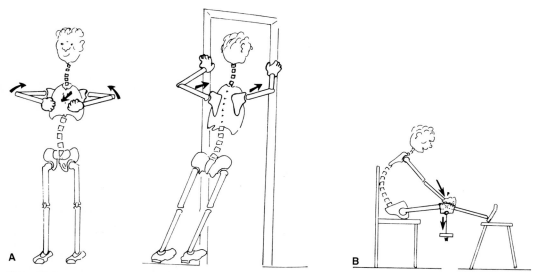

FIG. 19–4. Postural exercises. **A:** For tight pectoral muscles. **B:** Extension, to prevent contracture of knee joint. [From Cailliet, R. (1968): Rehabilitation in parkinsonism. In: *Rehabilitation and Medicine*, edited by S. Licht. Elizabeth Licht, New Haven.]

inforcement of speech patterns. With the help of the Vocalite, his vocal pitch and stress on syllables and words began improving noticeably after only 2 weeks of practice. He also practiced deliberately exaggerating syllables as he read in front of a mirror, recited in time to a slow, fixed beat recorded on tape, and played back these practice sessions on his tape player. An amplifier attached to his telephone improved his confidence in placing calls. In addition, the speech therapist referred him to a parkinsonian group in which they critiqued one another's performance as they practiced dialogues and short skits.

The speech instruction continued for 6 months. During this time, his physician contacted his employers about the illness. Although they had noticed marked improvement in his communication ability, they decided that he was still not quick enough to meet the demands of his position. Based on his premorbid exemplary performance and 30 years of service, however, they offered him an early retirement with full benefits in addition to paying him consultant fees on commission.

The patient was able to continue living alone. He had become socially reclusive after the death of his wife, throwing most of his energy into his work, but with his new free time, joined a church-associated singles group at the urging of his family physician. With the group, he was able to do some traveling and became more involved in a hobby, photography.

Accurate diagnosis of Parkinson's disease is often delayed by the similarity of early symp-

toms to other neurological disorders or to psychiatric problems. Diagnosis is therefore partially by exclusion. In this case, the patient's presenting symptoms initially suggested a reactivation of the endogenous depression. The previous history of depression in the absence of definite physical findings seemed to substantiate this diagnosis. However, depression often precedes, or coexists with, Parkinson's disease, which becomes evident with the onset of the more characteristic symptoms such as rigidity. Fortunately, as in this case, parkinsonism and depression can be treated simultaneously without drug interaction between the tricyclic antidepressant and levodopa. In fact, the anticholinergic properties of the antidepressant may help secondarily to alleviate the parkinsonian symptoms.

The levodopa, supplemented by speech therapy, also markedly improved this patient's communication ability. The common belief in the past was that parkinsonian speech impairment was resistant to treatment. Consequently, referral for speech therapy was rare. Recent studies indicate that new techniques of prosody management, such as the use of the Vocalite, have been successful when instituted early, with improvement documented to last for at least 6 months.

Despite this patient's improvement, the need for aggressive communication in his occupation forced him to modify his duties somewhat by becoming a consultant less involved in sales. Since Parkinson's disease typically strikes between the ages of 50 and 70, its victims are often retired or close enough to retirement to negotiate adequate severance terms with the employer. The handling of this case demonstrates how, through careful regulation of drug dosage, recognition of complicating emotional and vocational problems, and referral to appropriate rehabilitation specialists such as the speech pathologist, the primary care physician can play a crucial role in the maintenance of the parkinsonian patient's independence in the community.

MANAGEMENT OF DISABILITY IN AMYOTROPHIC LATERAL SCLEROSIS

Amyotrophic lateral sclerosis is a relentlessly progressive degeneration of motor units and pyramidal tracts. Its etiology is unknown and it is usually fatal within 3 to 5 years. The worldwide incidence is 1 per 100,000 and the prevalence rate is 2.5 to 7 per 100,000. Males are affected twice as often as females, usually in late middle age. In the presence of normal sensation, the clinical or electromyographic findings of denervation and fasciculation in both the upper and lower extremity muscles are fairly conclusive in making a diagnosis.

Prognosis and Preserving Function

Patients with bulbar symptoms at the onset of disease have the worst prognosis. However, there are relatively benign forms of degenerative motor neuron disease that may resemble amyotrophic lateral sclerosis at the onset. In these cases, rehabilitation potential is better because of the slower progression of the disease and the decreased severity of disability. In amyotrophic lateral sclerosis, treatment must anticipate inevitable progression of the disease and eventual loss of function. However, an attitude of pessimism and despair should not be conveyed to the patient. The physician should take both a practical and a supportive approach in trying to prevent complications and improve the quality of life. Prolongation of ambulation in the early stages of the disease is a reasonable goal, whereas in the later stages, prevention of deformity to facilitate nursing care takes precedence.

Alleviating Weakness and Cramps

Skeletal muscle weakness and atrophy are prominent and occur early. The location and progression of weakness dictate what therapy is appropriate. If electromyographic findings indicate a coexistent myasthenic state, administration of neostigmine or pyridostigmine can relieve weakness, at least temporarily. However, the doses must be carefully titrated. In such cases, guanidine hydrochloride, 25 mg/kg/day, may even modify the course of the disease. Calcium disodium edetate given intravenously may benefit patients with motor neuron disease associated with lead toxicity.

When the neck muscles become too weak to support the head, a soft, semirigid Philadelphia cervical collar should be prescribed. When more head support is needed, a rigid, custom-fitted, molded plastic orthosis can be constructed (Fig. 19–5). For shoulder girdle weakness, a sling or a balanced forearm orthosis can be prescribed to offset shoulder subluxation or improve upper extremity function. Weakness of the wrist extensors interfering with grip can be managed with a simple static wrist-hand orthosis that improves manual holding ability.

Footdrop caused by ankle dorsiflexor weakness is common. For patients with a relatively benign course, lightweight, plastic insert ankle-foot orthoses provide stability, improve gait pattern, and may prolong ambulation (Fig. 19–6). As paresis advances, canes, crutches, and walkers may improve balance and decrease falls. However, the patient should be taught to fall safely, since falls will inevitably occur. Eventually, a wheelchair and other special equipment will be needed. Help in the selection of hospital beds, adaptive devices, built-up toilet seats, and

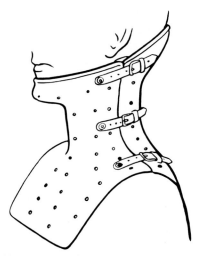

FIG. 19–5. Rigid plastic orthosis for head support. [From *Spinal Orthotics*, 1975. New York University Post-Graduate Medical School, New York.]

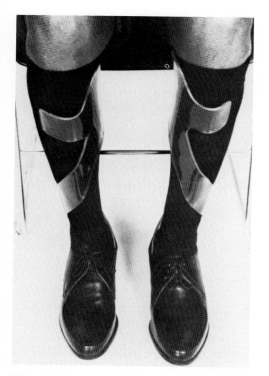

FIG. 19–6. Thermoplastic spiral ankle-foot orthosis for control of foot drop and medio-lateral ankle instability. [From Rusk, H. A. 1977. *Rehabilitation Medicine*, 4th edit., C. V. Mosby Co., St. Louis.]

other equipment, as well as financial support, should be sought from a local ALS Foundation chapter (see Appendix).

Therapeutic exercise seems to benefit most patients by forestalling disuse atrophy and joint contractures. Sustained periods of exercise, however, are contraindicated; instead, regular intervals of active exercise should alternate with passive range of motion exercises. Excessive exercise of involved muscles may increase weakness. Exhaustion can worsen amyotrophic lateral sclerosis and lead to painful cramps, which can be treated with massage or heat. Phenytoin, 100 to 400 mg/day, and quinine, 200 to 300 mg/day, are useful in relieving cramps.

Correcting Speech Problems

In patients with involvement of the bulbar nuclei, a dysarthria marked by hypernasality and progressive disintegration of articulation can result. Speech therapy for energy conservation techniques in speaking is indicated. For example, the patient is encouraged to express short ideas that can be articulated in a brief time period. In patients with diminished gag reflexes and nasal air loss but otherwise adequate articulation, a palatal lift may be tried.

If speech is no longer intelligible, the patient should be taught to employ his remaining motor functions to express himself, since communication may be the only means of influencing the environment. When writing or gesturing is impossible, alphabet word boards can be used. Severe communication problems may warrant the purchase of electronic communication systems activated by slight movements or vocalization to produce a prerecorded vocabulary or visual message. If the patient and the family have developed their own communication system, as often happens, it should be accepted and encouraged rather than replaced with another.

Overcoming Difficulty Swallowing

Oropharyngeal dysphagia, one of the most troublesome symptoms of bulbar involvement in amyotrophic lateral sclerosis, can make eating the most difficult activity of daily living to perform independently. Aspiration is a constant hazard. Typically, choking on saliva progresses to difficulty swallowing liquids and, eventually, to difficulty swallowing solid foods. Patients with bulbar symptoms should sit upright with the neck in flexion whenever they attempt to swallow food and liquids.

Choice of diet is important. Foods that form a bolus are best, while pureed foods should be avoided because they tend to fall apart. Soft foods such as casseroles and custard can be swallowed as a single bolus. Viscid mucus produced by the accumulation of saliva interacting with foods such as milk products and chocolate further impairs swallowing. These secretions can be liquified by taking papase sublingually before eating or by coating the tongue with meat tenderizer derived from papaya.

Because choking is sometimes unavoidable, the family should be taught emergency measures such as the Heimlich maneuver and the use of an aspirator to remove secretions. When swallowing becomes unsafe and the gag reflex is diminished, an orogastric tube can be used intermittently. Surgical creation of a stoma may eventually become necessary to ensure adequate nutrition. If so, cervical esophagostomy is preferred over gastrotomy or jejunostomy because it allows intermittent passage of a feeding tube while the patient is sitting. A tracheostomy with laryngeal closure or tracheal diversion may be carried out to prolong life when aspiration of secretions or vomit still remains a problem after stoma creation.

Relieving Impaired Breathing

In the final stages of amyotrophic lateral sclerosis, respiratory insufficiency inevitably occurs. Deep breathing and coughing exercises are prescribed to enhance gas exchange and to remove secretions. In more advanced cases, intermittent positive pressure breathing treatment and assisted cough techniques will be needed (see Chapter 13).

Annual influenza and pneumococcal vaccines are recommended to help prevent infection that will further compromise respiratory function. Eventually, life-threatening infection will occur, requiring vigorous antibiotic therapy and mechanical ventilation to maintain respiration. A discussion of these measures with the patient and the family before they become necessary is important to allow expression of personal desires concerning the quality of remaining life and the means of prolonging it.

Psychosocial Adjustment to Terminal Illness

Considering that amyotrophic lateral sclerosis is inevitably terminal, how soon should the patient be informed of the poor prognosis? Whether to tell the patient as soon as the diagnosis is established or to wait until the last possible moment must be determined on an individual basis for each patient. Give an anxious, questioning patient honest information, yet do not deprive a patient of hope who grasps for something to hang onto. The diffident or sanguine patient should not be pressed to comprehend the diagnosis. The physician should be responsive to patient cues, both obvious and subtle, that indicate either a desire for or aversion to more information. The family or those close to the patient must always be told of the prognosis and counseled concerning future plans. Eventually, personal care will have to be provided on a 24-hr basis.

Since intellectual function is rarely impaired, and most patients are painfully aware of their downhill course, reactive depression is common. Tricyclic antidepressants and tranquilizers are not helpful as a rule. Depression is best treated by supportive counseling and by allowing the patient to express his feelings on disability and death. Most importantly, the patient's sense of personal integrity should be reinforced and his participation in decisions regarding the management of his disease should be encouraged.

As the disease progresses inexorably, the patient must never be allowed to feel abandoned by the physician. In the end, an understanding and available primary care physician can help the patient and his family achieve acceptable management of the disease at home, even into the terminal phase.

MANAGEMENT OF DISABILITY IN MULTIPLE SCLEROSIS

Multiple sclerosis, a disease of unknown etiology, is characterized by the diffuse occurrence of circumscribed areas of demyelination in the white matter of the central nervous system, followed by gliosis and sclerotic plaque formation. Two-thirds of all cases occur in young adults between the ages of 20 and 40. The prevalence of this disease in the United States varies from 10 per 100,000 in the southern states to 60 per 100,000 in the north.

Diagnosis can be difficult, especially in the early stages. Because multiple sclerosis is diagnosed by exclusion and the prognostic implications are so important to the patient, this diagnosis should only be considered following a thorough work-up by a competent neurologist who is experienced in demyelinating diseases. Prognosis is complicated by the lack of knowledge about the specific etiology of the disease as well as pathogenic factors involved in its progression and remission. Because many patients are active and even employed a decade or more after diagnosis, a cautious but hopeful attitude should be taken in the long-term treatment of the patient.

Preventing Exacerbations of Neurological Symptoms

The lifestyle of the patient with multiple sclerosis may require adaptations to avoid physical or mental stresses that may worsen disability. The patient should be advised of these fundamental precautions:

1. Sleep regularly and avoid naps.
2. Maintain a nutritionally sound diet.
3. Avoid contact with people who have a cold or flu.
4. Take immunizations only when absolutely necessary.
5. Remain active in an enjoyable occupation.
6. Maintain a structured exercise program, including aerobics.

Both fatigue and heat exposure should be minimized, yet activity level must be sufficient to prevent the complications of immobility. Therefore, the prescription of exercise must specify intensity, duration, and frequency. Cold therapy that lowers body temperature 0.2°F to 1.3°F may temporarily improve function when applied prior to therapeutic exercises.

Heat Control

Even mild exertion may overheat the patient enough to worsen neurological symptoms or produce transient total disability. Lower the patient's body temperature by dipping terry cloth towels in water with ice shavings, then covering the body with the cold towels for at least a half hour, increasing the time interval with increasing body fat. Lukewarm or cold showers may also be helpful. Air conditioning in the patient's home is mandatory during the summer or whenever the climate is hot. The bedroom in particular should be kept cool. Confine vigorous activities to the cooler part of the day and avoid overdressing, as well as prolonged exposure to the sun.

Exercise

A program of hydrotherapy exercises performed at least once a day is ideal for preserving function while avoiding temperature increase that may aggravate weakness and other symptoms. Water also works the muscles harder and tones them more efficiently. Water exercise done with stretching movements increases flexibility and improves posture, while the resistance provided by water builds muscle tone and coordination. In addition, sense of balance, which is often compromised by multiple sclerosis, improves markedly in water. As exercise tolerance improves, an aerobics program on land should be added. Overheating while riding a stationary bicycle is avoided by using an electric fan. Walking may progress to jogging in an air-conditioned gym.

Controlling Spasticity

When spasticity is a significant manifestation of the disease, the goal of treatment is the maintenance of range of motion and strength of non-spastic agonist muscle groups. Active and passive exercise should be performed in conjunction with the aerobics program and according to functional capacity. Ice or cold packs should be applied locally before passive stretching to reduce spasticity (see Chapter 16).

Resting splints are used to maintain a neutral position and to prevent flexion contractures. In already existent flexion contracture, serial casting will stretch the spastic tendons progressively. Ultrasound applied to contracted periarticular tissues, at a dosage of 1.5 to 2.5 watts/cm^2 for 5 to 10 min twice daily, will enhance stretching.

Knee flexion contractures, the most disabling, are best prevented by regular walking or active standing, with assistance if necessary. Besides preventing contractures, ambulation maintains muscle tone and should be encouraged within the reasonable limits of fatigue and usefulness. Lower extremity spasticity and weakness interfering with gait in the ambulatory patient can be managed by a plastic ankle-foot orthosis (Fig. 19–6). Overwhelming gastrocnemius spasticity may require lengthening the Achilles tendon, arthrodesis of the subtalar joints, or surgical or chemical neurectomy.

Antispasticity drugs may help some patients. While effective at 10 to 40 mg/day, diazepam has the major drawback of sedation in therapeutic doses. Dantrolene, 100 to 800 mg/day, which acts directly on skeletal muscle, is useful but can increase weakness and potentially produce serious hepatotoxicity. Baclofen, 40 to 80 mg/day, is probably the safest and most effective drug that alleviates the symptoms of spasticity in patients with multiple sclerosis. Motor point blocks with alcohol or phenol may be necessary in recalcitrant cases.

Management of pressure sores and the neurogenic bladder and bowel are discussed, respectively, in Chapters 23 and 25.

Overcoming Motor Weakness

Muscle paresis is a major cause of disability in patients with multiple sclerosis. Weakness of the lower extremities is usually more pronounced than that of the upper extremities. Intensive efforts to increase strength during the acute phase of the disease are unrewarding. Strengthening exercises apparently cannot reverse the weakness resulting from the lesions of multiple sclerosis. However, strengthening exercises that are below the level of injurious exhaustion should be prescribed when associated disuse weakness is present.

Sensorimotor neurological function may improve following repeated electrical stimulation of the dorsal columns, although the method by which it increases voluntary motor power is unknown. Both spinal implants and transcutaneous stimulators have been used with success. The latter are safe and easy to use, and miniature units are available for continuous stimulation at home.

Compensating for Ataxia and Sensory Impairment

Cerebellar incoordination is highly resistant to therapy. Therapeutic exercise cannot reduce ataxia or tremor. The use of specially weighted devices in canes, walkers, bracelets, or eating utensils may permit functional activity in the presence of moderate ataxia. Gait retraining with a wider base of support, or a raised wheelchair seat, are also helpful. Ablative neurosurgery reduces severe tremor fairly successfully, but should be used only as a last resort.

Loss of position sense requires learning ways to compensate visually in order to control movements. Frenkel's exercise program (Table 19–1) for instability resulting from locomotor ataxia is worth trying in mild-to-moderate cases. The patient must also be taught to take precautions to avoid trauma to insensible limbs.

Unfortunately, there is no effective treatment for scotoma. Diplopia, however, can be managed by covering one of the patient's eyes with a patch or a frosted lens. Using the direction of gaze that gives the least difficulty helps compensate for visual disturbances. In cases of corneal insensibility, tarsorrhaphy may be required.

Correcting Dysarthria

Since the cranial nerves affecting the speech mechanism are often involved in multiple sclerosis, speech may become slurred and low in volume. Cerebellar disturbances can cause a dysmetric, scanning speech, and an inability to talk rapidly. Progressive resistive exercises of the muscles of phonation, as well as instruction by a speech therapist in articulation and breathing, may be beneficial.

Adjusting to Sexual Dysfunction

Sexual inadequacy is a very common, but often overlooked, complication of multiple sclerosis. In various surveys, nearly 50% to more than 90% of patients report either unsatisfactory or absent sexual activity. Men may be unable to achieve or sustain an erection or to ejaculate. Women complain of inability to attain orgasm, loss of libido, and spasticity interfering with sexual activity. Treatment that ameliorates neurological disturbances may improve sexual performance. The most useful intervention, however, is to initiate a candid discussion about sexuality between the patient and his or her sexual partner. Additional strategies and compensatory techniques of sexual intimacy are discussed in Chapter 26.

Psychosocial Adjustment

Premorbid personality, social environment, and organic changes in the brain resulting from disease activity may interact to produce emotional problems. Usually, these problems represent normal emotional reactions to the illness, and thinking processes remain intact. The patient typically progresses through several stages of adaptation:

1. **Denial**—Attempts to conceal symptoms and to seek a physician who will refute the diagnosis.
2. **Resistance**—Constant fight against the disease and unwillingness to accept help.
3. **Affirmation**—Process of learning to face the diagnosis and accept help.

4. **Integration**—Disease is fully accepted and no longer in the mainstream of thought, along with new identify and new lifestyle adjustments.

Frequent communication with the patient will facilitate the adaptation process. Reporting problems by telephone and having an annual neurological evaluation should be encouraged. The National Multiple Sclerosis Society sponsors supportive group therapy sessions in which patients with similar disabilities and family members discuss mutual problems. If one is available in your community, encourage your patient to try a session.

Most patients with multiple sclerosis exhibit concealed depression, which tends to increase as denial decreases. Therapy should emphasize verbalizing interpersonal relationships, while drug treatment is rarely indicated. Adaptation by the patient and family may be especially difficult because multiple sclerosis often strikes in the prime of life, when raising a family and establishing career goals are paramount. Self-image is compromised by the potential loss of somatic or intellectual function, and employment may be lost despite self-sufficiency if the employer is not understanding.

About 20% of patients with multiple sclerosis will need vocational counseling to retrain for another occupation. The selection of long- or short-term training should depend on whether disease progression is slow or rapid. In general, the ideal occupation is indoors, sedentary, and physically nondemanding, and requires minimal hand dexterity. Emotionally stressful occupations should be avoided, and the schedule should be flexible enough to enable scheduling of the most demanding activities early in the day.

SUGGESTED READINGS

Bauer, H. J. (1978): *A Manual on Multiple Sclerosis.* International Federation of Multiple Sclerosis Societies, Vienna, Austria.

Cailliet, R. (1965): Exercise in multiple sclerosis. In: *Therapeutic Exercise*, edited by S. Licht. Elizabeth Licht, New Haven.

Cailliet, R. (1968): Rehabilitation in parkinsonism. In: *Rehabilitation and Medicine*, edited by S. Licht. Elizabeth Licht, New Haven.

Gersten, J. W. (1982): Rehabilitation for degenerative diseases of the central nervous system. In: *Krusen's Handbook of Physical Medicine and Rehabilitation*, edited by F. J. Kottke, G. K. Stillwell, and J. F. Lehmann. W. B. Saunders, Philadelphia.

Hallpike, J. F., Adams, C. W. M., and Tourtellotte, W. W. (1983): *Multiple Sclerosis: Pathology, Diagnosis, and Management*. Williams and Wilkins, Baltimore.

Maloney, F. P., Burks, J. S., and Ringel, S. P. (1984): *Interdisciplinary Rehabilitation of Multiple Sclerosis and Neuromuscular Disorders*. J.B. Lippincott, Philadelphia.

Marsden, C. D., and Fahn, S. (1981): *Movement Disorders*. Butterworth Scientific, Boston.

Mulder, R. W. (1980): *Diagnosis and Treatment of Amyotrophic Lateral Sclerosis*. Houghton Mifflin, Boston.

Nimmer, W., and Kaplan, P. E. (1982): Progressive diseases of the central nervous system. In: *The Practice of Rehabilitation Medicine*, edited by P. E. Kaplan and R. S. Materson. Charles C Thomas, Springfield, IL.

Schneitzer, L. (1978): Rehabilitation of patients with multiple sclerosis. *Arch. Phys. Med. Rehabil.*, 59:430–437.

Sinaki, M., and Mulder, D. W. (1978): Rehabilitation techniques for patients with amyotrophic lateral sclerosis. *Mayo Clin. Proc.*, 53:173–178.

Wroe, M., and Greer, M. (1973): Parkinson's disease and physical therapy management. *Phys. Ther.*, 53:849–855.

Medical Rehabilitation,
edited by L. S. Halstead et al.
Raven Press, New York © 1985.

CHAPTER 20

Pediatric Rehabilitation

*Barry L. Bowser and **Itzel S. Solis

*Departments of Physical Medicine, Rehabilitation, and Pediatrics, Baylor College of Medicine, and The Institute for Rehabilitation and Research; and **Departments of Physical Medicine and Rehabilitation, Baylor College of Medicine, and Texas Children's Hospital, Houston, Texas 77030

Some of the more frequently encountered handicapping conditions of childhood are cerebral palsy, muscular dystrophy, spina bifida, developmental delays, and hypotonia. Diagnostic criteria, management principles, and frequently encountered complications are considered for the various disabilities associated with these medical conditions. The roles of the primary physicians, medical specialists, allied health personnel, educators, and parents are defined in relation to the diagnosis, as are the changing needs of the affected children at different ages and stages of development.

BASIC PRINCIPLES

Medical practitioners who encounter children with potentially handicapping conditions should keep in mind the following aspects of rehabilitation that are unique to treating children:

1. Do not treat children as though they are little adults; it is the job of parents and society to help children, including those with handicaps, to become mature adults capable of independent living. This responsibility should be shared by the health professionals concerned with their care.
2. Because children are largely products of their environment, educate parents about what would constitute a therapeutic environment for their children.
3. Rehabilitation of children, in contrast to that of adults, often does not mean relearning lost skills, but rather, learning appropriate

motor skills for age or developmental level under adverse conditions.
4. Knowledge of normal motor learning, growth, and development is essential for therapeutic intervention in the growing child. Understanding the emotional needs of the child at various ages is equally important.
5. Treatment must take into consideration decelerated bone growth in weakened extremities compared to the strong stimulus to bone growth in extremities with normal muscle activity. Asymmetrical muscle involvement may produce significant leg and arm length discrepancies. Carefully time surgical procedures to lengthen shortened extremities or slow the growth rate of normal extremities by monitoring the child's bone age through roentgenographic studies.

CEREBRAL PALSY

Cerebral palsy applies to symptoms resulting from nonprogressive brain damage that occurs any time before the brain has reached maturation, from conception to age 5 or 6 years. It has an incidence of approximately 5.5 per 1,000 live births and is distributed equally between the sexes, among the races, and across national boundaries.

To be classified as cerebral palsy, the brain damage must result in loss or impairment of control over voluntary muscles. The symptoms of cerebral palsy vary greatly, ranging from extremely mild and barely detectable to almost total lack of voluntary motor functions and profound retardation. Therefore, specification of the type and distribution of motor disturbance, the degree of involvement (mild, moderate, or severe), and the etiology, if known, is important before planning rehabilitation management. Table 20–1 describes the motor disturbances most commonly associated with cerebral palsy.

Etiology

The etiologies of cerebral palsy encompass all the causes of brain damage in the fetus, newborn, and young child. They can be divided into congenital (prenatal and perinatal factors) and acquired (postnatal factors). The most common prenatal causes are anoxia (maternal shock or anemia, placental disturbances, Rh incompatibility), maternal infections (rubella, toxoplasmosis, cytomegalovirus, herpesvirus, syphilis), trauma, metabolic factors, and congenital malformations of the brain. The perinatal causes include anoxia (respiratory obstruction, atelectasis, premature separation of the placenta, oversedation, breech delivery) and trauma (cephalopelvic disproportion, cesarean section,

prematurity). Postnatally, cerebral palsy may be caused by trauma (skull fracture, brain contusion), infections (meningitis, encephalitis), cerebrovascular accidents, anoxia (shock, poisoning, near drowning), or brain tumors. In many cases, more than one etiological factor is present.

Diagnosis

Diagnosing cerebral palsy may be extremely difficult in early infancy. Spasticity may not become manifest until 6 to 9 months of age, and athetoid movements may not occur until the second year of life. Comprehensive evaluation of the cerebral palsy patient is multidisciplinary. It requires an assessment of physical growth, developmental level of the child, and motor and neurological skills, a psychological evaluation for intellectual level or potential, as well as speech, visual, and hearing evaluations. In addition, the older child should receive language and learning assessments.

Taking a careful history of pregnancy, labor, delivery, and the immediate neonatal period, and repeating developmental assessments of the infant, are essential for arriving at a diagnosis of cortical damage. In general, failure to ac-

TABLE 20–1. *Motor disturbances associated with cerebral palsy*

Disturbance	Lesion site	Characteristics[a]
Spasticity	Motor cortex, area VI, pyramidal system	Increased muscle tone, hyperactive deep-tendon reflexes, easily elicited stretch reflexes, increased resistance to full range of motion of joints
Athetosis	Basal ganglia, extrapyramidal system	Slow, involuntary, continuous writhing movements of the extremities, trunk, face
Ataxia	Cerebellum or cerebellar tracts	Wide-based, unsteady gait; dysmetria; intention tremor in upper extremities; truncal titubation
Tremor	Basal ganglia	Often hereditary; fine tremulousness of musculature similar to that seen in parkinsonism; not seriously disabling
Rigidity	Diffuse; basal ganglia, cortex	Muscles contract slowly and stiffly; increased resistance to passive movement of muscle throughout range of motion; slow, laborious voluntary movements
Hypotonia	Motor cortex, area IV	Markedly decreased muscle tone, hyperelasticity of joints; hyperactive deep-tendon reflexes despite diminished muscle tone if central in origin

[a]With the exception of concurrent spasticity and hypotonia, mixtures of any of these motor manifestations are possible.

complish motor milestones at the expected time, persistence of primitive reflexes beyond the time at which they are expected to disappear, paucity of movement in affected extremities, and inappropriate muscle tone in affected extremities suggest cerebral palsy.

Viral antibody titers from the mother and infant for toxoplasmosis, syphilis, rubella, cytomegalovirus, and herpesvirus may identify prenatal infections as a possible cause. A CT scan of the brain may show cortical abnormalities or areas of damage.

Principles of Management

Management of cerebral palsy is truly a coordinated, multidisciplinary effort involving physical therapists, occupational therapists, speech therapists, educational psychologists, educators, social service personnel, pediatricians, family practitioners, physiatrists, orthopedic surgeons, ophthalmologists, ENT specialists, and dentists. The relative involvement of members of the various disciplines will depend on the child's problems and stage of development. In addition to the obvious motor dysfunction, approximately 50% of all children with cerebral palsy exhibit mental retardation. Convulsions are present in approximately 40%, speech and language problems in 80%, visual problems in 40%, and diminished hearing acuity in 20%. Almost 100% have significant dental problems, and a significant number may have leg length discrepancies. All of these areas must be watched expectantly and dealt with at appropriate times in the child's development.

Anticonvulsant medication may be necessary if the child has an associated seizure disorder. Spasticity may be reduced by carefully titrated doses of diazepam, baclofen, or dantrolene. Although these drugs do not abolish spasticity, they may reduce it to the point where increased voluntary control of spastic muscles is possible.

Rehabilitation Management

Birth to Three Years of Age

For the normal child, this is the age period when intense motor learning and basic language development occur. Accordingly, this is when intervention with physical therapy, occupational therapy, and speech therapy can be most beneficial in promoting the development of normal motor patterns (gross, fine, and oral) and inhibiting abnormal patterns. With a good program of early intervention, surgery is rarely necessary in this age group.

Therapists must teach the parent or caretaker specific play activities so that the child's daily environment encourages normal motor patterns while discouraging abnormal patterns. In addition, exercise programs are necessary to stretch tight muscles and prevent deformity resulting from tight muscles and joints (Fig. 20–1). Special positioning may be needed to support weak muscles and prevent deformity from the unopposed force of gravity. Special feeding techniques enable the child to learn to chew and develop normal control of the oral musculature so that speech will be possible at a later age.

Three to Seven Years of Age

Rarely is bracing required before 3 years of age, unless the child is standing or ambulating with severe leg, ankle, or foot deformity. Bracing is used to augment weak muscles and oppose strong muscles, thus preventing deforming forces on the bones and joints.

We tend to prefer minimal bracing; often a short leg brace to stabilize the ankle and prevent extreme plantar flexion of the foot is sufficient. If spasticity is extreme in the plantar flexors, a long leg brace may be needed to keep the heel in the brace. In some cases, the foot and ankle cannot be braced properly until the Achilles tendon is lengthened. For severe adductor spasticity, which causes scissoring on attempted ambulation, long leg braces, with or without a pelvic band, may be necessary to control the lower extremities.

If functional ambulation with minimal or no bracing has not been achieved by 5 to 7 years of age, refer the child for orthopedic surgery to release or lengthen spastic muscles, reduce the amount of bracing, and promote more normal patterns of ambulation. This recommendation

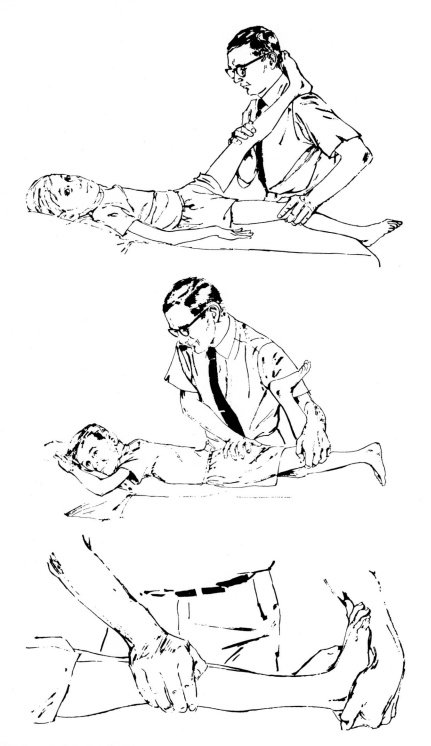

FIG. 20–1. **Top:** Passive stretching of hamstrings, with contralateral side of pelvis stabilized to prevent lifting of buttocks. **Middle:** Passive stretching of iliotibial band by pulling hip in toward examiner (adduction) while stabilizing pelvis. Lying prone while extending hip stretches tight hip flexors. **Bottom:** Passive stretching of heel cord. Knee is extended so that stretching occurs mainly at heel. [From Vignos, P. J. (1968): Rehabilitation in progressive muscular dystrophy. In: *Rehabilitation and Medicine*, edited by S. Licht. Elizabeth Licht, New Haven, Connecticut.]

presupposes that the child has the balance, voluntary motor control, and motivation to walk. Dislocation or subluxation of the hip is a frequent problem associated with adductor and flexor spasticity. Its mean age of occurrence in the spastic child is 7 years. When this occurs, reduction of the dislocation can be maintained only if it is accompanied by surgical release of the spastic muscles.

The occupational therapist will be concerned with improving fine motor control and independence in feeding, dressing, grooming, and toileting, as well as preventing deformities and enhancing function of the upper extremities. Night splints may be used to maintain muscle length of the wrist flexors and small muscles of the hand. Functional splints may be used during the day to improve position of the hand and facilitate fine motor function of the fingers, such as writing and eating.

Speech therapy should begin during this age period to continue language development, overcome articulation problems, and correct dysarthria. Therapeutic techniques to correct speech and language disorders are described in Chapter 8.

Eight Years of Age to Adulthood

Periodic monitoring of children or adults with cerebral palsy is necessary to prevent or correct deformity before permanent damage or pain results. If functional ambulation has not been achieved by 8 years of age, despite adequate therapeutic intervention, it is probably not a realistic goal.

Physical therapy should be limited to a maintenance program for preventing contractures and deformity and promoting independence at the wheelchair level. This will allow the child to direct his or her energies toward academic and social learning to acquire the intellectual and social skills needed for competition in the adult world. Occupational therapy may still be necessary to enable the child to reach a maximum level of independence in activities of daily living in accordance with abilities and limitations.

If speech has not developed by age 8, further speech therapy is probably a waste of the child's

and the therapist's time. Alternate forms of communication should be developed. Eventually, vocational assessment and counseling will be necessary to help the patient set realistic goals for employment and financial independence, if possible.

MUSCULAR DYSTROPHY

Muscular dystrophy applies to a group of relentlessly progressive diseases of voluntary muscle, characterized by increasing weakness and eventual loss of voluntary motor power in the muscles affected. While all muscular dystrophies are genetically transmitted, they differ primarily in their mode of inheritance, age at onset of clinical symptoms, rate of progression, and muscles first affected, as indicated in Table 20–2.

Incidence and Mode of Inheritance

Duchenné muscular dystrophy is the most common of the muscular dystrophies seen in childhood, and the most rapidly progressive. Therefore, comments on diagnosis and management will be directed mainly at this type of muscular dystrophy. Although the others progress at a much slower rate, the principles of management are the same as for Duchenné muscular dystrophy.

Duchenné muscular dystrophy affects only male children because of the sex-linked recessive mode of inheritance. The mother is an asymptomatic carrier of the recessive gene and each of her male offspring has a 50% chance of receiving the affected gene and thus manifesting the disease; each of her female offspring has a 50% chance of receiving the affected gene and being an asymptomatic carrier of the disease.

Diagnosis

History

The affected boys are usually normal at birth and reach their motor milestones at the appropriate time. It is not until between the age of 2 and 4 years that, compared to his siblings or

TABLE 20–2. *Classification of muscular dystrophies*

Diagnosis	Percentage	Genetic transmission	Age at onset
Duchenné	30%	Sex-linked recessive	3 to 5 years
Fascioscapular-humeral	10%	Autosomal dominant	Second or third decade
Limb-girdle	± 5%	Mixed, most are autosomal recessive	First to third decade
Myotonic	50%	Autosomal dominant	Second to third decade

peers, the child seems to fall more often and have more difficulty negotiating stairs and curbs and arising from the floor unassisted. A family history of affected males on the mother's side is extremely helpful, but not necessarily present, in diagnosing Duchenné muscular dystrophy.

Physical Examination

The first signs and symptoms of Duchenné muscular dystrophy involve increased fatique and weakness of the hip girdle muscles. However, a routine physical examination is unlikely to reveal such manifestations early in the disease. Deep tendon reflexes are still normal early in the disease, maintained until extreme muscle weakness occurs. Increased lumbar lordosis and hypertrophy of the calves may serve to make the child look stronger than he actually is. Other subtle signs are flatfootedness and a slightly waddling gait that is accentuated by having the child walk fast. These children also rise on their toes when they walk, which becomes more pronounced as the disease progresses. Signs of muscular dystrophy are best revealed by watching the child in motion—walking, rising from the floor, or stepping up on a low stool or chair.

Laboratory Examinations

In Duchenné muscular dystrophy, there is marked elevation of the creatinine phosphokinase (CPK) level in the blood, usually 30 to 60 times normal, and a slightly elevated CPK level in other forms of dystrophy. The electromyogram (EMG) is helpful in differentiating weakness caused by primary muscle disease from weakness resulting from anterior horn cell disease. Muscle biopsy with histochemical staining

also is helpful in differentiating the dystrophies from neuromuscular atrophy and congenital, infectious, and metabolic myopathies.

Principles of Management

Since the underlying defect in muscular dystrophy has not yet been identified, there is currently no treatment that will arrest or cure the disease. The basic philosophy of management is to maintain ambulation as long as possible, maintain maximum muscle strength by encouraging the family to allow the child to do as much as he can for himself, avoid immobilization and prolonged bedrest at all cost, and delay joint contractures and respiratory impairment by appropriate therapeutic intervention.

Surgical Intervention

Percutaneous tenotomies at hips, knees, and ankles on carefully selected patients may significantly prolong ambulation. These procedures, like any other surgical procedure on these children, must be followed by ambulation on the day after surgery. This is accomplished by applying lightweight casts. To continue ambulating after the casts are removed, the patients are placed in lightweight, plastic long leg braces. After surgery, these patients are only able to walk with their knees locked in long leg braces.

Genetic Counseling

All families of patients with muscular dystrophy should have genetic counseling as soon as the diagnosis is made. Since the mode of inheritance differs considerably among the various dystrophies, it is important that an accurate diagnosis be made. Search for carriers throughout the family, and inform family members at risk for having affected children of the risk factors and options available to them. Genetic counseling is available free of charge through clinics sponsored by the Muscular Dystrophy Association.

Rehabilitation Management

Management of the patient during the ambulatory phase of the disease is aimed at maintaining functional ambulation and muscle strength for as long as possible. The parents are instructed in range-of-motion exercises for the lower extremities, with gentle muscle stretching to delay joint contractures (Fig. 20–1). The child is encouraged to sleep on his abdomen to prevent hip flexion contractures. In addition, when ankle dorsiflexion becomes limited, the child may be placed in night splints with maximum dorsiflexion at the ankles to help delay ankle contractures. Some physicians prefer using long leg night splints that incorporate the knee. Specific exercise programs are unnecessary in ambulatory patients because their daily activity level is usually adequate to maintain muscle strength at an optimum level for their disease state. When ambulation becomes too slow and laborious to be functional, or when the patient suffers frequent falls or fractures, consider surgical treatment or placing the child in a wheelchair.

Management of the patient confined to a wheelchair is directed primarily at maintaining spinal alignment and maximum respiratory function. Lower extremity contractures develop quickly; to delay them, encourage the child to spend some time out of the wheelchair at home, on his abdomen on the floor, and crawling about as long as he can. Early in the period of wheelchair confinement, some children may delay the development of flexion contractures of the hips and knees by being upright in a standing table for several hours a day in school and at home. This tends to delay the flexion contractures of the hips and knees that occur very quickly after wheelchair confinement.

When the child becomes confined to a wheelchair, the spine must be watched very closely for signs of scoliosis. Fitting the child with a high lumbosacral corset with metal stays (see Chapter 6) helps maintain good posture in the wheelchair. Even while the child is in the corset, however, evidence of scoliosis may appear. It is then necessary to place the child in a molded body jacket to prevent rapid progression of the scoliotic curve and respiratory embarrassment.

Vital capacity must be monitored carefully in muscular dystrophy patients. Breathing exercises as well as postural drainage and assisted cough should be taught to the child and his family to help in dealing with respiratory secretions. (See Chapter 13 for a description of these therapeutic techniques.) Intermittent positive pressure breathing (IPPB) is used to maintain compliance of the thorax and lungs. Respiratory infections must be treated promptly and adequately. Toward the end of the disease, patients may exhibit evidence of CO_2 retention as manifested by morning headache and lethargy. Many patients need assistive respiratory devices when sleeping (see Chapter 13). Adequate respiratory treatment is critical because the cause of death in children with muscular dystrophy is usually respiratory infection and failure.

Psychosocial Adjustment

A high rate of emotional disturbance and some intellectual impairment, particularly verbal, is associated with Duchenné muscular dystrophy. Intellectual impairment, affecting from 8% to 30% of these patients, is nonprogressive. Passivity related to confinement to a wheelchair may produce self-image problems and agitated, aggressive, almost paranoid behavior. The latter is most common in patients who survive after age 20 and feel they are living on borrowed time, yet not fit vocationally for continued life. Typical personality traits of muscular dystrophy patients are superficial brightness, hysteria, and apathy. Minor dementia and other organic changes may result from pulmonary insufficiency associated with respiratory muscle weakness and scoliosis, with anoxic cerebral changes secondary to hypercapnia and infection. Typically, the I.Q. of the patient with Duchenné muscular dystrophy hovers at about 85 + .

Parental distress is most marked on diagnosis because usually the child had appeared normal during infancy only to begin deteriorating suddenly from 2 to 6 years of age. The parents are then faced not only with the physical handicaps of their disabled child but also with the need to acquire educational assistance, keep up with numerous medical appointments, become familiar with frequently changing assistive devices and appliances, and understand the language of the various medical disciplines involved to be able to supervise the child's home treatment. As a result, families often become so overwhelmed that they fail to prepare the child to cope with not only the ordinary events of childhood, such as school, but also the knowledge of probable premature death. Inadvertently, parents may interfere with the child's development of autonomy and associated persistence of effort, initiation of activity, and motivation to participate in interpersonal relationships. Lack of practice in applying steady effort and diligence toward completing a task often causes disabled children to perceive that they have less control over their environment than they actually have and thus avoid trying to perform some independent functions they could master with effort.

SPINA BIFIDA

Spina bifida is defined as the separation of the vertebral elements in the midline. The three major classifications—occulta, manifesta, and aperta—are described in Table 20–3. Associated congenital anomalies are micropolygyria, abnormalities of the aqueduct, Arnold Chiari malformation, vertebral anteroposterior and lateral wedges, myelovertebral disproportion, large fontanelles, shallow posterior fossa, and large foramen magnum.

There is a polygenically inherited predisposition to this disease. It is probably caused by environmental factors, which may or may not be specific, acting on a genetically susceptible embryo around the 28th day of gestation.

The incidence of this disease in the United States and England is 1:1,000 when there are no other family members affected, 5.5:100 after one affected child, 13:100 after two affected children, and 20.6:100 after three affected children.

Prenatal Diagnosis

Prenatal diagnosis of spina bifida is possible by measuring alpha-fetoproteins in amniotic fluid between 14 and 16 weeks of gestation. Because of the risks involved (amnionitis, spontaneous abortion), this procedure should not be done unless the parents will agree to an abortion if the diagnosis is positive.

Principles of Management

To receive adequate treatment, the patient with spina bifida must often consult many different specialists. It is not unusual for such patients to require the services of a neurosurgeon, pediatrician, orthopedist, urologist, ophthalmologist, and physiatrist. These patients may also require physical therapy and occupational therapy. Ideally, they should be treated in a multidisciplinary clinic where all of these services are provided.

TABLE 20–3. *Classification of spina bifida*

Type	Description	Manifestations
Occulta	Epithelialized skin covers hidden lesion	Hair tuft or skin dimple
Manifesta	Skin is incompletely epithelialized	Cystica—vertebral elements covered by poorly epithelialized membrane Meningocele—cystic lesion of meninges only, with or without dysplasia of neural contents Meningomyelocele—meninges around malformed neural tube
Aperta	No cover of neural tissue	Myeloschisis—neural tube is wide open

Such clinics allow specialists to share information and coordinate treatment, and often mean a decrease in the number of visits for the patients and their families.

Management of Complications

Unfortunately, a great many complications are associated with this disease.

Hydrocephalus

Hydrocephalus develops toward the end of intrauterine life. It is present in 80% of children affected with spina bifida in the first days or weeks of life even though the fronto-occipital circumference is normal. There is a high incidence of spontaneous arrest.

A shunting procedure (ventriculoperitoneal or ventriculoatrial) is necessary in the management of progressive hydrocephalus. Complications of shunting may include obstruction and ventriculitis, which are associated with a drop in I.Q. Intelligence is below average in children with spina bifida but no hydrocephalus, slightly lower in those with arrested hydrocephalus, and significantly lower in those with spina bifida requiring a ventricular peritoneal shunt.

Paralysis

There may be no motor weakness associated with lesions affecting the sacral segments, or motor weakness may be considerable as in the case of higher lesions in the thoracic and thoracolumbar segments. Paralysis may be either complete or incomplete. The deformities most often associated with paralysis and/or weakness are hip dislocation, knee contractures, and foot deformities. The management of weakness or paralysis includes the prevention of complications and bracing to improve function and enable ambulation. Figure 20–2 compares the motor development of the normal child and the child with spina bifida, indicating recommended assistive devices at each age level.

Hip Dislocations

Findings in spina bifida include decreased abduction, shortening of one leg, asymmetry of gluteal folds, and Ortolani click (felt when femoral head slides over acetabular rim). Hip dislocations can be present with lesions at any level but are more common when there is hip flexor function but no hip extensor function. The unilateral dislocation should be treated; however, there is much discussion as to whether bilateral dislocations should be treated. This is a decision that must be reached on an individual basis. The treatment can be conservative (traction and casting) or surgical.

Knee Flexion Contractures

Knee flexion contractures may be due to spasticity of the hamstrings in the case of weak or absent quadriceps function. They can also affect children who are flaccid across the knee and who do not receive daily passive range-of-motion exercise. In mild and early cases, stretching of the hamstrings (Fig. 20–1) will be sufficient treatment. In more severe cases, surgical procedures for lengthening or dividing the hamstrings are needed.

Foot and Ankle Deformities

The many deformities associated with spina bifida include equinovarus, calcaneovalgus, vertical talus, and pes cavus foot deformities, as well as valgus deformity of the ankle (Fig. 20–3). Mild conditions can be treated with conservative methods such as casting; however, most cases will require surgical correction.

Sensory Loss

Sensation is decreased in spina bifida, depending on the level of injury. The patient must be aware of the area of decreased or absent sensation in order to avoid complications such as burns and decubitus ulcers (see Chapter 23).

Spinal Deformities

About 5% to 20% of children with myelomeningocele are born with some degree of kyphosis. This is due to abnormalities of the vertebral bodies and weakness of dorsal muscles. Treatment by removal of the atypical ver-

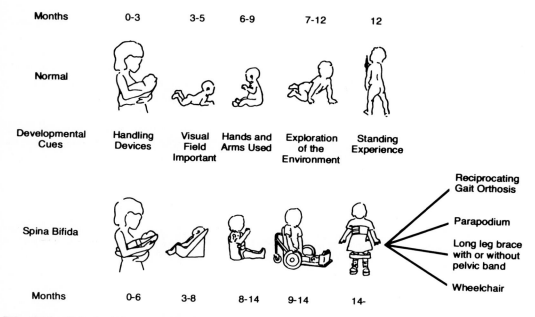

Months	0-3	3-5	6-9	7-12	12

Normal

Developmental Cues	Handling Devices	Visual Field Important	Hands and Arms Used	Exploration of the Environment	Standing Experience

Spina Bifida

Reciprocating Gait Orthosis

Parapodium

Long leg brace with or without pelvic band

Wheelchair

Months	0-6	3-8	8-14	9-14	14-

FIG. 20–2. Orthotic devices for the child with moderate spina bifida at progressive stages of development and ages, compared with crawling and standing of normal child. Child begins sitting stage with assistance of caster cart, uses reciprocating gait orthosis for standing and walking. Children ages 17 months to 14 years who have flaccid paralysis can wear a parapodium to facilitate rolling, standing from a prone position, and swivel walking. By age 10 years, many children will prefer the use of a wheelchair when walking becomes too energy consuming. [From Motloch, W. (1984): Orthotic philosophies of treatment. *Clin. Prosthet. Orthot.*, 8:10.]

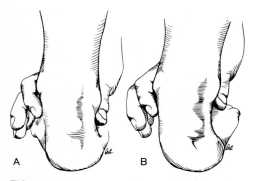

FIG. 20–3. A: Normal ankle. **B:** Valgus deformity in ankle of child with spina bifida. [From Schafer, M. S., and Dias, L. S. (1983): *Myelomeningocele: Orthopaedic Treatment.* Williams and Wilkins, Baltimore.]

tebral bodies may be necessary in the neonatal period to allow closure of the skin defect. In milder cases, surgery may be delayed. Scoliosis may be congenital and, in the case of spina bifida, associated with hemivertebra. Conservative management with the Milwaukee brace may be adequate to correct smaller curves if there is sufficient skin coverage to tolerate the brace. Correction of large curves will require surgical intervention.

Neurogenic Bladder

Neurogenic bladder is present in more than 90% of patients with spina bifida aperta. The neurogenic bladder may be either upper motor neuron or lower motor neuron type (see Chapter 25). If saddle anesthesia is present, there will be some disturbance of the child's bladder. The physical examination should include observation of the pattern of unaided micturition. Investigations during the neonatal period should include urine cultures and excretion pyelography.

Treat urinary tract infections promptly while avoiding overdistention. Some useful techniques for managing neurogenic bladder in children include Crede's maneuver, (which should be avoided in children with vesiculourethral reflux), vesicostomy, and early intermittent catheterization, which often becomes the ongoing treatment of choice.

Neurogenic Bowel

There is a very high incidence of neurogenic bowel in patients with spina bifida aperta. Some of the common problems associated with this condition are constipation, overdistention, incontinence, and rectal prolapse, the latter usually lessening with age. As in the case of neurogenic bladder, the neurogenic bowel may be either upper or lower motor neuron type.

Management should include the following:

1. Avoidance of overdistention.
2. Maintenance of soft stools with adequate bulk by adequate fluid intake, appropriate diet, and occasional stool softeners.
3. Use of suppositories and occasional enemas.

Upper Extremity Involvement

Because of the hydrocephalus, there may be upper motor neuron involvement of the upper extremities. Although this complication is often ignored, it may be significant. Typical manifestations are difficulties with fine motor coordination, muscle weakness, spasticity, and increased reflexes. The management of this condition should include strengthening exercises and activities to try to improve coordination.

DEVELOPMENTAL DELAY

The pediatrician, family physician, or general practitioner will see a number of children who fail to reach developmental milestones at the appropriate age. The parents may not be aware of the delay, especially if it is not marked, even though it invariably affects one or more areas of the child's behavior. Even a single disability may produce problems in different areas of the child's development, and the effects of multiple disabilities on development are exponential rather than additive. A child born prematurely should not be considered developmentally delayed if development is normal for his or her *gestational* age.

Occasionally, a specific cause of developmental delay cannot be determined, but the following are some possible causes:

1. Mental retardation.
2. Lack of stimulation, occurring sometimes in institutions or some homes.
3. Chronic illness, such as congenital heart disease.
4. Early neuromuscular disease, or peripheral nerve injuries such as brachial plexus injuries, associated with weakness.
5. Diseases associated with alteration of muscle tone and abnormal movements, as in the case of cerebral palsy.
6. Hearing deficits (delayed speech).
7. Visual deficits (motor delay).

Diagnosis

Since the normal child's development continues well after he or she learns to walk and talk, one screening test alone, without a complete examination, is insufficient for identifying developmental delays. Once you do suspect a delay, however, you must decide whether to refer the child to a developmental clinic or a pediatric neurologist, or to continue the diagnostic workup yourself.

The diagnosis of delayed development requires a complete examination on more than one occasion. In a busy practice, screening tests are of great value. There are several that offer different degrees of reliability. It is better to select screening tests that occasionally mislabel some uninvolved children as delayed than tests that fail to identify some delayed children. Preferred tests also divide rather than combine different areas of behavior. One of the more reliable tests is the Developmental Screening Inventory, which is standardized to 18 months of age. Unfortunately, there are presently no well-standardized tests that screen children beyond this age, although some are being devised.

The areas of behavior that should be measured are as follows:

1. Personal–social—the response of the child to his or her cultural habitat.
2. Adaptive—the child's use of resources in problem solving.
3. Speech—other forms of communication in addition to language.
4. Gross motor—head control, trunk control, standing balance, and ambulation.
5. Fine motor—the child's use of a hand to manipulate objects.

Rehabilitation Management

In planning treatment, note that tests of early development have poor correlation with future cognitive function; in other words, the child who performs poorly on these tests during infancy will not necessarily remain behind his or her peers in school. Nevertheless, parents will need support as well as information regarding the implications and prognoses of their child's condition that you can provide after making a diagnosis.

Most communities offer numerous programs for stimulating infants (<1-3 years) and young children (3-5 years). These programs provide the following kinds of help:

1. Support to parents and children.
2. Experiences appropriate to the child's maturity level.
3. Ways for parents to structure the child's activities.
4. Techniques for handling destructive behavior.
5. Reviews of parenting techniques.

These developmental programs suffer from two main disadvantages, however. First, overenthusiastic personnel may imply to parents that the programs are failure-proof and that if the child does not "catch up" with his or her peers, it is because the parents have not worked hard enough. This view places another burden on parents who already may feel guilty about their child's problem. Second, there is no definite proof that any of the techniques used in developmental programs will alter the ultimate performance of the child. There is evidence, however, that institutionalized children decline in their intellectual

functioning or do not progress as well as comparable children from good homes. Ultimately, learning can be compared to a reverse pyramid; the top of the pyramid, or the child's total knowledge capacity, is determined by the width of the bottom of the pyramid, or the breadth of the child's early experience.

HYPOTONIA

Often difficult to evaluate, hypotonia refers to decreased resistance to movement, sometimes including unusual postures and excessive joint mobility. The etiology of this condition is varied. Certain disorders of the central nervous system (perinatal brain insult, metabolic disorders, chromosomal abnormalities, e.g., Down's syndrome) and the peripheral nervous system (Werdnig-Hoffmann disease, neonatal myasthenia gravis, transient myasthenia gravis, congenital myopathies, glycogen storage disease) are some of the most common causes. Connective tissue disorders such as Ehler-Dahnlos syndrome, Marfan's syndrome, and congenital spinal cord injury are other causes.

Only those children who improve and who exhibit normal enzyme studies, EMG findings, and muscle biopsy results should be diagnosed as having benign congenital hypotonia.

Rehabilitation Management

In general, hypotonia may be managed in the following ways:

1. Genetic counseling of parents once the diagnosis has been established.
2. Range-of-motion exercises to prevent contractures, especially when the hypotonia is associated with weakness.
3. Bracing, when indicated, to improve function or to prevent deformity.
4. Instructing the caretaker in techniques of handling, including developmental stimulation programs (see section on Developmental Delay).

Management will be complicated in cases of congenital spinal cord injury by neurogenic bladder and bowel, decreased or absent sensation, respiratory difficulties, even in the presence of normal phrenic nerves, and difficulty regulating body temperature. Techniques for managing these complications are discussed in Chapters 13, 17, and 25, as well as earlier in this chapter.

SUGGESTED READINGS

Brooke, M. H. (1977): *A Clinician's View of Neuromuscular Disease*. Williams and Wilkins, Baltimore.

Brooke, M. H., Carroll, J. E., and Ringell, S. P. (1979): Congenital hypotonia revisited. *Muscle Nerve*, 2:84–100.

Downey, J. A., and Low, N. L. (1982): *The Child with Disabling Illness*, 2nd edit. Raven Press, New York.

Keele, D. K. (1983). *The Developmentally Disabled Child: A Manual for Primary Physicians*. Medical Economics Books, Oradell, N.J.

Levine, M. S. (1980): Cerebral palsy diagnosis in children over age 1 year: Standard criteria. *Arch. Phys. Med. Rehabil.*, 61:385–389.

Levitt, S. (1982): *Treatment of Cerebral Palsy and Motor Delay*. Blackwell Scientific, Boston.

Menelaus, M. B. (1980): *The Orthopedic Management of Spina Bifida Cystica*, 2nd edit. Churchill Livingstone, New York.

Motloch, W. (1984): Spina bifida: Orthotic philosophies of treatment. *Clin. Prosthet. Orthot.*, 8:9–11.

Rutten, M. (1980): The long term effects of early experience. *Dev. Med. Child Neurol.*, 22:800–815.

Schafer, M. F., and Dias, L. S. (1983): *Myelomeningocele: Orthopaedic Treatment*. Williams and Wilkins, Baltimore.

Scherzer, A. L., and Tscharnuter, I. (1982): *Early Diagnosis and Therapy in Cerebral Palsy: A Primer on Infant Developmental Problems*. M. Dekker, New York.

Thompson, G. H., Rubin, I. L., Bilenker, R. M., editors (1983): *Comprehensive Management of Cerebral Palsy*. Grune and Stratton, New York.

Medical Rehabilitation,
edited by L. S. Halstead et al.
Raven Press, New York © 1985.

CHAPTER 21

Geriatric Rehabilitation

*Thomas E. Strax and **Janice Ledebur

*Department of Rehabilitation Medicine, Temple University School of Medicine, and Moss Rehabilitation Hospital, Philadelphia, Pennsylvania 19141; and **Department of Physical Medicine and Rehabilitation, Philadelphia Geriatric Center, Philadelphia, Pennsylvania 19104

EPIDEMIOLOGY

The number of Americans older than age 65 has been growing at a rate three times faster than that of the general population. In 1900, one person in 25 was over 65; that ratio is now one in nine, and by the year 2000, it will be one in seven. By the year 1990, an estimated 27.5 million people over age 65 will be living in the United States.

Because no place has been reserved for slow, aging individuals in our mechanized society, the elderly person commonly moves from one level of care to another, from independence to dependence, from home health aide, to nursing home, to a maximum care unit—all in a relatively short period of time. This process usually begins when the spouse of an elderly family member dies or becomes unable to perform activities of daily living.

EVALUATION

Before evaluating the functional status of the geriatric patient, take a complete history and perform a complete medical work-up to rule out organic disease. Included in the history should be the goals of the patient and the family. Some questions the functional history should answer are posed in the following list:

1. Can the family unit survive if the elderly members remain at home?
2. Is the home suited for the elderly person's level of function? Are there architectural barriers in the home or community that will prohibit function? Can any of these barriers be removed?
3. Must the elderly member move into an institution or residential facility, or are there alternative living plans?
4. What services are needed to keep the elderly person at home?
5. What community services can be provided?

Cardiovascular, Pulmonary, and Urological Problems

Decreased work tolerance, with or without chest pain, may indicate cardiovascular dysfunction. In people over age 65, the cardiovascular system is almost universally impaired by a 25% decrease in coronary blood flow. Besides the problem of decreased work ability, evaluate the possibility of arrhythmias and conduction disturbances. Patients who complain of these symptoms and who do not have obviously abnormal electrocardiograms should be given a stress exercise test and a Holter monitor evaluation (see Chapter 14).

Many older men were blue collar workers in the early years of this century. They have been exposed to numerous toxic agents, which have reduced pulmonary function. If there is any evidence of shortness of breath, a pulmonary evaluation with spirometry and FEV_1 readings would be helpful (see Chapter 13).

The kidneys of older people should be thoroughly evaluated, since people in the eighth decade have as much as a 50% reduction in kidney function.

Musculoskeletal Changes

Decreased endurance in the elderly is also due to diminished bulk of skeletal muscle. Many muscle fibers are replaced through the aging process with noncontractile tissue. Despite this problem, remaining muscle mass can be conditioned through an exercise program.

Osteoporosis is extremely common in the elderly. Bones are brittle and fractures occur frequently. The causes of osteoporosis vary; decreased calcium intake and decreased exposure to the sun, with resultant diminished vitamin D reserves, are common. These problems are compounded in postmenopausal women by diminished estrogen levels.

Gait Dysfunctions

A variety of conditions may impair gait. For example, impaired ability to overcome a change in balance results in a wide-based and shuffling gait pattern. Patients with this type of gait should be evaluated for such problems as Parkinson's disease. Those with a combination of ataxic gait disturbance, mental confusion, and incontinence should be evaluated for the possibility of normal pressure hydrocephalus or other cerebral mass lesions. Gait disturbance can also be caused by vascular disease or metabolic problems.

Skin Changes

Skin changes usually involve all three layers. The epidermis no longer retains sufficient moisture, leading to dryness and cracking. The dermis becomes dehydrated and loses its elasticity. There are decreased numbers of fat cells and a diminished blood supply. The skin of the elderly also is more susceptible to infection and pressure sores. Areas of thin skin, especially over bony prominences, should be evaluated. The lower extremities must be examined carefully to identify atrophy of skin appendages; for example, loss of hair or brittle, cracking nails.

Failing Vision and Hearing

Most older people have failing vision and reduced ability of the lens to accommodate. The need for eyeglasses is almost universal, and failure to wear them can mimic certain organic problems. Cataracts and glaucoma are common causes of reduced vision and blindness in the elderly.

Hearing, especially at high frequencies, is seriously reduced in the older individual. For hearing deficits of 25 or 30 decibels or less, a hearing aid attached to the frame of the glasses may suffice. However, in the case of hearing deficits above 35 or 40 decibels, a body aid would be more useful. All patients with hearing loss should be evaluated by a competent audiologist for proper fit and training in the use of a hearing aid. Hearing deficits above 70 or 80 decibels usually are not correctable with any kind of hearing aid.

Since auditory deficits can mimic organic impairment, ENT and audiology screening evaluations should be considered. Hearing deficits are often severe enough to impair rehabilitation efforts. Many hearing-impaired people do not get the full benefit of their hearing aid because they have never been trained to use it properly. Aural rehabilitation consists of instructions on how to wear and maintain the aid and batteries, as well as supplemental lip reading to improve the effectiveness of the aid. One cue to the hearing-impaired regarding positioning is to avoid facing bright light when trying to lip read.

NUTRITIONAL DEFICITS

Because many elderly people cannot afford adequate meals, or they are not physically able to shop for or prepare their own food, their diets may be nutritionally incomplete. Some lack the skills for selection or preparation of a well-balanced meal, or the incentive to prepare a good meal alone. Therefore, food is often selected because of the patient's likes, the cost, and/or the ease of preparation.

The average resting metabolic rate decreases about 2% per decade in adults. Protein requirements, however, do not change with age, but remain about 1 g/kg/day. Vitamin deficiencies are rare in older patients because many take vitamin supplements. However, few older people take sufficient bulk in their diets, a deficiency associated with diverticulosis and cancer of the gastrointestinal system.

With aging, there is a decrease in the output of hydrochloric acid from the stomach, as well as in pancreatic secretion. This impairs the digestion and absorption of food. Older people frequently complain of indigestion, belching, or heartburn, and they tend to take antacids in abundance. They also tend to ingest great amounts of aspirin, contributing to gastritis and blood loss.

Deficits have been discovered even in those nursing homes that provide proper care for their patients. Although most elderly persons need about 2,000 calories per day, many of them in nursing homes receive more than 3,000 calories. Surveys have revealed that many nursing homes load residents with desserts to keep them happy, while special dietary needs are frequently disregarded.

Good nutrition must go hand in hand with good rehabilitation. A poor diet can lead to an anemic, osteoporotic, listless patient. Bleeding gums because of poor dentures or no dentures can lead to an angry disgruntled patient who cannot or will not proceed with rehabilitation efforts. While vitamin supplementation will protect the malnourished patient from vitamin deficiencies, it cannot substitute for inadequate carbohydrate and/or protein intake.

MANAGEMENT OF COMMON GERIATRIC PROBLEMS

Some of the more debilitating medical problems affecting the geriatric population are general deconditioning, stroke, heart disease, Parkinson's disease, peripheral vascular disease and amputation, visual impairment, pulmonary problems, pain, psychosocial impairment, and organic brain syndrome.

General Deconditioning

Coupled with normal reduced muscle bulk and tone and diminished endurance, inactivity

makes prolonged hospitalizations very dangerous for elderly people. Up to 3% of motor power can be lost per day with complete immobilization (see Chapter 22). Therefore, an individual who functions at 60% motor power who is kept at complete bed rest for 10 days, may decline to 30% or 40% of motor power. This reduction may prevent the individual from being strong enough to perform normal activities of daily living, or to climb up and down stairs in a multistory building. For this reason, a general conditioning program for all elderly individuals who are hospitalized for any period of time is recommended. These programs also decrease the possibility of the development of orthostatic hypotension and pneumonia. A conditioning program should include the following elements:

1. Instruction in proper breathing or coughing techniques, using abdominal splinting to augment a poor cough response.
2. Postural drainage with gentle vibration for all patients with pulmonary disease (see Chapter 13), except in cases of multiple fracture, osteoporosis, and primary or secondary lung lesions in the ribs.
3. Instruction in bedside mobility and bedside range of motion.
4. Sitting activities begun 72 hr after a cerebrovascular accident without hemorrhage and 7 days after a CVA with hemorrhage once the patient has been stabilized.
5. Short-distance ambulation begun as soon as the patient is allowed out of bed and able to sit for 1 hr.
6. Bedside bimanual activities up to a level of 2.4 METs started as soon as possible (see Chapter 14).
7. Complete activities of daily living evaluation for any patient who has been hospitalized for more than 2 weeks.

Deconditioned patients or elderly persons in the community should be started on a graduated exercise program of walking, stair climbing, or bicycling with cardiac precautions and limits set by the family physician.

These programs are very useful in geriatric patients who have long-term disabling illnesses, especially when coupled with energy conservation and joint preservation techniques. With modification, they can also be used for diabetics and patients with rheumatoid diseases.

Stroke

Most older people who have strokes have multiple concurrent problems, such as heart disease or peripheral vascular disease. Employ neurofacilitation techniques to focus the elderly patient's attention on the affected side. Neglecting the affected side often exacerbates problems with senses, balance, and skin. The management of stroke is covered in more detail in Chapter 15.

Parkinson's Disease

Encourage patients with Parkinson's disease (see Chapter 19) to use proper breathing techniques. Facial exercises, deep breathing exercises, and trunk extension and rotation exercises are essential for improving functional capacity. In addition to a general conditioning program, balance and posture can be improved through rocking, which employs the vestibular reflexes and postural responses. Lateral weight shifting should be stressed to improve ambulation and gait cadence; weights can be placed on distal portions of the body to facilitate phasic motion. Group education can be used to increase the patient's awareness of his or her problems and to develop self-monitoring techniques.

Peripheral Vascular Disease and Amputation

As one ages, the atherosclerotic process involving all parts of the vasculature tends to manifest clinically as venous and/or arterial insufficiency. Chronic long-standing edema is very common in older people, especially women with peripheral vascular disease. This nonpitting edema is not readily corrected with long-term Jobst therapy. The following are some practical suggestions for treatment:

1. Keep legs elevated when sitting for any prolonged period.

2. Exercise to the point of intermittent claudication or slightly longer.

3. Wear support stockings that induce flow from the superficial veins, thus increasing venous return in the deep system and decreasing stagnation in the superficial levels of the skin, which can lead to skin breakdown and pressure sore formation.

4. Take whirlpool baths for ulceration with infection, keeping water temperature within 10% of local skin temperature, usually below 94°F (in the patient with severe peripheral vascular disease, any increase in the temperature of an extremity creates a metabolic need exceeding the ability of the blood supply to handle tissue needs, which may lead to necrosis and possible amputation).

5. At home, bathe extremity in mild soap every evening, patting it dry and using corn starch in the summer and a mild skin lotion to lubricate the skin in the winter.

6. Wear comfortable shoes that accommodate the foot and foot deformities accurately, for example, a deep inlaid shoe with Plastiazote innersole conforming to any plantar deformities and providing toe contact during weight bearing.

Two major concerns of the geriatric amputee are the increased cardiovascular demands of walking, and survival of the remaining extremity in the unilateral amputee.

The energy expenditure of the unilateral below-knee amputee for ambulation is between 10% and 30% greater than normal; the upper limit is most frequently found in the geriatric patient. With bilateral below-knee amputation, this energy expenditure approaches 60%. In the case of unilateral above-knee amputation, energy expenditure for ambulation is almost 100%. This expenditure approaches 300% or 400% with bilateral above-knee amputation. Under such conditions, a patient with limited cardiovascular reserve is likely at some time to be pushed beyond his or her cardiovascular limit.

In making decisions about amputation in aged patients, you must realize that the preservation of the knee joint may make the difference between the patient being a functional or a non-functional amputee. Rehabilitation after above-knee amputation should include strict cardiac precaution; putting on an above-knee prosthesis uses a tremendous amount of energy.

Most of the amputations performed on geriatric patients result from peripheral vascular disease, which is rarely found in only one extremity. Consequently, the other leg is at great risk; 50% of unilateral amputees lose the other extremity in less than 2 years.

For psychological and cosmetic reasons, all patients who want a prosthesis should be given one. Those patients with sufficient cardiovascular reserve should be allowed to walk. Teach all patients proper care of the remaining extremity and advise them to limit ambulation in order to minimize the risk of increased trauma to it.

The outcome of rehabilitating a geriatric amputee depends on the type of amputation performed. Only 12% to 17% of bilateral above-knee amputees ever gain the ability to walk short distances with their prostheses. With above-knee and below-knee amputation, the results increase to 25% to 54%. In the case of bilateral below-knee amputations, between 30% and 100% of the patients become independent in the ability to ambulate short distances. In unilateral amputees, these figures are 80% for below-knee amputees and 60% for above-knee amputees.

Prosthetic restoration in the geriatric amputee has some special considerations. Prescribe the most stable knee and ankle available, usually a single-axis knee with a manual lock. If the amputations are above-knee, patients are usually given a manual locking knee or a Boch safety knee, which enables the individual to lock the knee during the stance phase of gait. Managing the amputee is covered in more detail in Chapter 11.

Visual Impairment

There are few programs in the country that offer training for the blind. Such training requires more than teaching an individual to ambulate with a cane or to make use of auditory stimuli.

Since vision training employs the adaptive use of other senses to compensate for visual impairment, successful vision training in the elderly may be somewhat limited. It is very difficult to teach a visually impaired person mobility or activities of daily living in the presence of other disabilities.

Before vision training is initiated, the type of visual loss, as well as when and how it occurred, should be known. Evaluate hearing, tactile discrimination, stereognosis, cognition, memory, coordination, and balance in order to set up a realistic training and treatment plan.

Also, ascertain the patient's motivational level. Many elderly people feel they are too "old" to learn. Some are resistant to change, and others are afraid of failure.

Most techniques for teaching activities of daily living and mobility to the elderly with visual impairments are the same as for teaching younger people. In teaching these techniques, make sure the instructions are clear, simple, and consistent. Each task should be relevant to the patient and taught in short time spans (15 to 30 min), and each training session should end on a successful note. Break down and structure activities, especially if the person is cognitively impaired, and allow adequate time for slowed processing ability. Those with diminished sensation should be given activities to facilitate tactile discrimination and stereognosis. Mobility training may not be feasible until gait deviations, balance, coordination, and strength have been improved.

For people with auditory and visual impairments, compensations such as speaking slowly, distinctly, and in a slightly raised voice may facilitate the learning process. If a body hearing aid is worn, speech should be directed at the body aid. Raised communication boards may also be helpful.

Pulmonary Disease

In the elderly patient with acute pulmonary disease, a specialized program should be instituted immediately, whenever possible. The patient should be comfortably placed in a side-lying position (Fig. 21–1) with pillows or bolsters

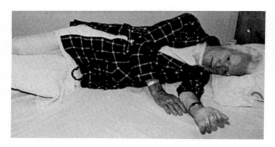

FIG. 21–1. Elderly patient positioned on side. [From Earls, K., Linville, L., Meltzer, M., Tornick-Bruch, H., and Wolfson, A. (1984): Occupational therapy. In: *Current Therapy in Physiatry: Physical Medicine and Rehabilitation*, edited by A. P. Ruskin. W. B. Saunders, Philadelphia.]

for support. If one lung is congested, the patient should spend more time lying on the opposite side so that gravity can help drain the secretions into the bronchi. This is also facilitated by proper positioning and using percussion or vibration to loosen secretions. The patient should be instructed to take deep breaths and give short, forceful, hacking coughs. In patients with weak abdominal muscles or in postoperative patients, the abdomen should be held firmly or splinted when the patient coughs, to accentuate discharge. The upper segments should be drained first, then lower, so as not to spread infection.

Once the patient has recovered from an acute event, conditioning exercises coupled with deep breathing and relaxation exercises are initiated. Relaxation is particularly important in patients with chronic obstructive pulmonary disease, since agitation will accentuate breathlessness.

Pulmonary therapy is not useful in patients with congestive heart failure because the fluid is usually interstitial and not in the bronchi. Therapy should be discontinued when less than 30 cc of fluid can be brought forth with therapy. All patients should be taught energy conservation techniques.

Pain

Etiology

Complaints of pain by the geriatric patient are frequently ignored. Instead of receiving a thorough investigation, many complaints are written off as ploys for attention or the inevitable results of an aging body. All too often it is assumed that nothing can be done. Pain may be a warning of physical or emotional distress, and should be recognized as such. Whether the cause is physical or emotional, the etiology of the pain should be determined and treated, if possible, in a multidisciplinary pain clinic (see Chapter 9).

As people get older, certain patterns of pain may change; headaches become less common in the elderly than they are in the younger age group. Migraine headaches are relatively rare and might warn the physician of subsequent development of transient ischemic attacks or strokes. The older patient is also less likely to have serious abdominal pain with life-threatening illness, and leukocytosis is less common than in the younger patient. From 1% to 2% of the geriatric population have pain secondary to herpes zoster. With poor skin healing and poor peripheral circulation, as well as a history of wearing tight shoes, foot pain is quite common.

Management

Conservative measures such as whirlpool bath, heat, ice, and massage, as well as exercise, improved muscle tone, posture, and function can eliminate most patients' pain. Others will need nerve blocks or transcutaneous electrical nerve stimulation (TENS) to help relieve the pain of herpes, phantom limb, or neuropathies.

The use of nerve blocks has been advocated for certain kinds of pain. Shoulder and arm pain may be reduced by giving multiple blocks to the stellate ganglion; this is usually coupled with physical therapy. TENS supplies a mild tingling sensation to the sensory fibers of the skin, which in turn, blocks the slower pain fibers. It is extremely effective in acute painful states, such as postoperatively. Its efficacy in chronic long-standing pain, however, has not been proved. Analgesics, steroids, mood elevators, antidepressants, and psychological support also are useful. At times, the use of protective orthoses will help to diminish pain by immobilizing and supporting affected joints (Fig. 21–2).

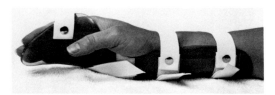

FIG. 21–2. Protective orthosis holds wrist joint at 15° extension with slight flexion of fingers and is easily applied and removed by patient. [From Bluestone, R. (1980): *Practical Rheumatology: Diagnosis and Management.* Addison-Wesley, Menlo Park, CA.]

Psychosocial Considerations

Isolation, depression, and loneliness are common and lead to inappropriate behavior and intensification of psychosomatic complaints. Motivating patients to achieve a higher functional level is difficult if they feel they have nothing to live for. Efforts to rehabilitate such patients are usually most effective when a team deals with the patient, family, and peers.

To enhance the effectiveness of this team, have them participate in an "instant aging program." Participants in such a program undergo activities that simulate disability:

1. Diminish vision by coating lenses with petroleum jelly.
2. Diminish tactile sensation by wearing cotton gloves.
3. Diminish auditory sensation by inserting ear plugs.

Participants are then required to do several tasks, such as:

1. Find a telephone number in a telephone directory.
2. Use a dial pay telephone.
3. Locate an unknown office in a strange building.
4. "Sit and wait" in an unknown area until a guide comes along.

After the staff has participated in these and various other tasks, discussing their feelings and ideas will help them understand their patients' problems.

Two aspects of treatment programs that should be stressed are patient control and patient performance. It is important to give the patient some control over his or her own therapy sessions, and respect should be shown for the patient's judgment. The staff is encouraged to place reasonable expectations on each patient and to expect appropriate behavior. Input from staff psychologists, physicians, social workers, nurses, and therapists is pooled to establish reasonable expectations and ways of achieving goals.

An important method used to motivate patients is peer pressure and interaction in a group, which facilitates increased awareness of the patient's problems through observing others with similar problems. Groups should be homogeneous. Individuals with skills that are too high or too low should be excluded, as should individuals who are disruptive. Group programs are designed so that patients will have some control over the environment. For example, the groups may designate their own leaders. In some, members decide which activities they will perform. This tends to increase the self-esteem of group members.

Organic Brain Syndrome

Rehabilitation and motivation of patients with organic brain syndrome is extremely difficult, since most rehabilitation programs depend on their ability to understand and follow one- or two-step commands, either verbalized or demonstrated, and carry over learned behaviors.

Special programs designed for these patients include a reality orientation program, sensory integration, and a progressive learning program in which activities are broken into components and patients are shown these activities in a stepwise sequence.

Sexuality

Many older people are still sexually active; almost all need and want companionship. Many centers separate people from their mates within a particular institution. Usually such separation occurs because one partner is functioning at a much higher level than the other. Occasionally, there are centers that allow such married couples to spend time with each other in quiet areas;

however, this is the exception and not the rule. Although helpful, this technique is only a partial solution. It is hoped that in the future, centers will be able to offer areas where patients may express their sexuality privately.

SPECIAL THERAPEUTIC ADAPTATIONS

In setting up treatment programs, the more functional a program is, the easier it is for a geriatric patient to participate. However, the modalities used are still essentially the same as for other age groups, even though at times equipment must be modified to insure the safety of the patient.

An example of a piece of equipment that has been modified for the elderly is the bicycle ergometer. Many older patients, because of balance and coordination problems, cannot use a treadmill for exercise and are afraid of using a bicycle. However, the bicycle can be modified in such a way that the patient feels secure riding it. This can be done by building a platform around the bike and having a special backrest to support the patient's back. The bicycle provides range of motion in the lower extremities with zero resistance, and builds up resistance for the patient's cardiac function. In practice, it is very difficult to exceed the patient's cardiac function using the bicycle ergometer. This is probably because most elderly patients have peripheral vascular disease, which limits the amount of work they can do before exceeding their cardiac capacity.

Another useful piece of equipment for a physical therapy program that deals with the geriatric patient is the Jobst compression therapy unit. This unit can be used to reduce leg edema and to decrease long-term foot pain in some patients. If both legs are edematous, care should be taken before treating the extremities simultaneously. If the patient has significant heart disease, treating both legs simultaneously might precipitate acute heart failure. Preoperative high-risk surgical patients should be taught bedside programs and deep breathing exercises. These can be continued into the postoperative period, to be fol-

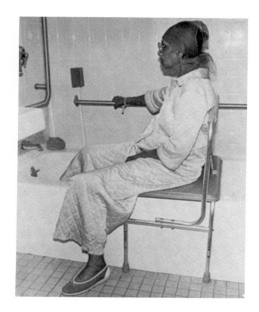

FIG. 21–3. Elderly patient transfers with assistance of tub seat and grab bars. [From Earls, K., Linville, L., Meltzer, M., Tornick-Bruch, H., and Wolfson, A. (1984): Occupational therapy. In: *Current Therapy in Physiatry: Physical Medicine and Rehabilitation*, edited by A. P. Ruskin. W. B. Saunders, Philadelphia.]

lowed by ambulation, stair climbing, and activities of daily living.

Gait training programs have to be tailored to the elderly. Most of these patients have some degree of ataxia (probably cerebrovascular) and numerous dizzy spells. Therefore, the appliance used should consider safety as well as cosmesis.

Suggest adaptive equipment for buttoning patients' shirts, pulling up zippers, or bathing. Evaluation of toilet and bath transfers (Fig. 21–3), as well as the use of a kitchen, is mandatory since direct evaluation will give valuable information which can be passed on to the family.

Comprehensive rehabilitation of the older patient does improve the quality of the patient's life by helping him or her achieve independence in the areas of ambulation and activities of daily living, which, in turn, enables living in a community setting for a longer period of time. Achieving this result requires a comprehensive rehabilitation team with special training in working with geriatric patients. This training should emphasize developing programs to motivate this particular patient population; however, most of the techniques used in geriatric therapy are standard ones that are also used in other rehabilitation programs.

SUGGESTED READINGS

Anderson, W. F. and Williams, W. B. (1983): *Practical Management of the Elderly,* 4th edit. Blackwell, Boston.

Covington, T. R. and Walker, J.I., eds. (1984): *Current Geriatric Therapy.* W. B. Saunders, Philadelphia.

Cutler, L. S. (1979): *The Mature Years: A Geriatric Occupational Therapy Text.* C. B. Slack, Thorofare, N J.

Ernst, N. S. and Glazer-Waldman, eds. (1983): *The Aged Patient: A Sourcebook for the Allied Health Professional.* Year Book, Chicago.

Gryfe, C. I. (1979): Reasonable expectations in geriatric rehabilitation. *J. Am. Geriatr. Soc.,* 27:238–248.

Hallas, G. (1979): Understanding aging, the physiology of growing older. *J. Practical Nursing,* 29:21–27.

Hamill, C. M., and Oliver, R. C. (1980): *Therapeutic Activities for the Handicapped Elderly.* Aspen Systems, Rockville, MD.

Liss, S. E. (1976): A graded and monitored exercise program for senior adults. *Tex. Med.,* 72:58–63.

Portnoi, V. A. (1980): What is a geriatrician? *JAMA,* 243:123–124.

Salsman, C., and Shader, R. I. (1978): Depression of the elderly. I. Possible drug etiologies: Differential diagnostic criteria. *J. Am. Geriatr. Soc.,* 26:303–308.

Strax, T., and Ledebur, J. C. (1979): Rehabilitation of the geriatric patient: Potentials and limitations. *Geriatrics,* 34:99–101.

Williams, T. F., ed. (1983): *Rehabilitation in the Aging.* Raven Press, New York.

and legs. Initially, the patient should do this once or twice a day by applying sustained pressure against the board for 5 sec, relaxing for 10 sec, and repeating the isometric contraction-relaxation three or four times. To achieve effective isometric contractions of the arm muscles, the patient should make a bilateral strong grip action for a few seconds with the arms extended. This exercise should take place at the same rate and frequency as the trunk and leg isometric exercises.

Skeletal System

The changes in the bones result mainly from the same functional disturbances affecting the muscular system. Metabolic activity in human bone relies heavily on the daily stresses and strains imposed by the pulling action of the tendons and by the force of gravity during the standing position. Inactivity and a prolonged stay in the horizontal position create profound changes in the skeletal system.

The most common changes are osteoporosis and joint fibrosis. Osteoporosis results not only from decreased muscular activity but also from complex endocrine and metabolic reactions (see section on Endocrine and Renal Systems). Fibrosis occurs whenever a joint is not subjected to active or passive motion. It becomes stiff, unable to go through a full range of motion, and, occasionally, irreversibly deformed. For example, the patient who has suffered a stroke frequently has trouble walking not because of paresis and spasticity but because of ankyloses of the hip and ankle that occur if the patient remains in a recumbent position with the hip slightly flexed and the ankle in plantar flexion.

Adequate positioning and range of motion exercises are necessary to prevent the skeletal changes that occur in immobilized, heavily sedated, or debilitated patients. Each joint of the extremities should be maintained in its functional position to avoid impaired range of motion and deformities. A judicious program of range of motion exercises consists of making three to five consecutive full range movements of each joint at least once (preferably twice) daily. The

bathing of the patient offers an excellent opportunity for the nurse or family member to achieve passive range of motion of nearly all the joints.

Cardiovascular System

The cardiovascular responses to immobilization are the consequences of autonomic, endocrine, metabolic, and physical influences. The net result is an impairment of the system's capacity to respond to metabolic demands above the basal state. Because physical deconditioning leads to the preponderance of the sympathetic or adrenergic system over the parasympathetic system, the basal heart rate increases and cardiac reserve decreases. Patients who remain in bed for several weeks, as well as paralyzed patients, typically show heart rates above 80 beats per minute. Maintaining a low basal heart rate is critical for sufficient coronary blood flow, which occurs mainly during the diastolic phase of the cardiac cycle, because only at low rates is the diastolic phase longer than the systolic phase. The opposite occurs at high rates. For example, at 60 beats per minute the systole time is 0.40 sec and the diastole 0.60 sec, whereas at 150 beats per minute the systole time is 0.25 sec and the diastole 0.15 sec. This greatly diminished cardiac reserve prevents even limited physical effort, which may cause marked tachycardia and anginal pain.

Orthostatic hypotension and phlebothrombosis both result from the insufficient constricture of the arterioles and venules of the legs during prolonged bed rest. Orthostatic hypotension occurs in spite of the increased adrenergic state. When a deconditioned person attempts to sit up or stand up, blood pools in the lower extremities, the circulating blood volume and the venous return decrease, and the stroke volume may be too small to achieve adequate cerebral irrigation. In some instances, the blood pressure reaches levels as low as 60/30 mm Hg within 10 to 20 sec of sitting with legs hanging unsupported at the side of the bed. Blood pools in the lower extremities because the arterioles and venules of the legs do not constrict sufficiently to offset the effect of gravity on the column of blood that falls from the heart to the feet. Thus, there is increased hydrostatic pressure in the capillary bed, extravasation of fluid in the interstitial tissue, and dependent edema. Venous stasis coupled with disturbed clotting are the major influences in the pathogenesis of phlebothrombosis.

The programs of muscular exercise previously described are helpful in preventing severe cardiovascular deconditioning. Yet, exhausting the patient by imposing excessive metabolic demands should be avoided. During bed rest, it is wise to maintain the patient's heart rate at less than 120 beats per minute while he or she is performing isotonic or isometric exercises.

Individuals who are not paralyzed should gradually assume the sitting and the standing postures as soon as feasible. The first attempts to sit up should consist of propping up the head of the bed at gradually increasing angles while keeping the patient's legs horizontal. As the patient begins to sit at the edge of the bed and to stand up, orthostatic hypotension is discouraged by wearing elastic stockings, which prevent stasis of the blood and edema.

If paralysis or some other disabling condition prevents sitting up, imposing the effect of gravity on the body through passive assumption of the upright posture on a tilt-table (Fig. 22–4) is advised. Initially, the patient should remain at a slight degree of tilt (30°) for 1 min, then the duration of tilt should be gradually increased to 30 min twice a day. As the patient's tolerance improves, the degree of tilt is increased by 5 to 10 degrees every week until the 70° position is maintained for 30 min twice a day.

Respiratory System

Changes accompanying those in the cardiovascular system include decreased vital capacity and maximal voluntary ventilation. Often reflecting an overall decrease in muscle strength, general deconditioning of the respiratory muscle results in decreased vital capacity. Indeed, supine patients seldom contract the intercostals, diaphragms, and abdominal muscles to accomplish a maximum inspiration or a forceful expiration. The capacity of the chest to achieve

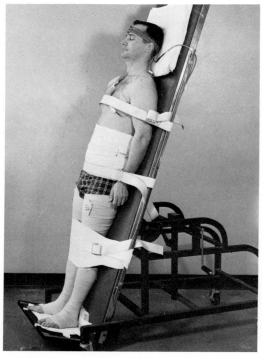

FIG. 22–4. Gradual elevation on the tilt-table helps patient develop cardiovascular tolerance to the upright position. [From Kottke, F. J. (1982): Therapeutic exercise to develop neuromuscular coordination. In *Krusen's Handbook of Physical Medicine and Rehabilitation*, edited by F. J. Kottke et al. W. B. Saunders, Philadelphia.]

maximum inspiration may decline even further if, in addition, the costovertebral and costochrondral joints are not submitted to a full range of motion and they become fixed in an expiratory position. Thus, there is a marked reduction in the total lung capacity, including vital capacity, inspiratory capacity, expiratory reserve volume, functional residual capacity, and residual volume. A nonparalyzed person who does not carry out a program of respiratory exercises may experience a 25% to 50% decrease in vital capacity and in maximal voluntary ventilation after several weeks of bed rest.

The prescription of respiratory exercises is essential in the treatment of immobilized patients. The bedridden patients should take three to five slow, deep breaths at least every hour while awake. Forced expiration should accompany each maximum inspiratory effort to maintain all lung compartments at a normal level. The intercostals and the diaphragms must be used equally to achieve full inspiration. By concentrating on expanding the abdomen during inspiration, the individual learns to contract both diaphragms, which lowers their position and pushes the viscera against the abdominal wall. If the abdominal muscles are weak, a good contraction of the diaphragms significantly expands the abdomen because the flabby abdominal wall provides little resistance. If the patient has respiratory muscle paralysis with a decrease in vital capacity below 60% of normal, three to five passive lung inflations should be performed twice daily with a positive pressure apparatus at high settings of pressure, flow, and volume.

Digestive Apparatus

An overall decrease in gastrointestinal activity affects not only the motility but also the secretory functions of the salivary glands, pancreas, and other digestive glands. Common gastrointestinal problems caused by immobilization include anorexia and constipation. Decreased caloric demand, as well as endocrine changes, anxiety, and depression often interact to produce anorexia. Constricted sphincters and inhibited peristalsis, compounded by increased intestinal absorption of water and a diet low in fluid and fiber content, contribute to constipation. Frequently, constipation is severe enough to cause fecal impaction.

Adequate nutrition and fluid intake are the prophylactic mainstays of severe digestive and metabolic complications of immobilization. The caloric intake should be commensurate with the metabolic needs of the bedridden patient. Excessive caloric intake is rare because the patient's inactive state inhibits appetite. The diet should have a high fiber content to facilitate bowel movements. A stool softener such as dioctyl sodium sulfosuccinate may help prevent constipation and fecal impaction.

A daily diet containing approximately 10 mg/kg of calcium and 1 g/kg of protein helps minimize osteoporosis and hypoproteinemia in the non-paralyzed individual. In cases of hypoproteinemia, the protein content should be raised to approximately 1.5 g/kg/day. Paralyzed patients inevitably experience extensive, unpreventable osteoporosis. These patients, who frequently have a concomitant urinary tract infection and renal stasis, do not require a calcium supplement since excessive calcium intake may contribute to hypercalciuria and to renal lithiasis.

Endocrine and Renal Systems

In the immobilized patient, diuresis and natriuresis increase initially due to a temporary rise in intravascular volume, hypercalciuria occurs, and renal lithiasis may result, in conjunction with the other systemic changes. As diuresis increases, natriuresis also increases to maintain the plasma osmolality at a normal level. Hypercalciuria results from the active mobilization of calcium from the bone matrix into the blood and the eventual urinary excretion of the excess calcium. Also contributing to hypercalciuria is the excessive release of adrenal corticosteroids when, trying to sit or stand, the immobilized patient develops orthostatic hypotension. These conditions, aggravated by an attempt to compensate for the decrease in circulating blood volume, trigger the release of fluid-retaining hormones (ADH, aldosterone, cortisol).

Increased calciuria, urinary stasis, and urinary tract infection constitute a dangerous triad that may lead to the production of calculi in the renal pelvis or lower urinary tract. Renal lithiasis is magnified in paralyzed persons who have had catheter drainage for several days or weeks because preventing or controlling a urinary tract infection is difficult.

An adequate diet and fluid intake will help minimize endocrine and renal problems in the immobilized patient. The caloric intake must be proportional to the patient's level of activity, body temperature, and general nutritional status. In the absence of depression or anxiety, the patient's appetite usually is proportional to the required caloric intake. If the diet is nutritious and varied, there is little need for vitamin supplements. To prevent urinary complications, fluid intake should be increased unless the heart muscle would be taxed by cardiac problems. The initial diuresis of immobilization may be negligible if the patient is receiving intravenous fluid replacement. Since increased natriuresis is often transient sodium supplements are unnecessary.

Integumentary System

Immobilization affects the skin and adnexa by producing atrophy and pressure sores. Structural changes affecting the consistency of the subcutaneous tissues and dermis gradually diminish turgor. Insufficient appetite and inadequate nutrition may exacerbate the loss of subcutaneous fat and changes in skin turgor. Poor hygiene may lead to bacterial or fungal infections and to ingrown toenails.

Pressure sores, one of the most common manifestations of prolonged immobilization, are discussed in detail in Chapter 23. Extensive bed sores severely diminish serum protein, especially albumin. At the capillary level, the decrease in serum protein represents a drop in oncotic pressure. This facilitates extravasation of fluid to the extracellular space in dependent areas of the body or in the feet and ankles when the individual gets up from the bed. The extravasation in turn leads to a decreased circulating blood volume and to orthostatic hypotension.

Scrupulous skin hygiene of the immobilized patient is crucial. Cleansing and massaging the skin thoroughly will help maintain good turgor and avoid infections, particularly in the skin of the dependent areas that undergo constant pressure against the lying surface. Fingernails and toenails should be trimmed frequently. When immobilization is due to paralysis, the patient's position should be changed periodically in order to prevent prolonged, excessive pressure on the skin of the dependent areas. An accepted schedule is to shift the body from one side to the back and from the back to the other side every 2 to 4 hr.

SUGGESTED READINGS

Asher, R. A. (1983): The dangers of going to bed. *Crit. Care Update*, 10:40–41,50.

Claus-Walker, J., and Halstead, L. S. (1981, 1982): Metabolic and endocrine changes in spinal cord injury, Parts I–IV. *Arch. Phys. Med. Rehabil.*, 62:595–601, 63:569–580, 63:628–631, 63:632–638.

Convertino, V. A., Hung, D. J., Goldwater, D. J., et al. (1982): Cardiorespiratory responses to exercise in middle-aged men following 10 days of bed rest. *Circulation*, 65:134–140.

DeBusk, R. F., Convertino, V. A., Hung, J., and Goldwater, D. (1983): Exercise conditioning in middle-aged men after 10 days of bed rest. *Circulation*, 68:245–250.

Greenleaf, J. E., and Kozlowski, S. (1982): Physiological consequences of reduced physical activity during bed rest. *Exerc. Sport Sci. Rev.*, 10:84–119.

Greenleaf, J. E., VanBeumont, W., Convertino, V. A., and Starr, J. C. (1983): Handgrip and general muscular strength and endurance during prolonged bedrest with isometric and isotonic leg exercise training. *Aviat. SpaceEnviron. Med.*, 54:696–700.

Krølner, B. and Toft, B. (1983): Vertebral bone loss: An unheeded side effect of therapeutic bed rest. *Clin. Sci.*, 64:537–540.

Kottke, F. J. (1966): The effects of limitation of activity upon the human body. *JAMA*, 196:117–122.

Schneider, V. S. and McDonald, J. (1984): Skeletal calcium homeostasis and countermeasures to prevent disuse osteoporosis. *Calcif. Tissue Int.* 36(Suppl.):S151–S164.

Spencer, W. A., Vallbona, C., and Carter, R. E. (1965): Physiologic concepts of immobilization. *Arch. Phys. Med. Rehabil.*, 46:89–100.

Steinberg, F. U. (1980): *The Immobilized Patient. Functional Pathology and Management.* Plenum Publishing Co., New York.

Whedon, G. D. (1984): Disuse osteoporosis: physiological aspects. *Calcif. Tissue Int.* 36(Suppl):S146–S150.

Medical Rehabilitation,
edited by L. S. Halstead et al.
Raven Press, New York © 1985.

CHAPTER 23

Pressure Sores

Katie D. Irani

Physical Medicine Service, Ben Taub General Hospital, and Department of Physical Medicine, Baylor College of Medicine, Houston, Texas 77030

Pressure sores or ischemic ulcers are areas of cellular necrosis, usually occurring over bony prominences, caused by external pressure exceeding the capillary pressure for prolonged periods of time. They are often called decubitus ulcers, a misnomer because the patient does not have to be lying down to develop these ulcers.

EPIDEMIOLOGY

The occurrence of pressure sores is rising as the number of elderly people with associated dementia and chronic illnesses increases and more patients survive spinal cord and brain injuries. The healing of pressure sores may require many months of preventable hospitalization. The treatment of a pressure sore can cost from $10,000 to $50,000 in 1982 dollars.

Although pressure sores can affect anyone, certain types of patients are predisposed to ulceration. At high risk are geriatric patients with a broken hip, individuals with a tight-fitting, poorly applied plaster cast, or patients with anesthetic skin and poor cerebration who do not respond to undue pressure by changing position. The risk is considered chronic when the cause of immobility is persistent and transient when immobility is temporary. Therefore, the recurrence rate of pressure sores is very high in patients with brain damage, spinal cord injury, or multiple sclerosis. Younger individuals who are obtunded with drugs or have ill-fitting splints, casts, or shoes tend to develop transient sores.

CLASSIFICATION

Pressure sores are classified by site and by the depth of the tissue involved. The typical site

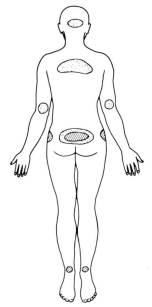

FIG. 23–1. Areas of immediate risk *(striped)* from pressure sores and areas that may also break down *(stippled)* when potentiating factors are strong. [From Barton, A. A. (1976): The pathogenesis of skin wounds due to pressure. In: *Bedsore Biomechanics*, edited by R. M. Kennedi, J. M. Cowden, and J. T. Scales, University Park Press, Baltimore.]

is over an underlying bony prominence against which external pressure compresses the intermediate skin and soft tissues (Fig. 23–1). Although the sacral ulcer (Fig. 23-2A) is the most common type occurring in the recumbent patient, breakdown can occur at the heels (Fig. 23-2B) and the inferior angle of the scapulae in a severely debilitated patient. Lying on the side may break down the skin over the greater trochanters and

TABLE 23–1. *Pathophysiology of decubitus ulcers*

Primary factors	Contributing factors
Pressure	Malnutrition
Shear forces	Anemia
	Edema
	Sensory loss
	Motor paralysis
	Dementia
	Maceration
	Sepsis

lateral malleoli, while prolonged sitting often breaks down the skin over the ischial tuberosities. Figure 23–3 shows the classification of pressure sores according to the depth of tissue involvement.

ETIOLOGY

Effects of Time, Pressure, and Friction

The primary causes of pressure sores are prolonged pressure exceeding the normal capillary pressure from about 25 to 32 mm Hg and shearing forces (Table 23–1). Patients who shift position often, either consciously or subconsciously, seldom develop pressure sores, even during sleep, because pressure is insufficient in duration to produce ulceration.

When external pressure rises beyond the normal capillary pressure, ischemia and anoxia of the tissues result. This leads to acidosis, which increases capillary permeability and extravasation. Further increases in the intensity and/or duration of the pressure escalate interference with tissue metabolism. Eventually, necrosis of the underlying soft tissues occurs.

These effects of the pressure force increase as the surface on which pressure is exerted becomes smaller. A pressure gradient exists from the surface, or skin, to the bone in a cone-shaped manner, resulting in a relatively smaller area of skin necrosis with a much wider area of the soft tissue breakdown in the deeper layers of fat and muscle tissue (Fig. 23–4).

While pressure exerts a perpendicular force on the soft tissues, shearing produces a parallel force similar to the sliding or pulling that creates friction. In normal daily activities, the elasticity of the soft tissues, enabling them to stretch, compensates for the applied shear forces. In a disabled person, however, these shear forces may also tear tissue; hence, capillary destruction with resultant ischemia and tissue necrosis occurs.

Predisposing Factors

Although the factors listed in Table 23–1 alone do not cause ulceration, they predispose the debilitated patient to tissue breakdown.

Malnutrition

A well-nourished tissue, more viable than poorly nourished tissue, can better withstand the effects of pressure and ischemia. Any illness or injury profoundly alters body metabolism. Negative nitrogen balance is even more pronounced in a severe insult, which may lead to hypoproteinemia, anemia, and emaciation. The resultant loss of protective soft-tissue covering increases susceptibility to pressure sores in the bony prominences.

Anemia

When pressure causes ischemia, the possibility of this ischemic tissue surviving is greatly enhanced if the impoverished blood supply is offset by normal hemoglobin content and oxygen supply. In the presence of anemia, the oxygen content of the blood decreases, further compromising cellular metabolism.

Edema

With edema, the extra interstitial fluid increases the distance between the capillary and the cell. Because the rate of diffusion of oxygen and food from the capillary to the cell decreases with increasing distance, edema further depletes cellular nutrition and potentiates tissue breakdown.

Sensory Loss and Motor Paralysis

Pressure ulcers are common in patients with neurological deficits. Patients with a sensory

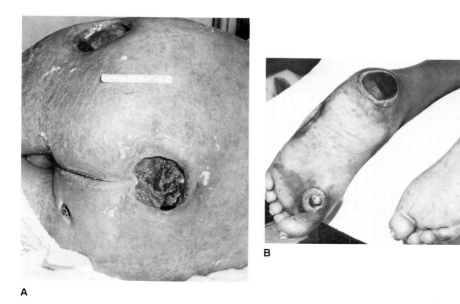

FIG. 23–2. Typical sites of pressure sores. **A:** Sacral ulcer. [From Scales, J. T. (1976): Pressure on the patient. In: *Bedsore Biomechanics*, edited by R. M. Kennedi, J. M. Cowden, and J. T. Scales. University Park Press, Baltimore.] **B:** Lateral malleolar, heel, and plantar ulcers. [From Constantian, M. B. (1980): *Pressure Ulcers: Principles and Techniques of Management.* Little, Brown, Boston.]

loss fail to change positions because they cannot perceive the pressure and pain, whereas patients with a motor loss may be able to feel the pressure and pain but cannot move to shift position. Sensory loss is more critical than motor loss; ulcers are rare in poliomyelitic patients, who can respond to discomfort by asking a caretaker to move them, compared with the high occurrence in patients with spinal cord injuries.

Maceration and Senile Dementia

Maceration and senile dementia often interact to produce pressure sores. These conditions are frequently seen in nursing homes, where patients often cannot think clearly and where nursing care may be less than optimal. Incontinent or profusely perspiring patients may lie for long periods of time in wet areas. When severe maceration of the skin results, minimal shearing or pressure breaks down the skin.

PREVENTION

Most pressure sores can be prevented through meticulous care of the patient, as well as edu-cation of the patient, family, and health care staff. The patient should be turned frequently and lifted gently, never dragged. The skin should be kept clean and dry and inspected with each turn for early signs of impending skin breakdown. The sheets should be clean and free of wrinkles. Good nutrition is also essential.

Recognition of Imminent Skin Breakdown

Erythema of the skin, which blanches when pressed, is the earliest sign of imminent skin breakdown. Unless pressure on the area is relieved immediately, the condition progresses to include inflammation and erythema that does not blanch when pressed, and the skin and underlying tissue become indurated. Frank breakdown is still preventable at this stage by turning the patient or shifting weight. However, these signs of imminent breakdown are not always predictive; some ulcers present no visible warning signs until extensive internal tissue destruction has already occurred.

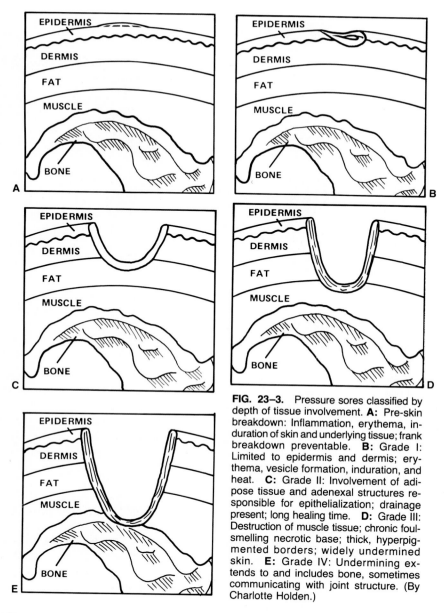

FIG. 23–3. Pressure sores classified by depth of tissue involvement. **A:** Pre-skin breakdown: Inflammation, erythema, induration of skin and underlying tissue; frank breakdown preventable. **B:** Grade I: Limited to epidermis and dermis; erythema, vesicle formation, induration, and heat. **C:** Grade II: Involvement of adipose tissue and adenexal structures responsible for epithelialization; drainage present; long healing time. **D:** Grade III: Destruction of muscle tissue; chronic foul-smelling necrotic base; thick, hyperpigmented borders; widely undermined skin. **E:** Grade IV: Undermining extends to and includes bone, sometimes communicating with joint structure. (By Charlotte Holden.)

Skin Hygiene

Agents chosen for skin hygiene should keep the skin clean and dry, but without depleting the natural, protective oils. Alcohol is commonly used for its drying effect. If a skin lotion such as Alpha Keri or Vaseline Intensive Care Lotion is used for dryness, it must be rubbed in thoroughly so that the skin does not remain wet and susceptible to maceration. If a plastic or rubber sheet is used over the mattress, which tends to cause excessive perspiration, special care must be taken to avoid maceration of the skin.

Relief of Pressure

Prolonged pressure should be avoided. If the patient is sitting, he must do push-ups in the

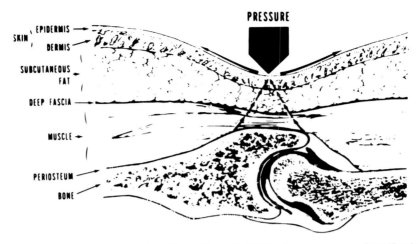

FIG. 23–4. Cone effect of pressure gradient. [From Shea, D. (1975): Pressure sores—Classification and management. *Clin. Orthop.*, 112:90, with permission of J. B. Lippincott.]

chair or move from side to side as often as every 10 to 15 min. If the patient is in bed, he should turn often; if unable to turn himself, he should be turned to all four positions (front, back, and each side), in sequence, every 2 hr. Patients with multiple risk factors should be turned more frequently. Mechanically operated beds such as the Stryker frame and Roto-Rest bed (Fig. 23–5A) facilitate turning the patient but too often lead to negligence in turning the patient often enough. For example, patients often develop pressure sores on the heels if left upright in the CircOelectric bed for more than 2 hr.

Cushions and Beds

Various kinds of cushions, mattresses, and beds are available to help prevent pressure sores by distributing the pressure more evenly over a large surface (Fig. 23–5). The simplest cushion is an air cushion. Other cushions are made with silicone, platinum silicone gel, foam rubber, water, and combinations of these. Some flotation devices are effective in distributing pressure, but moving around is difficult, and some patients complain of seasickness or experience sensory deprivation syndrome. These problems can be minimized by using beds that can be adjusted to remove the patient from flotation temporarily. A few of the available cushions and

mattresses are described in Tables 23–2 and 23–3.

Pads

Pads in a variety of shapes and contours for different parts of the body, such as the heels and elbows, are available for home as well as institutional use.

Sheepskin, acrylic, and lamb's wool pads can be placed over an ordinary mattress, with the woolly side contacting the patient's skin. These pads remain wrinkle-free, allow air to circulate, and prevent shearing more than they distribute pressure. A simple water cushion can be made by half filling rubber gloves or a beach ball with water to cushion small areas such as the heels. Similarly, a standard camper's mattress can be nearly filled with water and placed over a regular mattress. Relatively inexpensive and readily available, this water mattress is well-suited for use in nursing homes or in the patient's home.

With or without a cushion, the wheelchair should be adjusted so that the posterior part of the thighs bears some weight. If the foot plates are too high, the thighs are raised off of the seat and the pressure is concentrated in a small area over the ischial tuberosities. This greatly increases the danger of early breakdown of the tissue and resultant pressure sores.

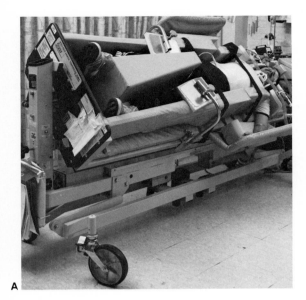

FIG. 23–5. Beds that reduce pressure build-up. **A:** Roto-Rest bed turns from one side to other to shift patient's weight away from high-pressure areas. (By Gordon Stanley.) **B:** Lobuoy hydrofloat water bed, in addition to promoting healing of pressure sores by regulating temperature to reduce metabolic demand, is also at same height as standard wheelchair to facilitate independent transfers. (Courtesy of The Jobst Institute, Inc., Toledo, OH 43694.)

A

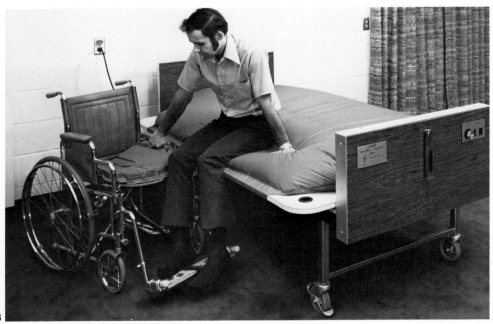

B

TABLE 23–2. *Comparison of cushions commonly used to prevent pressure sores*

Brand	Type	Weight	Cost (1983 $)	Comments
Bye-bye decubiti	Air-filled	2–4 lb	26	Balancing difficult for quadriplegics, but suitable for paraplegics; easily punctured, especially by pets; quadriplegics may not notice air leakage; not always easy to transfer
ROHO	Multiple air-filled pouches	Light	230–250	Same as above; can be filled in halves
Aquaseat	Flotation	7 lb	65	Heavy, durable, cumbersome; can be punctured
Comfort	Flotation	Heavy	60	Punctures easily; heavy
Stryker	Gel flotation	14 lb	250–290	Expensive; heavy
Action	Gel flotation	12 lb	130	Heavy; difficult to adjust to other cushions after this one is used
Temper foam	Polymer foam	3–4 lb	40–60	Easy to transfer; cracks, especially in warm, humid climate; can be wedged
Scimedics	Polymer foam	3 lb	35–45	U-shaped, factory cut-out
Vasio-para	Sheepskin-covered foam	Light	50	Contoured to redistribute weight away from bony prominences of sitting areas to muscle-covered areas; reduces urethral blockage; deters abductor and extensor spasticity; easy to transfer
Hydro-float	Water-filled	22–25 lb	100	Contoured cut-out; heavy

TREATMENT

Nutrition

Good nutrition with a high-calorie diet rich in proteins, vitamins, and minerals should be maintained. To maintain hemoglobin levels at 12 g/100 ml or above, blood transfusions may occasionally be required when dietary supplements are inadequate.

Local Care

An ulcer needs daily local care to remove necrotic tissue, prevent infection, contract the wound, and promote epithelialization (Fig. 23–6). Several remedies have been used with varying degrees of success. However, the agent selected is not as important as the persistence and care with which these ulcers are dressed. Saline, potassium permanganate, boric acid, pHisoHex®, Betadine®, Daykins® solution, magnesium sulphate, antibiotic ointments, and multiple enzymatic (e.g., Elase®) and mechanical debriding agents may be used in the care of pressure sores.

The simplest treatment for wounds requiring minor debridement is to wet a Kerlix bandage with normal saline, pack the ulcer, let it dry from 4 to 6 hr, and then remove the dry dressing. The necrotic material is removed as it sticks to the dry dressing. To discourage bacterial contamination, this wet-to-dry dressing needs to be changed at least three or four times a day. It should be discontinued once the wound has begun to epithelialize, however, to avoid stripping new epithelial cells from the sore.

If the surface of the ulcer looks shiny, it is probably infected with *Pseudomonas* and requires soaking in a weak (0.25%) acetic acid solution. Actual scraping of the granulation tissue, rather than merely swabbing the area, is necessary to obtain an adequate culture.

Local antibiotics, which tend to keep the skin soft, moist, and maceration-prone, are useless in the treatment of pressure sores. Because systemic antibiotics do not reach the granulation tissue, they are indicated only in the presence of cellulitis or systemic infection, which may progress to life-threatening sepsis.

Hydrotherapy in the whirlpool or Hubbard tank accelerates the removal of necrotic debris, as well as the resolution of any induration in

TABLE 23–3. *Comparison of beds commonly used to prevent or treat pressure sores*

Brand or type	Description	Weight	Cost (1983 $)	Comments
Water bed	Big bath tub filled with water	Very heavy	4,000	Most effective in treatment, but sensory deprivation and seasickness; some patients become mildly psychotic; nursing care difficult
Mud bed	Filled with oil-well drilling, mud-like material	Very heavy, 1,800 lb	Expensive	Good results; nursing care difficult
Foam egg-crate mattress	Foam	Light	60–80	Good distribution of pressure with 4-inch thickness; not very satisfactory results with 2-inch thickness; nursing care easy; good aeration
Stryker frame	Horizontal turning frame	Light		Easy to turn patient; no spine loading; side-lying impossible
CircOelectric bed	Electrically operated		Expensive	Patient brought to vertical position with spine loading and pressure on damaged vertebra; breaks down heels
Foam mattress and mattress with gel pad in center		Light	Relatively inexpensive	Effective treatment
Hydro-float bed	Water-filled	Heavy	3,500–4,000	Patient buoyed up by regulated amount of water
Camper's mattress	Water-filled	Medium	Inexpensive	Water buoyancy; easy nursing care; no nausea
Akros DFD (damped fluid displacement) mattress	Gel-controlled flotation	Light	Relatively inexpensive	Eliminates motion sickness; self-adjusts to weight shifting; allows patient better bed mobility than water or air mattress

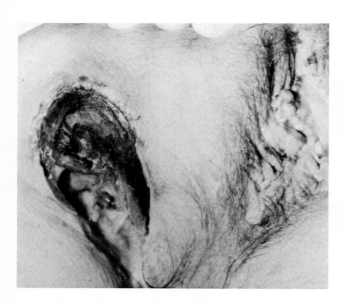
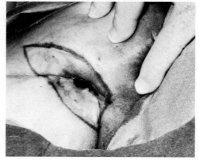

FIG. 23–6. Daily local care of grade III pressure sore prepares wound for successful ischiectomy. **Left:** Deep ischial ulcer with erosion into bursa. **Right:** Contraction of ulcer to more easily managed size. [From Constantian, M. B. (1980): *Pressure Ulcers: Principles and Techniques of Management.* Little, Brown, and Co., Boston.]

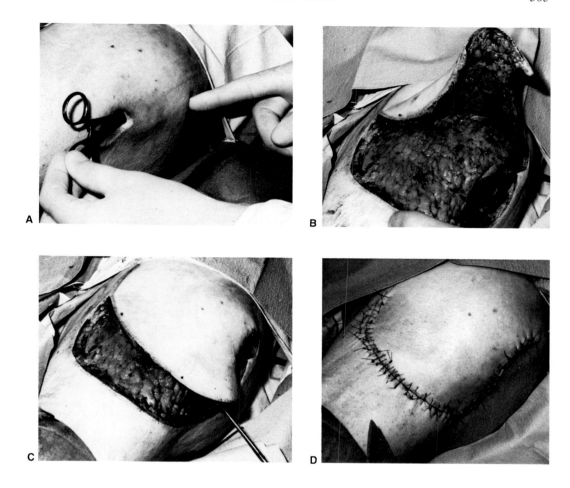

FIG. 23–7. Surgical closure of trochanteric ulcer. **A:** 10-cm proximal extension of ulcer from hemostat to surgeon's fingertip. **B:** Ulcer excised and flap elevated. **C:** Transfer of flap. **D:** Closure of wound. [From Constantian, M. B. (1980): *Pressure Ulcers: Principles and Techniques of Management.* Little, Brown, Boston.]

big, deep, and multiple ulcers. PHisoHex® or Betadine® may be added to the water.

Infrared lamps are beneficial for drying the wound. At home, an electric hair dryer can be substituted. The hose is directed at the ulcer, about 6 to 8 inches away, for 15 to 20 min. Although this technique accelerates healing, caution should be taken to avoid over-drying, which can crack the surrounding skin.

Ultraviolet lamps promote the healing of pressure sores by sterilizing and exfoliating the skin.

Sun lamps are available for home use. The dose should be regulated carefully to prevent burning.

Stages of Healing

The outcome of conservative treatment can be gauged by monitoring the progress of healing. There are three stages of healing in grades I and II pressure sores:

1. **Stage 1:** Exudative—Infiltration of tissues with edema and an inflammatory reaction.

2. **Stage 2:** Phagocytic—Formation of granulation tissue.
3. **Stage 3:** Reparative—Occurrence of reepithelialization. Depending on the initial depth of destruction, this area of repair is often void of hair and sweat glands.

Surgical Therapy

Grade III and grade IV ulcers usually require surgical treatment. If the eschar is slightly elevated above the skin, the ulcer is likely to be superficial with epithelialization taking place underneath. If the eschar is below the wound, the ulcer is deep and the only epithelialization is from the periphery. This type of ulcer requires a graft. The following are general indications for surgical repair of pressure sores:

1. Extensive undermining of skin.
2. Meager subcutaneous tissue.
3. Large ulcer extending into chronically inflamed, thick-walled ischial or trochanteric bursa.
4. Unusual local bony anatomy.

The following preparations are necessary before the patient undergoes surgery. The skin should be clean, and granulation tissue must be present. The patient should be in a good nutritional state, although sometimes hypoproteinemia cannot be corrected because of excessive loss of protein from a big ulcer. An attempt should be made to eliminate spasm with antispasmodic drugs such as diazepam (Valium®), dantrolene sodium (Dantrium®), or baclofen (Lioresal®). Spasms tend to increase the chance of postoperative hematoma formation under the flap.

The basic purposes of surgery for pressure ulcers are to cover the area, increase the blood supply, and pad the area to discourage recurrence of ulcers. The usual surgical procedures are split-thickness skin grafts, rotational flaps with neurovascular supply intact, and, in the case of extensive ulceration, salvage surgery often involving amputation. The flap should be large enough to be used again to cover secondary ulcers, which tend to recur. If enlarged, thick-walled, or calcified bursae underlie the sore, they must be excised to discourage the recurrence of ulcers over the ischial tuberosities or greater trochanters. Figure 23–7 shows a typical surgical flap procedure to close a trochanteric ulcer.

SUGGESTED READINGS

Blincharz, M. (1979): Interventions that promote decubiti healing. In: *Current Practice in the Nursing Care of the Adult.* edited by M. S. Kennedy, and G. M. Pfeifer. C. V. Mosby, St. Louis.

Constantian, M. B., editor (1980): *Pressure Ulcers: Principles and Techniques of Management.* Little, Brown and Co., Boston.

Dindsdale, S. M. (1974): Decubitus ulcers: Role of pressure and friction in causation. *Arch. Phys. Med. Rehabil.,* 55:147–152.

Enis, J., and Sarminento, A. (1973): The pathophysiology and management of pressure sores. *Orthop. Rev.,* 2:25–34.

Horsley, J. A., editor (1981): *Preventing Decubitis Ulcers.* Grune and Stratton, New York.

Kennedy, R. M., Cowden, J. M., and Scales, J. T., editors (1976): *Bedsore Biomechanics.* University Park Press, Baltimore.

Kosiak, M. (1982): Prevention and rehabilitation of ischemic ulcers. In: *Krusen's Handbook of Physical Medicine and Rehabilitation,* edited by F. J. Kottke, G. K. Stillwell, and J. F. Lehmann. W. B. Saunders, Philadelphia.

Moolten, S. E. (1972): Bedsores in the chronically ill patient. *Arch. Phys. Med. Rehabil.,* 53:430–438.

Parish, L. C., Witowski, J. A., and Crissey, J. T. (1983): *The Decubitus Ulcer.* Masson, New York.

Pierce, D., and Nickel, V., editors (1977): *The Total Care of Spinal Cord Injuries.* Little Brown and Co., Boston.

Zacharkow, D. (1984): *Wheelchair Posture and Pressure Sores.* Charles C Thomas, Springfield, Illinois.

Medical Rehabilitation,
edited by L. S. Halstead et al.
Raven Press, New York © 1985.

CHAPTER 24

Spasticity

Paul C. Sharkey

Department of Rehabilitation, Baylor College of Medicine, Houston, Texas 77030

Spasticity is characterized by hyperactive deep tendon reflexes, abnormal spinal reflexes, hypertonic muscles, and muscle spasms in flexion or extension. When involved muscles are manipulated rapidly, increased resistance to stretch occurs. Commonly observed in patients with upper motor neuron dysfunction, this condition may also produce such signs as muscle cramps, spasms, fasciculations, rigidity, dystonia, athetosis, and ataxia. Findings associated with spasticity imply the existence of an underlying neurological disorder. Spasticity is an expected component of most cases of spinal cord injury, but may also accompany the following medical disorders:

1. Cerebrovascular disorders involving cortex or brain stem.
2. Head injuries resulting in cortical or brain stem damage.
3. Spinal cord injuries: any lesion, complete or incomplete, traumatic or otherwise, above the conus medullaris.
4. Demyelinating disorders, such as multiple sclerosis or transverse myelitis.
5. Amyotrophic lateral sclerosis.
6. Cerebral palsy.
7. Metabolic disorders, such as Tay-Sachs disease or metachromatic leukodystrophy.
8. Vitamin B_{12} deficiency, with subacute combined degeneration.

Decisions about managing spasticity are difficult: a method that improves the functioning of one patient may prevent another from performing essential everyday activities. Similarly, a method that is effective 3 months after injury or in the early stages of a disease may be counterproductive a year later. The constant muscle contraction stimulates the periosteum and retards osteoporotic activity, but, paradoxically, may lead to the formation of immobilizing joint contractures. While spastic lower limb and trunk muscles help improve balance for transfers and ambulation, spasticity is often so severe that it impedes exercise programs, self-care and hygiene, and wheelchair transfers. Therefore, when selecting a therapeutic modality, consider not only the initial cause of spasticity but also its severity and the likely functional consequences.

CLINICAL CLASSIFICATION

To facilitate the selection of an appropriate treatment plan, spasticity can be classified as cerebral or spinal in origin and as mild, moderate, or severe. The neurological and functional consequences of the mildest to the most severe spasticity associated with cerebral and spinal lesions are described in Tables 24–1 and 24–2. The pathophysiological differences among the different types of spasticity cause differences in the degree of muscle resistance to passive stretch and affect the presence or absence of clonus and tendon jerks.

Mild spasticity, which affects only muscles that normally contract reflexively, is characterized by slight muscle resistance or catch toward the end of rapid stretching. Because of slight hypertonia, more generalized or less stimulation is required to elicit tendon jerk. Resistance to stretch is greatly increased in severe spasticity.

TABLE 24–1. *Neurological and functional consequences of spasticity associated with cerebral lesions*

	Neurological consequences		Resistance of muscle to passive stretch	Functional consequences
	Tendon jerks	Clonus		
Mild	Absent or hypoactive	Absent	Minimal	In absence of volitional activity, lack of reflex muscular tone may impede upright postural support needed for transfers and may lead to shoulder subluxation
	Active or mildly hyperactive	Absent or unsustained	Moderate	Diminished reflex muscular tone may affect postural support; mild to moderately increased reflex activity may cause early dysfunctional effects, e.g., equinovarus posture during gait
	Hyperactive	Sustained	Marked	Severe irradiating clonus can interfere with transfers and dressing and cause psychological distress; postural shortening of physiological extensors (antigravity muscles) may result in dysfunctional deformities such as equinovarus of foot and severe wrist and finger flexion; synergy patterns often helpful in locomotor activities; marked resistance to passive stretch can hinder therapeutic exercise programs and compromise volitional movement
Severe	Active or hypoactive	Mild or absent	Marked	Impaired use of braces; cosmetic deformities

TABLE 24–2. *Neurological and functional consequences of spasticity associated with spinal lesions*

	Neurological consequences		Resistance of muscle to passive stretch	Functional consequences
Type	Tendon jerks	Clonus		
Mild	Absent	Absent	Minimal	Absent reflex support of postural activities; absent protective withdrawal reactions to noxious stimuli
	Hypoactive to active	Absent or unsustained	Minimal	Mainly phasic flexor limb movements that intermittently impede transfers, sleep, dressing, sexual function, use of braces; limb manipulation may be aided by triggering flexor responses
	Active to hyperactive	Sustained or unsustained	Moderate (usually flexor muscle predominance)	Mainly phasic responses of greater duration, intensity, and frequency, and mainly tonic (sustained) activity can cause major hindrances in transfers, dressing, bed positioning, wheelchair activities, therapeutic exercise programs, sexual function, bracing, and ambulation; tonic muscular spasms may be used for postural support
	Hypoactive to hyperactive (dependent on degree of rigidity)	Sustained, unsustained, or absent	Marked (proximal flexor and/or extensor muscle predominance)	
Severe	Active or hypoactive	May be present in distal muscles	Marked	Proximal muscle contracture impairing bed positioning, wheelchair transfers, and brace use

As a result of increased tonic stretch reflex, stimulation produces prolonged muscle contraction with widespread irradiation to other muscle groups, including antagonistic muscle pairs. Paradoxically, tendon jerks are slight or even absent. In addition to increased tendon jerks, clonus, and irradiation to other muscle groups, moderate spasticity includes the clasp-knife response, the sudden relaxation of a muscle toward the end of passive stretch.

EVALUATION

Once you have decided that spasticity sufficiently interferes with function to warrant treatment, periodic evaluations will be necessary to determine when the management plan should be revised. To assess whether the patient is benefiting from a specific treatment, observe his or her ability to perform activities of daily living and conduct neurophysiological laboratory tests to assess physiological capacities.

Functional Capacity

Keep careful records of the patient's ability to perform various functional activities. If standing, transfer, walking, or wheelchair use have become inefficient or unsafe, more aggressive treatment may be warranted. Is spasticity interfering with intermittent catheterization or the patient's bowel program? Do leg spasms interfere with driving? Other indications for altering treatment include inadequate grooming and hygiene, as well as predisposition to skin breakdown. Also note the presence of stressors that can exacerbate spasticity: pressure sores, urinary tract infection, fractures, poorly fitting clothes, fecal impaction, fatigue, or anxiety.

Serial measurements of joint range of motion may reveal an insidious loss that could compromise function. Manual testing of muscle strength, however, may be unreliable; rapid testing may give the illusion of voluntary strength at a joint if stretch reflexes are excited.

Neurophysiological Tests

Useful neurophysiological tests include a polyelectromyographic examination, ischemic test, and muscle infiltration with 2% lidocaine. Electromyographic studies of the motor control of the lower extremities indicate the reflex response of tested muscle groups to tendon jerk, clonus, passive stretch, vibratory reflex, Jendrassik maneuvers, and the Babinski reflex. These measures are particularly useful for predicting the effects of spasticity on ambulation. They also help differentiate true spasticity from local muscle spasm caused by trauma or contractures caused by prolonged immobilization and positioning of the joints in a shortened position.

Simulated Deafferentation

The ischemic test is designed to assess the degree to which spasticity should be reduced. Particularly for patients with severe paralysis, preservation of some spasticity assists circulation in the legs, thereby helping to reduce abnormally swollen ankles and to avoid thrombophlebitis. Most of these patients are wheelchair-bound, so the goal is optimal capacity for wheelchair activities rather than ambulation. Application of a pneumatic cuff to the extremity, with the pressure increased above the systolic blood pressure for 20 min, enables evaluation of the effects of transitory deafferentation on muscle hypertonia. The last 10 min reveal the status of the patient when hypertonia is removed and other abnormal motor phenomena that were hidden by hypertonia. Is volitional control improved when hypertonia is removed? Another method of artificially reducing muscle hypertonia is by infiltrating the muscles with a 2% lidocaine solution. These tests demonstrate whether nerve or motor blocks would improve functional capacity.

PRINCIPLES OF MANAGEMENT

The three primary approaches to managing spasticity are physiological, pharmacological, and surgical. Physiological measures, based on properties of neural control mechanisms that augment impaired control of muscle tone, emphasize prevention of nociceptive input and stimulation of nerve trunk, spinal cord, and cerebellar structures. At the foundation of the physiological approach is a home stretching program. These techniques form the basic management program to be instituted before other methods are tried.

When additional measures are necessary to improve function, diazepam, dantrolene sodium, or baclofen is prescribed, according to the cause of the patient's spasticity and how the drug's side effects will affect the patient's functioning. As these three drugs have increasingly displaced less effective medications, surgical treatment of spasticity has become less prevalent. Surgical procedures now represent the last line of treatment, reserved for patients who would need toxic doses of the drugs to control spasticity. The management of spasticity can thus be conceptualized as a pyramid (Fig. 24–1), in which foundation procedures are established first and additional levels of treatment added only when the lower levels alone no longer control spasticity sufficiently to preserve function.

Physiological Approaches

In addition to control of nociceptive stimuli, changes in posture, inhibitory positions, application of cold, stretching and other exercise, vibration over antagonist tendons, functional electrical stimulation, and spinal cord stimulation may temporarily modulate spasticity.

Controlling Nociceptive Stimuli

Any patient who complains of increased spasticity should be checked for urinary tract infections, fecal impaction, pressure sores, and deep vein thrombosis. Appropriate treatment of these conditions often diminishes spasticity without resorting to medications or surgery. Make sure the patient is complying with instructions for self-care of skin, bowel, and joints. In addition, loosen tight clothes, external catheters, or leg bands and replace aged or underinflated wheelchair cushions.

Local Cooling

Application of cold packs or immersion in ice water for 25 to 30 min can reduce spasticity for

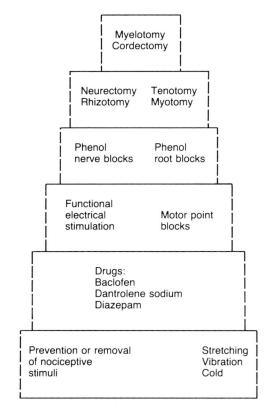

FIG. 24–1. Pyramidal approach to management of spasticity. Try first level techniques first. If these alone are insufficient, add second level treatments, and so on, using the surgical methods only when those on the lower levels fail. [Adapted from Merritt, J. L. (1981): Management of spasticity in spinal cord injury. *Mayo Clin. Proc.,* 56:616.]

as long as 3 or 4 hr. During this period, mobility can be facilitated by going through the range of motion of the joints. This treatment can also be used as a therapeutic test to check the efficacy of baclofen and diazepam; patients who respond to cryotherapy, which reduces gamma rather than alpha spasticity, probably will also respond to drugs that diminish muscle spindle activity.

Changing Posture

Positioning the body in certain ways can control spasticity by inhibiting undesirable spinal and supraspinal reflexes. Flexion of the neck may reduce extensor spasms in the lower extremities, as may changing position from supine to prone. Extension and abduction of the shoulder and extension of the elbow and wrist during ambulation may reduce flexor spasms in hemiplegic patients. Tapping, vibration, or other sensory stimulation over the antigravity muscles improves muscle contraction, enabling the patient to exert some control over undesired movements. These techniques are especially helpful in treating cerebral palsy and stroke patients.

Stretching and Exercise

Maximum contraction of the extrafusal muscle fibers helps unload stimulation of muscle fibers. A home stretching program should supplement a program of active, active-assistive, or passive range of motion exercise. Stretching is performed by the patient, a family member or assistant, or by standing frames or bracing. Caution patients to avoid sudden changes in force or direction, as well as bouncing or oscillating, which counteract the therapeutic benefits of stretching by stimulating muscle spindle activity. In addition to muscles, stretch joint capsules that have become contracted. Stretching performed at least once daily, twice in severe cases, may modulate spasticity for several hours.

Braces or splints provide constant stretch that can also facilitate autogenic inhibition of muscle spindles. For example, use of a below-knee brace to prevent plantar flexion often reduces the spastic equinus deformity that typically inhibits the hemiplegic patient's ambulation. Splinting and bracing also help prevent contractures resulting from prolonged spasticity, such as the extreme flexion contracture of the wrist and finger joints often occuring after a stroke.

Pharmacological Approaches

Selection of the most efficacious drug to control spasticity depends on whether the origin is spinal or cerebral, the impact of the drug's side effects on the patient's functioning, the dosage reguired to control symptoms, and concurrent medical conditions that would contraindicate the drug's use. These factors are compared in Table 24–3 for the three drugs most commonly prescribed for spasticity: dantrolene sodium, diazepam, and baclofen.

Diazepam is one of the most frequently prescribed medications for spasticity associated with hemiplegia, multiple sclerosis, cerebral palsy, and spinal cord injury. Its antispastic effects are more marked, however, with incomplete myelopathy than with complete spinal cord injuries. Diazepam is most appropriate for the temporary treatment of nociceptive-induced painful flexor spasticity in patients with incomplete myelopathies, where rapid resolution and the sedative effect are especially advantageous to the patient.

Baclofen, available in the United States only for the past 7 years, has comparable antispastic effects, but is usually preferred because it is much less likely to produce sedation or reduce voluntary power. In addition, baclofen seems to be more effective in relieving intermittent, painful flexor spasms. It would not be the drug of choice, however, for some elderly patients and those with a history of hallucinations or seizures.

Dantrolene sodium and baclofen are effective in both complete and incomplete myelopathies. Compared to dantrolene sodium, baclofen does not cause generalized muscle weakness or compromise other organ systems. However, dantrolene sodium may benefit patients with cerebral lesions who are not helped by baclofen or diazepam. Often, side effects from any of these drugs will subside after several days of administration.

Chemical Blocks

Injection with sclerosing agents, such as alcohol or phenol, intrathecally or into the peripheral nerves, represents a transitional stage in the management of spasticity. With effects lasting 6 to 12 months, this treatment may suggest which surgical techniques, if any, would, for example, improve gait. A 5% to 7% solution of phenol in distilled water is usually preferred over alcohol because the effects are less permanent, sexual function and sphincter function may not be lost, and it can be injected either into the motor points of the muscle or into the peripheral nerves.

TABLE 24–3. *Clinical effects of pharmacological agents on spasticity*

Drug	Site of action	Optimal safe dose	Side effects	Clinical effectiveness	Contraindications
Dantrolene sodium	Peripheral; sacroplasmic reticulum in muscle fiber; inhibits calcium release	100–400 mg in four doses/day; start 25 mg b.i.d., increase every 1 or 2 weeks to 6 weeks	Weakness in nonspastic muscles, drowsiness, nausea, diarrhea, fatigue, dizziness, possible hepatic injury and hepatitis in women and patients over 35	Complete or incomplete spinal cord injury; most helpful in cerebral lesions; tolerance does not develop; reduces hyperactive reflexes, clonus, dystonia, muscle stiffness, phasic abnormal movements; does not prevent development of contracture	Severe myocardial disease; liver disease; estrogen therapy; borderline pulmonary function
Diazepam	Presynaptic inhibition in reticular formation of brain stem and at spinal segmental level	20–40 mg in two or three doses per day; start 2–5 mg b.i.d., increase every 2–5 days	Sedation, drowsiness, fatigue, ataxia, weakness, anxiety, lightheadedness	Incomplete spinal cord injury with mild to moderate spasticity; some cases of cerebral palsy; most effective for continuous painful or disabling spasms; ineffective for most patients with cerebral lesions	Narrow angle glaucoma; third trimester of pregnancy; depression; liver, kidney, or hematological disorders; with diuretics or antihypertensive drugs; alcoholism; may reduce pulmonary function
Baclofen	Inhibits release of excitatory transmitters in spinal cord; acts on presynaptic mechanisms	40–80 mg in four doses/day; start 5 mg b.i.d., increase every 5–7 days	Sedation, drowsiness, weakness, nausea, dizziness, confusion, muscle ache, headache, constipation, ankle edema; hallucinations or confusion in patients with cerebral lesions	Paraplegia or quadriplegia with spinal cord lesions from trauma or multiple sclerosis; reduces frequency and severity of painful flexor or extensor spasms, either spontaneous or induced by various cutaneous stimuli; reduces protracted tonic flexor dystonia of lower extremities in patients with spinal cord injury; overall, most effective drug with fewest side effects; relaxes tightly flexed and adducted legs; may improve bladder and bowel control	Ineffective in cerebral lesions; seizure disorders; children under age 12; does not improve stiff gait or increase manual dexterity

Blocking the peripheral nerve, though easier than injecting the motor point, has the possible disadvantages of destroying sensation or producing uncomfortable dysesthesia. On the other hand, this technique enables the selective reduction of spasticity in a particular group of muscles; blocking the obturator nerve, for instance, would facilitate nursing and hygienic care compromised by severe hip adductor spasm. Motor point blocks are even more selective than nerve infiltration and do not disturb sensation. Muscles commonly injected include the pronator teres muscles, the short flexor of the toes, the flexor-extensor of the fingers, the brachialis, or certain heads of the triceps brachii. This procedure is recommended particularly in cerebral palsy and stroke. Motor or nerve blocks have marked positive effects on cerebral or spinal spasticity of moderate severity (see Tables 24-1 and 24-2). Like the systemic agents, however, they are unable to prevent the development of contractures.

A more effective procedure for patients with severe flexor spasm of the lower extremities is chemical rhizotomy, in which a 2% to 20% solution of phenol and glycerol is applied subarachnoidally using a spinal tap approach. The treatments are given at intervals of at least 1 week, and the effects of the procedure usually last for about 3 months. Placing the patient with the shoulders and pelvis higher than the mid-lumbar level in a side-lying position enables selective lesion of the lumbar roots without affecting bladder innervation. Chemical rhizotomy is preferred over surgical rhizotomy in treating spasticity associated with multiple sclerosis to avoid exacerbations after surgery and general anesthesia.

Electrical Approaches

Functional Electrical Stimulation

When ankle clonus interferes with ambulation, functional electrical stimulation (FES) can help maintain the foot in a position of slight tonic dorsal flexion and eversion. An external stimulator is connected to electrodes placed over the peroneal nerve. As the patient walks, a heel switch triggers the FES unit each time the heel contacts the floor. This treatment offers the advantage of being local and selective; when properly applied and adjusted, it does not interfere with other muscle groups or spinal segments. Unfortunately, using FES may be difficult if clinical engineers and experienced physical therapists are not available for maintenance and readjustment of the units as the patient's needs change.

Spinal Cord Stimulation

Implanting spinal cord stimulation (SCS) systems can modify disturbed motor control by activating afferent volleys and long loop reflexes, particularly in patients with multiple sclerosis. An externally worn transmitter, with electrodes attached to a passive internal receiver, provides power and control for stimulating sensory pathways. The result is improved endurance and motor control for many patients, often enabling the resumption of a more active lifestyle and return to gainful employment. Patients may gain the ability to suppress ankle clonus, improve coordination, and walk longer distances without fatigue.

Surgical Approaches

Surgical treatment of spasticity is reserved primarily for wheelchair-bound patients, especially those whose spontaneous flexor or extensor spasms interfere with bed-wheelchair transfers or remaining in a seated position. Like chemical neurolysis, surgical procedures should rarely be considered until spasticity has fully evolved, usually no earlier than a year after injury. Surgery may help reduce the marked dystonia resulting from cerebral lesions, since no medication is effective when the upper extremities are tightly flexed and adducted and the lower extremities stiffly extended and adducted. Occasionally after surgery, the patient becomes responsive to SCS or drugs that were previously ineffectual.

Surgical managment of spasticity consists of orthopedic or neurosurgical procedures. Some common orthopedic procedures are hamstring

TABLE 24–4. *Comparison of neurosurgical approaches to controlling spasticity*

Procedure	Description	Advantages	Disadvantages
Neurectomy	Sectioning of peripheral nerve		
Obturator		Strong hip adductor spasticity interfering with peroneal hygiene, sitting balance, or walking; may be combined with iliopsoas myotomy to reduce hip flexor and hip adductor spasticity simultaneously; improves positioning of patient to prevent pressure sores and frequent urinary tract infections	
Pudendal		Helps resolve significant detrusor-sphincter dyssynergia interfering with bladder retraining program	
Rhizotomy			
Posterior root	Sectioning of posterior root to abolish afferent impulses entering reflex arc; usually done at L2 to S2 level or C4 to T1 level	May spare sacral roots	Recurrence of spasticity and severe sensory disturbances in affected extremity; no effect on alpha spasticity
Anterior root	Sectioning of anterior root to prevent efferent impulses from reaching muscle; usually done at T11 to S1 level	Reduced spasticity in areas innervated by root sections	Results in permanent paralysis and flaccidity; residual voluntary sphincter may be lost; technically difficult; may add to spinal instability; muscle atrophy and reduced muscle padding
Myelotomy	Longitudinal division of spinal cord into anterior and posterior half from T12 to S1	Low recurrence rate of spasticity; interrupts both monosynaptic and polysynaptic reflex arcs while preserving all long tracts	Possible loss of any residual bladder or motor function; no effect on alpha spasticity
Cordectomy	Excision of spinal cord, resulting in totally flaccid paraplegia	Enables simultaneous conversion of upper motor neuron bladder control to lower motor neuron control	Loss of muscle mass; atrophy of pelvic, thigh, and calf musculature; exposure of bony prominences directly to subcutaneous tissue, may increase pressure sores.

tenotomy, heel cord tenotomy, heel cord lengthening, iliopsoas myotomy, and adductor tenotomy. In addition to rhizotomy, neurosurgical procedures include neurectomy, myelotomy, cordotomy, and cordectomy. The type of procedure selected depends on the type of spasticity, presence of contractures, and functional capabilities of the patient. Indications for the various procedures are compared in Table 24–4.

Orthopedic procedures carry the disadvantage of requiring static splints or casting up to several weeks. However, tenotomy is usually preferred over neurectomy if contractures have already developed. Hamstring release is indicated for severe spasticity complicated by knee flexion contractures. Nerves most commonly subjected to peripheral neurectomy are the obturator and posterior tibial. Myelotomy is the preferred procedure for abolishing spasticity in the lower extremities while preserving all long spinal tracts. Cordectomy, the most drastic procedure, is reserved for patients whose spasticity is uncontrollable by any other method and who would benefit from simultaneous conversion of upper motor neuron bladder control to lower motor neuron control. The result of this procedure is a totally flaccid paraplegia.

SUGGESTED READINGS

Davidoff, R. A. (1978): Pharmacology of spasticity. *Neurology*, 28:46–51.

Dimitrijevic, M. R. (1980): Spasticity: Medical and surgical treatment. *Neurology*, 30:19–27.

Feldman, R. G., Young, R. R., and Koella, W. P. (1979): *Spasticity: Disordered Motor Control.* Symposia Specialists, Miami.

Merritt, J. L. (1981): Management of spasticity in spinal cord injury. *Mayo Clin. Proc.*, 56:614–622.

Sharkey, P. C. (1981): Medical and surgical management of spasticity. *Clin. Neurosurg.*, 28:589–596.

Varghese, G., and Redford, J. B. (1980): Spasticity: Current concepts of management. *J. Kans. Med. Soc.*, 81:109–114.

Young, R. R., and Delwaide, P. J. (1981): Spasticity, parts I and II. *N. Engl. J. Med.*, 304:28–96.

Medical Rehabilitation,
edited by L. S. Halstead et al.
Raven Press, New York © 1985.

CHAPTER 25

Neurogenic Bladder and Bowel

Martin Grabois

Department of Physical Medicine, Baylor College of Medicine, Houston, Texas 77030

Neurogenic bladder and bowel, a group of disorders caused by partial or complete disturbance of the neurological control of normal bladder and bowel function, are frequent complications of neuromuscular disorders. Primary neurological impairment may result from trauma, infection, or degenerative, vascular, or neoplastic processes. The central nervous system at the spinal or supraspinal level, or the peripheral nerves, may be involved.

Successful management of these syndromes reduces not only possible mortality and morbidity, but also psychosocial and nursing problems. Neurogenic bladder and bowel are better understood and treated today because of the comprehensive, interdisciplinary approach to their management. With the help of a knowledgeable primary care physician, urologist, nurse trained in proper techniques, and a patient who is motivated to adapt to this disability, neurogenic bladder and bowel can be successfully managed within the patient's community.

The principal goals of managing neurogenic bladder are preventing urinary tract infection and overdistention of the bladder and implementing a satisfactory method of urinary elimination. Normal bowel function is attained when incontinence, diarrhea, and impaction are minimized or eliminated.

NEUROANATOMY

The spinal center for control of bladder and bowel function is S_2-S_4. Coordination of the motor and sensory nerves of the somatic and autonomic nervous system enables normal functioning of the urinary tract and bowel. Parasympathetic efferent nerves supply the bladder's detrusor muscle and the sphincter of the bowel while sympathetic efferent nerves supply the smooth muscles of the urinary tract. Somatic efferent nerves supply the striated muscle of the external urethral sphincter and pelvic floor as well as the external sphincter of the bowel. There are afferent fibers in the visceral and somatic systems of the urinary tract and bowel. These nerves mediate pressure, function, and stretch, as well as sensory modalities such as temperature.

CLASSIFICATION

While many cases of neurogenic bladder or bowel are not pure representations of any one type, usually patients exhibit predominant characteristics of one or another and can be classified and managed accordingly. Table 25–1 describes the five primary types of neurogenic bladder and bowel: uninhibited neurogenic, sensory paralytic, motor paralytic, autonomous neurogenic, and reflex neurogenic.

NEUROGENIC BLADDER

Physiology of Voiding

Although the reflex of voiding is automatic, it can be inhibited or facilitated by brain centers. As the bladder expands with increased urine volume, stretch receptors in the detrusor muscles of the bladder send nerve impulses to the spinal cord center by way of the visceral afferent

TABLE 25–1. *Classification of neurogenic bladder and bowel*

Type	Lesion	Anatomic level	Possible etiology	Effect on function
Uninhibited neurogenic	UMN	Cortex	Cerebrovascular accident, multiple sclerosis	Resembles bladder or bowel of infant; when bladder or bowel fills, patient is unable to inhibit voiding or defecation; frequent incontinence results
Sensory paralytic	LMN	Posterior S_2, S_3 S_4 roots, cells of posterior horns of spinal cord	Diabetes mellitus; tabes dorsales	Patient is unaware of bladder or bowel filling and does not receive sensory stimulus to initiate reflex; can lead to incontinence
Motor paralytic	LMN	Anterior horn cells or anterior S_2, S_3, or S_4 roots	Poliomyelitis, peripheral neuropathy, trauma, tumor	Patient is aware of bladder or bowel filling, but cannot initiate reflex; result is retention and overflow incontinence
Autonomous neurogenic	LMN	Spinal cord level S_2–S_4	Spina bifida or other congenital defect; trauma, tumor, spinal shock period after spinal cord injury	No sensation or sustained contraction possible; results in retention and overflow incontinence
Reflex neurogenic	UMN	Spinal cord above S_2–S_4	Trauma, tumor, vascular disease, multiple sclerosis, infection	Reflex is intact, but no cerebral control; no sensation is lost, but insufficient motor contraction for complete emptying; retention of urine or feces

pelvic nerves. The desire to void is then projected to the brain. When the time for voiding is appropriate, the facilitory fibers are activated, leading to increased parasympathetic activity with resultant increased detrusor muscle activity, relaxation of the sphincter through inhibition of the pudendal nerve, and voiding. However, if the time for voiding is inappropriate, the brain will send inhibitory nerve signals to the spinal cord center to inhibit the voiding reflex.

Evaluation

The physical examination includes, besides the routine examination, a detailed neurological evaluation, careful evaluation of the genitalia and prostrate, perineal sensation, and anal tone. There are a number of bedside reflex evaluation techniques that are helpful in determining the type of condition the patient has.

Ice Water Test

The ice water procedure tests the autonomic function of the bladder by way of the pelvic nerves. Three ounces of 38°F saline are injected into a catheter that is in the bladder. If the saline is rapidly expelled, the test can confirm previous findings of an upper motor neuron lesion.

Bulbocavernosus Reflex

The bulbocavernosus reflex tests the somatic function of the bladder by way of the pudendal nerve. A finger is placed in the rectum and the glans penis or clitoris is squeezed or the catheter pulled. If the rectal sphincter contracts, reflex activity is present and a lower motor neuron lesion is unlikely.

Residual Urine

The residual urine test provides information about the completeness of bladder emptying. After emptying the bladder as completely as possible a patient is catheterized. Residual urine is normally negligible. Values greater than 10 to 20%, commonly seen in neurogenic bladder, are usually not considered acceptable. They indicate incomplete bladder emptying, the residual possibly serving as a reservoir for infection.

Radiographic Tests

The most common radiographic techniques employed are the static cystogram to examine the anatomy of the urinary tract, voiding cystourethrogram to test urethra and bladder function during voiding, retrograde urethrogram to detect stricture, reflex, or diverticuli, and sphincterometry, which measures the resistance offered by the sphincter.

Urodynamic Tests

A cystometrograph is a useful guide for treating neurogenic bladder as well as for classification. It provides a pressure-volume curve pattern that will give information on sensation, filling pressure, capacity and detrusor contraction. Table 25–2 summarizes the physical examination and cystometrographic findings in normal and various types of neurogenic bladder.

Principles of Management

The primary goal, regardless of the etiology and stage at which the diagnosis is made, is the preservation of renal function. This can be accomplished by restoring the cyclical function of the bladder and by complete emptying. Prevention of urinary tract infections and overdistention of the bladder are an integral part of the rehabilitation program, as is finding a method of urinary elimination that suits the patient's individual needs.

An internal catheter (intermittent or indwelling) should be used only if urine is being retained in the bladder. Incontinence can often be handled in the male by external condom drainage and in the female by the use of diapers initially. If catheterization becomes necessary, intermittent catheterization is preferred to an indwelling catheter because of the reduction of infections and complications, and the acceleration of bladder retraining.

Intermittent Catheterization

Intermittent catheterization is the treatment of choice, especially if some bladder recovery can be expected and the patient is alert and sufficiently dexterous to learn self-catheterization. It can be started 24 to 48 hours after spinal cord injury, and may also benefit some patients with multiple sclerosis or after stroke. Three to five times a day, a soft rubber catheter is inserted using clean technique, all urine is drained, and the catheter is removed when the bladder is empty. This technique can be performed by a urology-trained technician or nurse, and eventually, by a relative or the patient at home. To be continued successfully, the technique must be performed frequently enough to maintain bladder urine at 500 cc or less, typically every four hours initially. Fluid intake should be limited to no more than 2500 cc in 24 hours. As voluntary or reflex voiding returns, the frequency of catheterization can be reduced. The intermittent catheterization program can be discontinued when residual urine is consistently less than 100 cc. Treat any infections that develop vigorously and immediately.

Indwelling Catheter

Chronically disabled persons are already predisposed to urinary tract infections. Since indwelling catheters are a major cause of such infections, they are usually reserved for patients with sphincter damage, detrusor sphincter dyssynergia, and reflux.

The risk of infections can be reduced by taking the following precautions.

1. Use the smallest size needed to obtain adequate drainage and select one of the silastic types; these are inert and less apt to form encrustation and bladder calculi as rapidly as the latex Foley catheter.

TABLE 25–2. *Physical examination and cystometrographic findings for various types of neurogenic bladder*

		Bladder type				
Findings	Normal	Uninhibited neurogenic	Sensory paralytic	Motor paralytic	Autonomous neurogenic	Reflex neurogenic
Bladder sensation	N	N	D	N	D	D
Saddle sensation	N	N	D	N	D	D
Bulbocavernosus reflex	N	N or I	N	0	0	I
Intravesical pressure	N	I	D	D	D	I
Uninhibited bladder contractions	0	+	0	0	0	+ +
Bladder capacity	N	D	I	I	I	D
Residual urine	N	N or I	I	I	I	I
Urinary incontinence	0	+ +	+	+	+ +	+ + +

I = increased; D = decreased; N = normal; 0 = absent; + = mild; + + = moderate; + + + = severe.

2. Maintain a closed collecting system, avoiding continuous irrigation.
3. Cleanse the meatus, perineum, and area around the catheter with a Betadine® solution two or three times a day and apply a thin film of Neosporin® ointment around the external meatus and on the catheter as it exits.
4. Change the catheter frequently, every one or two weeks for latex and four to six weeks for inert catheters.
5. Tape the catheter to the abdomen of the male to avoid penoscrotal fistula and check for periurethral induration along the underside of the scrotum.
6. Observe urine for changes in amount, color, and formation of crystals.
7. Maintain acidity of the urine by favoring an acid-ash diet, and prescribe ascorbic acid and mandelamine; routinely monitor urine pH with nitrazine paper.

Pharmacologic Treatment

Medications to control neurogenic bladder may be prescribed to stimulate or inhibit detrusor activity or sphincter tone, or for antiseptic antibiotic properties (Table 25–3).

Bladder Training Program

Bladder training is started as soon as the patient is medically stable and there are no renal complications, usually when he or she is partially mobilized. Bladder training consists of teaching the patient techniques that optimize normal bladder function, regulating fluid intake, and facilitating bladder emptying by triggering reflex activity (stroking, massage, or Crede maneuver).

To start the bladder program, discard the indwelling catheter and encourage the patient to try voiding hourly. After voiding takes place, measure residual urine levels. If the level is unacceptable, recatheterization will be necessary. The trial is repeated at select intervals in conjunction with using the medications previously discussed in Table 23–3. Thereafter, time intervals should be gradually increased to four hours and prolonged as bladder tolerance improves. Fluids should be forced about one-half to one hour before each voiding attempt in order to produce sufficient urine. Help the patient begin voiding by tapping over the bladder, rubbing the thigh, stimulating the anus for patients with upper motor neuron lesions, and manually applying suprapubic pressure (Crede maneuver) for

Medical Rehabilitation,
edited by L. S. Halstead et al.
Raven Press, New York © 1985.

CHAPTER 26

Sexuality and Disability

Lauro S. Halstead

Departments of Rehabilitation, Physical Medicine, and Community Medicine, Baylor College of Medicine, and The Institute for Rehabilitation and Research, Houston, Texas 77030

Even without specialized training in sexual counseling, the primary care physician can play a crucial role in helping the disabled patient achieve a more satisfying sex life. Frequently, all that are needed to sanction a patient's desire to resume sexual activity or try alternative modes of sexual expression are a show of interest, an understanding and nonjudgmental attitude, and straightforward information about sexual function. Counseling the disabled patient about sexuality should not be limited to discussion about genital activity. Behavioral and social issues that also directly affect sexual fulfillment include nongenital physical contact, self-pleasuring and pleasuring of a sexual partner, intimacy, caring, and verbal and nonverbal communication.

BARRIERS TO INCLUDING SEXUALITY AS PART OF HEALTH CARE

Attitudes

There are a number of barriers that impede the delivery of effective sexual health care to disabled persons. Two of the most common are negative attitudes about sexuality and lack of information about normal sexual function in the presence of a specific disease process. Negative attitudes and lack of information lead to, and are perpetuated by, a third barrier—myths. These myths imply that disabled persons are disinterested in sex, do not function normally anyway, and might hurt themselves. Of all these barriers, negative attitudes are the most formidable obstacle because they tend to determine what we think, say, and do as professionals and patients.

Because most physicians feel more anxious about sexuality than about any other area of medicine, your own inhibitions, anxieties, or prejudices are easily projected onto your patients. Therefore, being aware of these inhibitions and biases is an important first step in opening a productive dialogue with patients. An effective tool for evaluating your personal and professional feelings about sexuality is the Sexual Attitude Reassessment (SAR) program developed by the National Sex and Drug Forum in San Francisco. This program has been adapted for use by many rehabilitation centers throughout the United States, as well as by churches and other community groups.

Like the physician's attitudes, the patient's attitudes about sexuality are determined by upbringing, moral and ethical values, personal experience, and level of satisfaction. In addition, these attitudes may be seriously altered by the disability, especially if it involves altered neuromuscular control or physical appearance.

Social institutions—including family, friends, schools, and churches—have set up various legal and moral sanctions that permit or condemn various sexual practices. These sanctions have influenced policies in hospitals, extended health care facilities, and nursing homes that affect the kinds of sexual interactions patients are permitted. How many hospitals are willing to provide a privacy room where patients can do whatever they choose without being disturbed? As a physician, how do you feel about masturbation being provided by a member of the hospital staff for patients who are unable to do it for themselves? If questions like these make you feel uncomfortable, you might want to explore why, and whether your discomfort might interfere with providing full health care to your patients.

Information About Sexual Response

In contrast to the abundant information available about sexual response in able-bodied men and women (Fig. 26–1), such information about

persons with physical disabilities is scarce. Tables 26–1 and 26–2 indicate the physiological changes during sexual response cycles in men and women with spinal cord injury. It is evident from these tables that information about female response is particularly incomplete. There are comparable gaps in knowledge about other disabled groups, either because they have not yet been investigated or because techniques that would permit adequate assessment have not been developed. As a result, the counseling physician may be ill-prepared to provide information that is specific enough to be helpful to diagnosis and treatment. Nevertheless, as more primary care physicians help their disabled patients become as sexually active as they would like, clinical

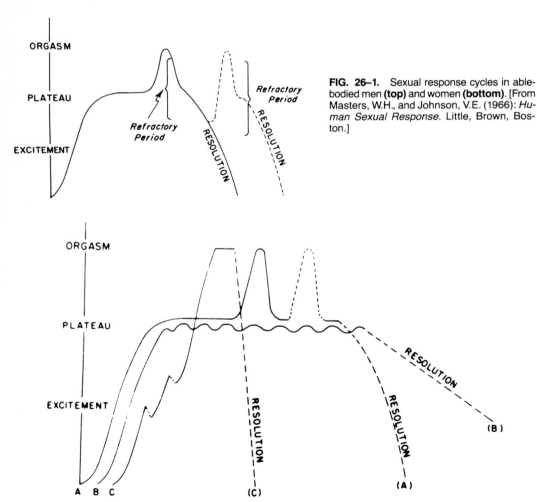

FIG. 26–1. Sexual response cycles in able-bodied men **(top)** and women **(bottom)**. [From Masters, W.H., and Johnson, V.E. (1966): *Human Sexual Response.* Little, Brown, Boston.]

TABLE 26–1. *Sexual response cycles in able-bodied and spinal cord injured men*

Response cycle	Able-bodied	Spinal cord injured
Penis erects	Yes	Yes, usually
Skin of scrotum tenses	Yes	Yes, usually
Testes elevate in scrotum	Yes	Yes, usually
Emission	Yes	No, not usually
Ejaculation	Yes	No, not usually

knowledge about sexual response should grow, and the success of therapeutic intervention should improve.

ASSESSMENT OF SEXUAL PROBLEMS

Classification of Disability

Three characteristics of physical disability have the greatest impact on the sexual adjustment of a given disabled patient—time of onset, stability of the lesion, and visibility of the impairment to others. How these three factors will affect sexuality in each patient depends on individual differences in sexual attitudes and experiences, as well as on unique ways of coping with physical limitations. As shown in Table 26–3, whether the disability is stable or progressive and whether it occurs pre- or postpuberty, strongly affect sexual development.

TABLE 26–2. *Sexual response cycles in able-bodied and spinal cord injured women*

	Able-bodied	Spinal cord injured
Wall of vagina moistens	Yes	—
Clitoris swells	Yes	Yes
Labia swells and opens	Yes	Yes
Uterus contracts	Yes	—
Inner two-thirds of vagina expands	Yes	—
Outer one-third of vagina contracts	Yes	—

Sex History

A thorough history of sexual function and enjoyment, taken with tact and candor, can be therapeutic as well as diagnostic. For many patients, this sexual history may be the first any physician has ever taken. The simple fact that you are sufficiently concerned to ask questions can relieve the patient's sense of anxiety, isolation, and frustration. The following are some practical guidelines for taking a sexual history:

1. Ask questions about sex during the review of systems, after inquiring about genitourinary and gastrointestinal functions, during the physical examination, or during some other appropriate context.

2. Be systematic; ask about sexual adjustment during three time periods: before disability onset (if appropriate), during exacerbations or complications, and presently. For example, ask the patient: Are you as active sexually as you would like to be? Has your disability caused any change in sexual activity or satisfaction? What are the reasons for decreased satisfaction? When did these begin?

3. Explore feelings of loss and how the patient's physical limitations affect view of oneself. Ask the patient: What do you feel you have lost? Has disability changed your self-image? Do you feel less masculine or less feminine?

4. Set realistic goals according to how knowledgeable the person is about sexual function, the level of satisfaction and areas of dissatisfaction, and the patient's willingness to explore new lovemaking options.

When interpreting the results of the sexual history, keep in mind that the level of sexual activity normally varies with the age of the patient, as well as the type of disability. In one study of 640 disabled and able-bodied persons for the behaviors of masturbation, intercourse, and oral/genital activity, disabled adults reported 20% to 30% less activity than persons without disability. By contrast, the level of satisfaction (approximately 40%) and reasons for dissatisfac-

TABLE 26–3. *Effects of disability on sexual development*

Onset	Medical conditions	Effects
Prepuberty		
Stable	Congenital loss of limb or sight; traumatic amputation	Normal psychological and psychosocial sexual development is difficult, perhaps impossible
Progressive	Cystic fibrosis; muscular dystrophy	Children tend to be overprotected, denied sexual experiences and information other nondisabled children obtain
Postpuberty		
Stable	Spinal cord injury; traumatic amputation; coronary heart disease; stroke	Adults with significantly altered body image may not see themselves as sexually attractive or as potential sexual partners
Progressive	Multiple sclerosis; arthritis; progressive blindness	Disorder that is visible to others has more profound impact than does disability that is less conspicuous

tion were surprisingly similar for both groups. Reasons for dissatisfaction included lack of partners, communication problems, and lack of interest on the part of the respondent and/or the partner.

Physical Examination

Focus the physical examination on detecting physical limitations that might require adaptations of sexual activity. These include strength, endurance, coordination, mobility, range of motion, sensation, and pain.

Assess whether the patient can control movement sufficiently to assume an active role in lovemaking. What is the extent of arm and hand dexterity? If a male patient is having difficulty with erections, assess wrist, hand, and finger function, which can be used effectively to stimulate and gratify the partner.

Loss of range of motion, particularly about the hips, and especially for a woman, can make normal coitus difficult, if not impossible. Therefore, check for hip flexion contractures and abduction, and assess the patient's "mechanical barrier." The FABER maneuver (flexion, abduction, and external rotation of the hips) performed with the patient supine will help identify mechanical limitations that might interfere with coitus. These limitations are often amenable to surgery. Testing for hip and pelvic mobility presents another appropriate time to initiate questions

about sexual activity and satisfaction, or to raise additional questions about your physical findings.

Identify areas of preserved or normal sensation in patients with sensory deficits. Many patients with sensory deficits report shifting of erogenous zones away from the genitals to the axilla, neck, or other areas. Even areas of diminished sensation, especially around the genitals or anus, can become highly erotic and play an important role in sexual stimulation and foreplay. Also identify painful areas and those movements and positions that relieve discomfort.

Differential Diagnosis

Your decision to treat a sexual dysfunction yourself or refer the disabled patient to a specialist will depend partly on whether the dysfunction is primary or secondary. Primary dysfunction refers to any long-standing problem that has been present for most of an individual's adolescent and adult life (for example, a male who has never had an erection). Patients with primary dysfunctions should be referred to a specialist. Secondary dysfunction refers to problems that have a fairly recent onset, such as intermittent or situational impotence. Such sexual problems may or may not be related to, or aggravated by, the patient's physical disability. Patients with a secondary dysfunction, which constitute the largest group, often can be treated quite successfully by the primary care physician.

MANAGEMENT OF SEXUAL DYSFUNCTIONS

A simple therapeutic approach designed for patients with secondary sexual dysfunctions is the P–LI–SS–IT model:

P —Permission: Sanction by authority figure to become sexually active or explore new ways to adjust to disability.

LI —Limited Information: Simple explanation of sexual anatomy and physiology to help patient make informed decisions and allay fears.

SS—Specific Suggestions: Tailoring sexual activity to each patient's specific limitations, such as barriers to mobility, as well as problems related specifically to the disorder, such as heart disease.

IT —Intensive Therapy: Referral of patients with primary sexual dysfunction, or those who do not respond to the above strategies, to a sex therapist.

A management program might also include the following solutions to some problems that frequently interfere with sexual activity:

1. Timing: Plan sexual activity around time of day when pain, spasticity, and other symptoms are least severe; alter medication schedule so period of maximum effectiveness coincides with planned sexual activity.
2. Position: Experiment with variety of positions to discover which requires the least energy expenditure and provides the most comfort; side-by-side positions (Fig. 26–2) are especially helpful when spine and hip mobility are problems.

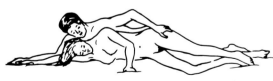

FIG. 26–2. Side-by side position—face-to-face or back-to-front, as shown—to compensate for spine immobility. [From Anderson, F, Bardach, J., and Goodgold, J. (1979): *Sexuality and Neuromuscular Disease.* Rehabilitation Monograph No. 56. The Institute of Rehabilitation Medicine, New York, and The Muscular Dystrophy Association.]

3. Barriers to mobility: Reduce spasticity, pain, and other barriers by taking warm bath with partner before sexual activity; reduce friction and fatigue by using water beds and massage oils; apply techniques that relieve discomfort during nonsexual activity to relieving discomfort during sexual activity.
4. Unrealistic expectations for performance: Encourage couples to discuss expectations of each other candidly; assign activities that minimize focus on genital play or on achieving orgasm.
5. Demands on nondisabled partners: Encourage open, honest communication with partner alone and then together with patient; determine partner's perceptions and attitudes about dysfunction and degree of satisfaction with his or her sex life; have third person take over the role of care provider when partner needs more time to concentrate on sexual role.
6. Myths: Provide basic information about disability, as well as anatomy and physiology of sexual function, to dispel myths about certain sexual activities being harmful.
7. Attitudes: Help patient reassess sexual attitudes.
8. Drugs: For drugs that interfere with sexual function (Table 26–4), try other drugs or adjust dosage.

In addition to these general solutions, specific therapeutic techniques can enhance sexual enjoyment in patients with heart disease, stroke, arthritis, or neuromuscular disorders.

Adaptation to Heart Disease

The major concerns in advising patients with heart disease about sexual activities are energy expenditure and oxygen consumption. The best way to develop a specific prescription for any physical exertion, including sexual activity, is with one of the standard exercise stress tests, using either a treadmill or bicycle ergometer (see Chapter 9). As a general rule, activities should be limited to heart rates that stay below 75% to 85% of the maximum recorded during the stress test.

TABLE 26–4. *Drugs that interfere with sexual function*

Antihypertensives

Diuretics

Spironolactone	Decreases testosterone; gynecomastia
Methyldopa	Impotence

Others

Guanethidine	Decreases erection, ejaculation, vaginal lubrication
Hydralazine	Decreases erection, vaginal lubrication
Glycosides	Decrease testosterone; gynecomastia

Tranquilizers

Phenothiazines	Decrease erection, ejaculation
Benzodiazepines	Galactorrhea, impotence (side effects greater with chlordiazepoxide than with diazepam)

Antidepressants

Tricyclic

Amitriptyline	Decreases libido and intensity of orgasms; galactorrhea, testicular swelling, breast swelling

Miscellaneous

Mecamylamine	Impotence
Phenoxybenzamine	Decreases ejaculation
Propantheline	Impotence

Another common method for prescribing a person's activity level is in terms of METs, which correlate well with the heart rate; this is a simple method of determining oxygen consumption. One MET is the energy expenditure per kilogram of body weight per minute for an individual sitting quietly in a chair or lying at rest. Walking 3 to 4 miles per hour is equivalent to 5 to 6 METs. During intercourse, energy expenditure usually reaches 5 METs for less than 30 sec during orgasm and is approximately 3.7 METs just before and after orgasm. Therefore, a cardiac patient who can walk on a treadmill at 3 to 4 miles per hour without symptoms or significant changes in blood pressure or the electrocardiogram (ECG), should be able to engage safely in sexual activity.

If necessary, a more specific prescription can be developed by employing the Sexercise Tol-erance Test. For this test, a Holter monitor is worn for 24 hr, including a period of usual sexual activity. With the aid of a diary kept by the patient, ECG changes can be correlated with specific activities and levels of exertion.

Patients with heart disease can be given the following guidelines for enhancing sexual enjoyment:

1. Resume sexual activity from 4 to 6 weeks following coronary artery surgery and 6 weeks after myocardial infarction.
2. There is no need to limit position to the male inferior one, since energy expenditure is not significantly greater in the male superior position; the side-by-side positions (see Fig. 26–2), however, may be less strenuous.
3. Counsel the patient and partner together to facilitate their communication with each other and help them understand each other's needs; alleviate stress by dealing with marital conflict.
4. Engage in sexual activity when well-rested.
5. Wait at least 3 hr after a heavy meal to engage in sexual activity because of demands of digestion on the heart.
6. Prior to sex, reduce alcohol intake, which reduces coronary circulation, may inhibit sexual desire, and may increase the amount of work required to accomplish sexual fulfillment.
7. Avoid extremes of temperature; high humidity especially increases cardiac work.
8. Improve level of physical fitness through cardiac conditioning programs.
9. Reduce the dosage or change the schedule of medications that may exacerbate sexual problems; guanethidine may cause retrograde ejaculations; pentolinium, mecamylamine, guadethidine, and methyldopa may delay or inhibit ejaculation.
10. Note warning signs: chest pains during or after sex; palpitations or breathlessness that continues 15 min after coitus; severe exhaustion that persists into the day after sexual activity.

Adaptation to Stroke

In contrast to heart disease, there is much less information available about the physiological changes and metabolic demands associated with sexual activity following a stroke. As a result, it is more difficult to provide patients with specific guidelines or suggestions. Unless cerebral damage is very severe, the sexual response, both anatomically and neurologically, is usually spared. The level of sexual interest and activity in stroke victims has not been studied extensively. However, in one group of 105 stroke patients under 60 years of age, the majority reported having some subjective sexual desire but a decreased opportunity to satisfy that desire. Of the patients in the study, 60% had the same or greater sexual interest following the stroke compared with their level of interest before the onset of disability; 43% had a decreased frequency of coitus, while 22% had an increased frequency of intercourse.

The following are some specific suggestions for enhancing the sexual gratification of stroke patients:

1. Focus erotic stimulation and love play on those areas of the body with normal sensation.
2. Experiment to discover what provides the most pleasure.
3. Inform partner of any visual deficits, such as homonomous hemianopsia, so that appropriate adjustments in positions or movements can be made.
4. Use positions of maximum comfort that place minimum stress on weakened muscles.
5. Use an overhead trapeze, a handle on the headboard, and firm pillows or cushions to facilitate moving in bed.

Adaptation to Arthritis

Differential diagnosis of a sexual dysfunction is likely to be more difficult in chronic arthritis, since it is frequently complicated by the underlying medical condition. Likewise, fluctuating physical and emotional conditions often associated with arthritis make successful intervention more elusive. Because arthritic patients have had to deal more directly with adapting to other problems caused by their disability, it is often easier for them than for their partners to accept limitations or explore alternative forms of sexual expression. Thus, involving the partner is especially critical in assessing and managing sexual dysfunctions in arthritic patients.

Since pain is a predominant problem in all forms of arthritis, most of the following suggestions refer to that symptom; however, the principles may apply to other symptoms as well:

1. Do simple warm-up exercises to prepare body for extra exertion of sexual encounter.
2. Apply moist heat for analgesia and relaxation.
3. Reduce friction and fatigue with use of water bed and massage oils.
4. Restore mobility with total joint replacements if arthritis is advanced.
5. Plan sexual activity around times when pain and other symptoms are least severe and time medications accordingly.
6. Use side-by-side positions (see Fig. 26–2) to compensate for inadequate spine and hip mobility.

Adaptation to Neuromuscular Disorders

The numerous neuromuscular disorders that have a lasting effect on sexual function include multiple sclerosis, amyotrophic lateral sclerosis, muscular dystrophy, spina bifida, cerebral palsy, and spinal cord injury. Although each of these disorders has a characteristic set of complications, some sexual issues are common to these and other neuromuscular disorders. With the exception of multiple sclerosis and spinal cord injuries, there is relatively little information available about physical and neurological changes that affect sexual functioning in these disorders. Most of the data that do exist are based on studies of men.

In a study of 37 men, changes in both potency and sweating correlated with clinical remissions and relapses of multiple sclerosis. Patients who were totally impotent sweated normally to the waist, but not below; subjects who were partially impotent sweated normally to the groin and perineum, but not in the lower extremities.

TABLE 26–5. *Sexual function in men with spinal cord lesions*

Lesion	Psycho erection	Reflex erection	Exterior ejaculation	Coital success	Orgasm	Progeny
Upper motor neuron						
Complete	0	90–95%	<7%	70%	Rare	1–3%
Incomplete	25%	95–100%	30%	80–85%	Occasional	5–10%
Lower motor neuron						
Complete	25%	25%	20%	70%	Occasional–common	5–10%
Incomplete	80–85%	90%	70%	90%	Common	10%

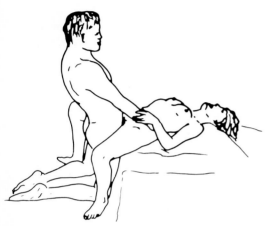

FIG. 26–3. Position for intercourse in limited range of motion at the hips and/or knees. [From Anderson, F., Bardach, J., and Goodgold, J. (1979): *Sexuality and Neuromuscular Disease.* Rehabilitation Monograph No. 56. The Institute of Rehabilitation Medicine, New York, and the Muscular Dystrophy Association.]

By contrast, patients with good potency exhibited normal sweating throughout the body.

Sexual functioning has been studied fairly extensively in men with spinal cord injuries. Table 26–5 summarizes several reports about reflex erections, anteriograde ejaculation, coital success, and fertility. Patients with incomplete lesions (sparing motor and/or sensory function below the level of injury) are more likely to have preserved function in these areas than are patients with complete lesions, regardless of whether they are upper motor neuron or lower motor neuron lesions. Reflex erections are more common in patients with upper motor neuron lesions, regardless of completeness; that is, in

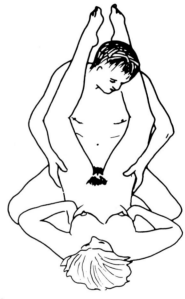

FIG. 26–4. Alternative position to compensate for reduced strength, endurance, or coordination. [From Anderson, F., Bardach, J., and Goodgold, J. (1979): *Sexuality and Neuromuscular Disease.* Rehabilitation Monograph No. 56. The Institute of Rehabilitation Medicine, New York, and the Muscular Dystrophy Association.]

lesions which are more likely to spare the reflex arc mediated by the sacral cord (S2–S4).

Ejaculation, which is mediated by sympathetic and somatic fibers, occurs most commonly in patients with incomplete lower motor neuron injuries, while coital success generally parallels the figures reported for reflex erections. In this group of men, the percentage who fathered offspring ranges from 1% to 10%.

As indicated in Table 26–2, information regarding the sexual response in female patients with spinal cord injury is incomplete. However, you should counsel patients that the spinal injury does not alter ability to conceive; these patients have the same physiological potential for becoming pregnant as they had before injury. For this reason, women with spinal cord injury who are contemplating becoming sexually active should take appropriate precautions to avoid unwanted pregnancies.

The following are some practical suggestions for spinal cord injured patients to improve their sexual functioning:

1. Incontinence: Plan bowel and bladder evacuation prior to sexual activity to minimize the possibility of an accident.

2. Indwelling catheter: Man can bend and fold catheter along shaft of penis; whether left uncovered or covered with condom, penis and catheter can be inserted into vagina without irritation. Female can position catheter to one side to avoid interference with foreplay or intercourse.

3. External catheter: Remove catheter; empty bladder using Crede maneuver or other technique before initiating foreplay.

4. Inadequate strength and physical dexterity: Have trained attendant assist in positioning and in removing or donning condoms or catheters; use water bed to facilitate movement; pleasure partner with vibrator strapped to forearm if use of hands and fingers is impaired; try other positions, such as female-astride if man is disabled, or man kneeling as disabled woman lies supine (Fig. 26–3).

5. Foreplay: Create environment conducive to sexual enjoyment, including privacy, lighting (candles), special smells (incense), sound (music), and tastes (food, drink).

6. Impotence: Facilitate and prolong erections by stimulating scrotum or by mildly irritating the testicular sac, inner thigh, pubic hair, or anal area; stuff flaccid penis into vaginal opening with help of partner; woman thrusts hips forward and squeezes vaginal muscles around penis to help produce reflex erection.

7. Decreased lubrication: Use lubricant like K-Y jelly to compensate for decreased lubrication of vagina.

8. Contraception: Usually avoid use of oral contraceptives due to risk of thrombophlebitis; impaired function of fingers and hands may make insertion of diaphragm impractical; IUDs are contraindicated in women with impaired genital and pelvic sensation; most sensible approach may be condom worn by man.

9. Contractures: Woman with contractures at hips and knees can position herself with legs over partner's shoulders (Fig. 26–4).

SUGGESTED READINGS

Anderson, F., Bardach, J., and Goodgold, J. (1979): *Sexuality and Neuromuscular Disease*. Rehabilitation Monograph No. 56. The Institute of Rehabilitation Medicine, New York, and the Muscular Dystrophy Association.

Boller, F., and Frank, E. (1982): *Sexual Dysfunction in Neurological Disorders: Diagnosis, Management, and Rehabilitation*. Raven Press, New York.

Cole, T. M. (1975): Sexuality and the spinal cord injured. In *Human Sexuality: A Health Practitioner's Text*, edited by R. Green. Williams and Wilkins Co., Baltimore.

Comfort, A. (1978): *Sexual Consequences of Disability*. George F. Stickley Company, Philadelphia.

Freedman, G. R. (1983): *Sexual Medicine*. Churchill Livingstone, New York.

Halstead, L. S., Halstead, M. G., Salhoot, J. T., Stock, D. D., and Sparks, R. W. (1978): Sexual attitudes, behavior and satisfaction for able-bodied and disabled participants attending workshops in sexuality. *Arch. Phys. Med. Rehabil.*, 59:497–501.

Lister, L. and Shore, D. A., eds. (1984): *Human Sexuality in Medical Social Work*. Haworth Press, New York.

Mooney, T. O., Cole, T. M., and Chilgren, R. A. (1975): *Sexual Options for Paraplegics and Quadriplegics*. Little, Brown and Company, Boston.

Munjack, D. J., and Oziel, L. J. (1980): *Sexual Medicine and Counseling in Office Practice: A Comprehensive Treatment Guide*. Little, Brown, and Co., Boston.

Sadoughi, S., Leshner, M., and Fine, H. L. (1971): Sexual adjustment in a chronically ill and physically disabled population: A pilot study. *Arch. Phys. Med. Rehabil.*, 52:311.

Woods, N. F. (1984): *Human Sexuality in Health and Illness*, 3rd edit., C. V. Mosby, St. Louis.

Appendix

Since disability is long-term, and often lifelong, physicians and other health care providers will need to educate their patients frequently about the nature of their illness, how to adjust to sometimes irreversible disabilities, and how to function as independently as possible in the community. Referring patients and their families to the following organizations, self-help books, and periodicals will encourage them to participate in their own health and lifestyle management. Manufacturers and suppliers of adaptive equipment are also listed.

ORGANIZATIONS

General

These organizations typically provide brochures, newsletters, videotapes, films, conferences, and information about local chapters, if available.

Center for Independent Living
2539 Telegraph Ave.
Berkeley, CA 94704

Channing L. Bete Co., Inc.
200 State Road
South Deerfield, MA 01373
(scriptographic booklets, health education)

Disabled American Veterans
National Headquarters
P.O. Box 1403
Cincinnatti, OH 45214

Disabled Resources Center
330 East Broadway St.
Long Beach, CA 90802

Handicapped Employment and Economic
    Development, Inc. (HEED)
115 East 57th St.
New York, NY 10022

International Society for Rehabilitation of the
    Disabled
432 Park Ave. S.
New York, NY 10016

National Association of the Physically Handicapped
2810 Terrace Rd. S. E.
Washington, DC 20020

National Center for Law and the Handicapped
1235 N. Eddy St.
South Bend, IN 46617

National Congress of Organizations of the
    Physically Handicapped
6105 North 30th St.
Arlington, VA 22207

National Easter Seal Society for Crippled Children
    and Adults
2023 West Ogden Ave.
Chicago, IL 60612

National Rehabilitation Information Center
    (NARIC)
4407 Eighth St. N.E.
The Catholic University of America
Washington, DC 20017

National Rehabilitation Association
1522 K Street N.W.
Washington, DC 20005

Office of Special Education and Rehabilitative
    Services
National Institute of Handicapped Research
Department of Education
Washington, DC 20202

People-to-People Committee for the Handicapped
1522 K Street, N.W.
Suite 1130
Washington, DC 20005

Programs for the Handicapped
Office for Handicapped Individuals
Switzer Building, Room 3517
330 C St. S.W.
Washington, DC 20201

Rehabilitation Information Round Table
Helga Roth
3107 Kent St.
Washington, DC 20795

Rehabilitation International
20 West 40th St.
New York, NY 10018

Specialized

Amputation

Amputees' Service Association
Suite 1504
520 North Michigan Ave.
Chicago, IL 60611

National Amputation Foundation
12-45 150th St.
Whitestone, NY 11357

Amyotrophic Lateral Sclerosis

Amyotrophic Lateral Sclerosis Society of America
15330 Ventura Blvd. Suite 315
Sherman Oaks, CA 91413

Arthritis

Arthritis Foundation
1212 Avenue of the Americas

New York, NY 10036*Cerebral Palsy*

American Academy for Cerebral Palsy and
    Developmental Medicine
P.O. Box 11083
Richmond, VA 23230

The Spastics Society
12 Park Crescent
London W1N 4LQ, England

United Cerebral Palsy Associations, Inc.
66 E. 34th St.
New York, NY 10016

Cerebrovascular Disease

Cardio-Vascular Disease
American Heart Association
4 East 23rd St.
New York, NY 10010

Stroke Clubs of America
805 12th St.
Galveston, TX 77550

Head Injury

National Head Injury Foundation
18A Vernon St.
Framingham, MA 01701

Multiple Sclerosis

Association to Overcome Multiple Sclerosis
79 Milk St.
Boston, MA 02109

National Multiple Sclerosis Society
205 East 42nd St.
New York, NY 10017

Parkinson's Disease

American Parkinson's Disease Association
116 John Street
New York, NY 10038

United Parkinson Foundation
220 South State St.
Chicago, IL 60604

Pediatric and Congenital Defects

Council for Exceptional Children
1920 Association Drive
Reston, VA 22091

National Foundation/March of Dimes
P.O. Box 2000
White Plains, NY 10605

Recreation

National Foundation of Wheelchair Tennis
3855 Birch St.
Newport Beach, CA 92660

Sexuality

American Association of Sex Educators,
    Counselors & Therapists
(AASECT)
5010 Wisconsin Ave., N.W., Suite 304
Washington, D.C. 20016

Sex Information and Education Council of the
    United States
(SIECUS)
1855 Broadway
New York, NY 10028

Speech Pathology

American Speech and Hearing Association
9030 Old Georgetown
Washington, DC 20014

Spina Bifida

Spina Bifida Association
The Texas Medical Center
1333 Moursund Ave.
Houston, TX 77025

Spina Bifida Association of America
104 Festone Avenue
New Castle, DE 19720

Spinal Cord Injury

National Paraplegia Foundation
333 North Michigan Ave.
Chicago, IL 60604

Paralyzed Veterans of America
7315 Wisconsin Ave N.W.
Washington, D.C. 20014

BOOKS

Addresses are provided for ordering books directly from the publisher.

General

Bowe, F. (1980): *Rehabilitating America: Toward Independence for Disabled and Elderly People.* Harper and Row, 10 East 53rd St. New York, NY 10022.

Bowe, F. (1981): *Comeback: Six Remarkable People Who Triumphed Over Disability.* Harper and Row, 10 East 53rd St., New York, NY 10022.

Chatham, M. A. F. (1982): *Patient Education Handbook.* Robert J. Brady, Routes 197 and 450, Bowie, MD 20715.

Cousins, N. (1979): *Anatomy of an Illness as Perceived by the Patient: Reflections on Healing and Regeneration.* W. W. Norton and Co., 500 Fifth Ave., NY 10036.

Cox-Gedmark, J. (1980): *Coping with Physical Disability.* The Westminster Press, 925 Chestnut St., Philadelphia, PA 19107.

De Graff, A. H.: *Attendees and Attendants: A Guidebook of Helpful Hints.* College and University Personnel Association, Suite 120, 11 Dupont Circle, Washington, DC 20036.

Ginther, J. R. (1978): *But You Look So Well.* Nelson-Hall, 111 N. Canal St., Chicago, IL 60606.

Hale, G. (1981): *The Source Book for the Disabled.* Paddington Press, 95 Madison Ave., New York, NY 10016.

Institute of Rehabilitation Medicine, New York University Medical Center. (1978): *Mealtime Manual for People With Disabilities and the Aging.* Essandoss Special Editions, Div. of Simon & Schuster, 630 5th Ave., New York, NY 10020.

Kraemer, D. G. (1980): *Driver Education for the Handicapped Manual.* Materials Development Center, Stout Vocational Rehabilitation Institute, University of Wisconsin, Stout, Menomonie, WI 54751.

Lane, J. (1980): *Wheelchair Bowling,* Wheelchair Bowlers of Southern California, 6512 Cadiz Circle, Huntington Beach, CA 92647.

Laurie, G. (1977): *Housing and Home Service for the Disabled.* Harper and Row, 2350 Virginia Ave., Hagerstown, MD 21740.

Megenity, J. (1982): *Patient Teaching: Theories, Techniques and Strategies.* Robert J. Brady, Routes 197 and 450, Bowie, MD 20715.

Ogg, E. (1979): *Recreation for Disabled Persons.* Public Affairs Committee, 381 Park Ave. S., New York, NY 10016.

Roback, H. B., editor. (1984): *Helping Patients and Their Families Cope with Medical Problems: A Guide to Therapeutic Group Work in a Clinical Setting.* Jossey-Bass, 433 California St., San Francisco, CA 94104.

The Saunders Health Care Directory. (1983): W. B. Saunders, West Washington Square, Philadelphia, PA 19105.

Van Meter, J. (1981): *Neurologic Care: A Guide for Patient Education.* Prentice-Hall, P.O. Box 500, Englewood Cliffs, NJ 07632.

Specific Disorders

Amputation

Kammerer, P., et al. (1978): *Pre-Prosthetic Care for Above-Knee Amputees.* Rehabilitation Institute of Chicago, 345 E. Superior St., Chicago, IL 60611.

Kammerer, P., et al. (1978): *Pre-Prosthetic Care for Below-Knee Amputees.* Rehabilitation Institute of Chicago, 345 E. Superior St., Chicago, IL 60611.

Madruga, L. (1979): *One Step at a Time.* McGraw-Hill, 1221 Avenue of the Americas, New York, NY 10020.

Arthritis

Engleman, E. P. (1979): *The Arthritis Book: A Guide for Patients and Their Families,* Painter Hopkins, Sausalito, CA 94966.

Hurdle, J. F. (1980): *A Medical Doctor's Home Guide for Arthritis, Muscle and Bone Ailments.* Parker Publishers, Div. of Prentice-Hall, P.O. Box 500, Englewood Cliffs, NJ 07632.

Kahn, A. P. (1983): *Arthritis.* Help Yourself to Health Handbooks., Contemporary Books, Inc., 180 N. Michigan Ave., Chicago, IL 60601.

Porter, S. F. (1984): *Arthritis Care: A Guide for Patient Education.* Appleton Century Crofts, 25 Van Zant St., East Norwalk, CT 06855.

Rosenbert, A. L., editor. (1979): *Living With Your Arthritis: A Home Program for Arthritis Management.* Arco Publishers, Div. of Prentice-Hall, 215 Park Ave. S., New York, NY 10003.

Swezey, R. L. (1978): *Arthritis: Rational Therapy and Rehabilitation*. W. B. Saunders, West Washington Square, Philadelphia, PA 19105.

Cancer

Donavan, M. (1981): *Cancer Care: A Guide for Patient Education*. Prentice-Hall, P.O. Box 500, Englewood Cliffs, NJ 07632.

Madruga, L. (1979): *One Step at a Time*. McGraw-Hill, 1221 Avenue of the Americas, New York, NY 10020.

Cardiac and Cerebrovascular Accident

American Heart Association. (1973): *Rehabilitation After Myocardial Infarction*. 44 East 23rd St., New York, NY 10016.

Freese, A. (1980): *Stroke: The New Hope and the New Help*. Random House, 201 E. 50th St., New York, NY 10022.

Johnstone, M. (1980): *Home Care for the Stroke Patient: Living in a Pattern*. Churchill Livingstone, 12 W. 44th St., New York, NY 10036.

Karch, A. M. (1981): *Cardiac Care: A Guide for Patient Education*. Prentice-Hall, P.O. Box 500, Englewood Cliffs, NJ 07632.

Cerebral Palsy

Cruickshank, W., editor. (1976): *Cerebral Palsy, A Developmental Disability*, 3rd ed. Syracuse University Press, 1600 Jamesville Ave., Syracuse, NY 13210.

Schleichkorn, J. (1983): *Coping with Cerebral Palsy: Answers to Questions Parents Often Ask*. University Park Press, 300 N. Charles St., Baltimore, MD 21201.

Communication Disorders

Broida, H. (1979): *Communication Breakdown of Brain Injured Adults*. College Hill Press, PO Box 35728, Houston, TX 77035.

Multiple Sclerosis

Birrer, C. (1979): *Multiple Sclerosis, A Personal View*. Charles C Thomas, 2600 S. First St., Springfield, IL 62717.

Chaffin, B. (1979): *Creative Living with M. S.*, Brad Chaffin, 5500 Monroe Ave., Evansville, IN 47715.

Forsythe, E. (1979): *Living with Multiple Sclerosis*. Faber and Faber, 99 Main St., Salem, NH 03079.

Scheinberg, L. C., editor. (1983): *Multiple Sclerosis: A Guide for Patients and Their Families*. Raven Press, 1140 Avenue of the Americas, New York, NY 10036.

Pain

American Medical Association. (1982): *Book of Back Care*. Random House, 201 E. 50th St., New York, NY 10022.

Florence, D., Hegedus, F., and Reedstrom, K. (1982): *Coping with Chronic Pain: A Patient's Guide to Wellness*, Publication No. 705. Sister Kenny Institute, 800 E. 28th St., Minneapolis, MN 55407.

White, A. A. (1983): *Your Aching Back: A Doctor's Guide to Relief*. Bantam, 414 E. Golf Rd., Des Plaines, IL 60016.

Parkinson's Disease

Dorros, S. *Parkinson's: A Patient's View*. (1981): Seven Locks Press, P.O. Box 72, Cabin John, MD 20818.

Duvoisin, R. C. (1984): *Parkinson's Disease: A Guide for Patient and Family*, 2nd ed. Raven Press, 1140 Avenue of the Americas, New York, NY 10036.

Stern, G. and Lees, A. (1982): *Parkinson's Disease: The Facts*. Oxford University Press, 16-00 Pollitt Dr., Fair Lawn, NJ 07410.

Poliomyelitis

Halstead, L. S. and Wiechers, D. (1985): *Late Effects of Poliomyelitis*. Symposia Specialists, P.O. Box 611587, Miami, FL 33161.

Laurie G., et al. (1984): *Handbook on the Late Effects of Poliomyelitis for Physicians and Survivors*. Gazette International Networking Institute, 4502 Maryland Ave., St. Louis, MO 63108.

Strauss, E. M. (1979): *In My Heart I'm Still Dancing*. Elaine and Simon Strauss, 597 Pine Brook, New Rochelle, NY 10804.

Pulmonary Disease

Modrak, M., editor. (1975): *Better Living and Breathing: A Manual for Patients*. CV Mosby, 11830 Westline Industrial Dr., St. Louis, MO 63141.

Sexuality

Becker, E. F. (1981): *Female Sexuality Following Spinal Cord Injury*. Accent Special Publications, P.O. Box 700, Bloomington, IL 61701.

Rabin, B. J. (1980): *The Sensuous Wheeler: Sexual Adjustment for the Spinal Cord Injured*. Multi Media Resource Center, 1525 Franklin St., San Francisco, CA. 94109.

Schover, L. (1984): *Prime Time: Sexual Health For Men Over 50*. Holt Rhinehart Winston, 521 5th Ave., New York, NY 10175.

Spina Bifida

Pieper, B. (1979): *The Teacher and the Child with Spina Bifida*. Spina Bifida Association of America, 104 Festone Ave., New Castle, DE 19720.

Pieper, B. (1977): *When Something is Wrong with Your Baby*. Chicago, Spina Bifida Association of America, 104 Festone Ave., New Castle, DE 19720.

Spinal Cord Injury

Chasin, J. *Home in a Wheelchair*. Paralyzed Veterans of America, 4330 East-West Hwy, Washington DC 20014.

Corbett, B. *Options, Spinal Cord Injury and the Future*. National Spinal Cord Injury Foundation, 369 Elliot St., Newton Upper Falls, MA 02164.

King, D. B. *Spinal Cord Injury Information Directory*. Roosevelt-Warm Springs Rehabilitation Center, Warm Springs, GA 31830.

Norris, W. C., Koble, C. E., and Strickland, S. B. (1981): *SILS: Spinal Injury Learning Series*. University Press of Mississippi, 3825 Ridgewood Rd., Jackson, MS 39211.

PERIODICALS

Accent on Living
PO Box 726
Gillum Rd. and High Dr.
Bloomington, IL 61701

ALLSSOAN (newsletter)
Amyotrophic Lateral Sclerosis Society of America
15330 Venture Blvd., Suite 315
Sherman Oaks, CA 91403

The AMP (newsletter)
National Amputation Foundation
12-45 150th St.
Whitestone, NY 11357

Crusader
United Cerebral Palsy Association
6 E. 34th St.
New York, NY 10016

Disabled, USA
President's Committee for Employment of the Handicapped
Washington, DC 20210

The Exceptional Parent
PO Box 4544
Manchester, NH 13108

The Independent
Center for Independent Living
2539 Telegraph Rd.
Berkeley, CA 94704

International Rehabilitation Review
219 East 44th St.
New York, NY 10017

Journal of Rehabilitation
Media Resources Branch
National Medical Audiovisual Center
Annex-Station K
Atlanta, GA 30324

The Mainstream
861 6th Ave.
Suite 610
San Diego, CA 92101

New World for the Physically Handicapped
PO Box 22552
Sacramento, CA 95822

Paraplegia Life
333 North Michigan Ave.
Chicago, IL 60601

Paraplegia News
5201 N. 19th Ave.
Suite 108
Phoenix, AZ 85015

Polling
United Cerebral Palsy Associations
122 East 23rd St.
New York, NY 10010

Rehabilitation Gazette
4502 Maryland Ave.
St. Louis, MO 63108

Rehabilitation World
20 West 40th St.
New York, NY 10018

Spina Bifida News
229 Smythe Dr.
Summerville, SC 29483

Sports 'N Spokes
5201 N. 19th Ave.
Suite 108
Phoenix, AZ 85015

MANUFACTURERS AND SUPPLIERS OF ADAPTIVE EQUIPMENT

Automotive Equipment

Drive-Master Corp.
61 N. Mountain Ave.
Montclair, NJ 07044

Blatnik Precision Controls, Inc.
1523 Cota Ave.
Long Beach, CA 90813

Ferguson Auto Service
1112 N. Sheppard St.
Richmond, VA 23230

Gresham Driving Aids
P.O. Box 405
Wixom, MI 48096

Thompson Hand Control
4333 N.W. 30th St.
Oklahoma City, OK 73112

Bath Fixtures and Aids

Bradley Corp.
Washroom Accessories Div.
Church & Fellowship Rds.
P.O. Box 321
Moorestown, NJ 08057

Eljer Plumbingware
(Wheelchair lavatories)
Three Gateway Center
Pittsburgh, PA 15222

Ondine Div. of Interbath, Inc.
427 N. Baldwin Park Blvd.
City of Industry, CA 91746

Universal-Rundle Corp.
217 N. Mill St.
P.O. Box 960
New Castle, PA 16103

Breathing Aids

Life Care Services, Inc.
(Portable ventilators)
5505 Central Avenue
Boulder, CO 80301

Strom Corp.
(Mechanical percussion)
11857 Judd Court, Building 206
Dallas, Texas 75243

Thompson Respiration Products Inc.
1925 55th St.
Boulder, CO 80301

Door Hardware Products

Amerock Corp.
4000 Auburn St.
Rockford, IL 61101

Stanley Hardware Div.
The Stanley Works
New Britain, CT 06050

Weslock
13344 S. Main St.
Los Angeles, CA 90061

Environmental Control Systems

C. R. Bard, Inc.
731 Central Ave.
Murray Hill, NJ 07974

Down East Electronics
44 Bucknam Rd.
Falmouth, Maine 04105

Scientific Systems International
506 B Oakwood Ave., N.E.
Huntsville, AL 35811

Western Technical Products
923 23rd Ave., E.
Seattle, WA 98112

Kitchen Appliances

Chambers Corp.
(Magnawave induction cooktop)
Oxford, MS 38655

In-Sink-Erator Div.
(Hot water dispenser)
Emerson Electric Co.
4700 21st St.
Racine, WI 53406

Munsey Products, Inc.
(Air Flo convection oven)
PO Box 9830
Little Rock, AR 72219

White-Westinghouse Appliance Co.
(Space Mates front-loading washer and dryer)
930 Fort Duquesne Blvd.
P.O. Box 716
Pittsburgh, PA 15230

Mobility Equipment and Aids

American Stair-Glide Corp.
4001 E. 138th St.
Grandview, MO 64030

Braun Corp.
1014 S. Monticello
Winamic, IN 46996

Cascade Medical Equipment
6500 6th N.W.
Seattle, WA 98117

Barrier-Free Design Equipment
and Aids Catalog by Miriam King
and Robert Williams
Michigan Center for a Barrier
Free Environment
6879 Heather Heath
West Bloomfield, MI 48033

Center for Orthotic Design
325 Princeton Rd.
Menlo Park, CA 94025

Earl's Stairway Lift Corp.
2513 Center St.
Cedar Falls, IA 50613

Everest & Jennings, Inc.
1803 Pontius
Los Angeles, CA 90025

Fidelity Electronics, Inc.
5445 Diversey Ave.
Chicago, IL 60639

General Teleoperators, Inc.
P.O. Box 3584
Los Amigos Station
Downey, CA 90242

Helper Industries
932 N.W. First St.
Fort Lauderdale, FL 33311

Howard Mobility-Plus, Inc.
124 W. S. Boundary
Perrysburg, OH 43551

Mobility Engineering and Development, Inc.
15936 Blythe St.
Van Nuys, CA 91406

Mobility Dynamics, Inc.
21029 Itasca Ave., Unit D
Chatsworth, CA 91311

Motorette Corp.
6014 Reseda Blvd.
Tarzana, CA 91356

The Chair Concern
11825 Alondra Blvd.
Norwalk, CA 90650

Self-Help Devices

Abbey Medical
Division of Abbey Rents
600 S. Normandie Ave.
Los Angeles, CA 90005

Barrier-Free Design Equipment
and Aids Catalog by Miriam King
and Robert Williams
Michigan Center for a Barrier
Free Environment
6879 Heather Heath
West Bloomfield, MI 48033

Carters Rehabilitation Equipment
Alfred Street
Westbury, Wilts BA 13 3D2
Great Britain

Cleo Living Aids
3957 Mayfield Rd.
Cleveland, OH 44121

Help Yourself Aids Catalog
PO Box 192
Hinsdale, IL 60521

Maddak, Inc.
Industrial Rd.
Pequannock, NJ 07530

Medical Equipment Distributors, Inc.
1701 S. First Ave.
Maywood, IL 60153
or,
1215 S. Harlem Ave.
Forest Park, IL 60130

G. E. Miller, Inc.
484 S. Broadway
Yonkers, NY 10705

Nelson Medical Products
5690 Sarah Ave.
Sarasota, FL 33581

J. A. Preston Corp.
71 Fifth Ave.
New York, NY 10003

Fred Sammons, Inc.
Box 32
Brookfield, IL 60513

Subject Index